DATE			
NOV 23 '94			
MAY 2 '95			
APR 13 '96			
MAY 12 '96			
AP 17 '98			
NO 27 '99			
OCT 10 '00			
DEC 15 '00			
1/06/05			

The Ends of Human Life

The Ends of Human Life

MEDICAL ETHICS IN A LIBERAL POLITY

Ezekiel J. Emanuel

HARVARD UNIVERSITY PRESS
Cambridge, Massachusetts
London, England
1991

Library of Congress Cataloging-in-Publication Data
Emanuel, Ezekiel J., 1957-
The ends of human life: medical ethics in a liberal polity /
Ezekiel J. Emanuel.
p.   cm.
Includes index.
ISBN 0–674–25325–6 (alk. paper)
1. Medical ethics. 2. Liberalism. I. Title
[DNLM: 1. Ethics, Medical.   2. Health Policy.   3. Political
Systems.   W 50 E53e]
R724.E5   1991
174'.2—dc20
DNLM/DLC
for Library of Congress   91–7090
CIP

To my parents
*a contribution toward fulfilling
the Fifth Commandment*

Contents

Acknowledgments

The ideas contained in this book have been created and nurtured with the contributions of many other people. The impetus for this work began in conversations on the relationship between science and ethics with Adam Schulman in the summer of 1978 when we were both Undergraduate Research Participants at Cold Spring Harbor. The actual work has been shaped by many subsequent conversations during our studies together at Oxford and Harvard.

Many graduate students at Harvard have been invaluable both in and outside the classroom. I am especially indebted to the generosity and insights of Greg Keating, Henry Richardson, and Liz Anderson, who spent many hours talking and reading with me on subjects ranging from Aristotle to Rawls and everything in between. They have made me wiser and saved me from many errors.

Over the years many teachers have knowingly and unwittingly shaped my thoughts on subjects related to this book. Tim Scanlon and John Rawls have been patient teachers, always willing to listen, to read, and to offer their suggestions. My understanding of many issues in political philosophy has grown immeasurably from their brilliance, and they have made me appreciate the many virtues of liberalism through both their words and their deeds. Many years ago at Amherst College George Kateb ignited my interest in political philosophy and has continued to encourage me. His warmth and elegant insights have never let me forget the importance of individualism and truth. Judith Shklar has been a warm and wonderful teacher, always forcing me to consider issues from a unique perspective.

Special appreciation goes to Dennis Thompson, director of the Program in Ethics and the Professions at Harvard University. Not only was he willing to risk a fellowship position in the program on me, he spent numerous hours reading and criticizing every page of this work. His criticisms have always been in the most generous spirit: an attempt to make my words more true to my vision.

I was uniquely privileged to have Michael Sandel as an adviser when this work was originally written. It could not have been written without his guidance. He gently shepherded me through each stage of graduate work, and every piece of advice he gave was filled with wisdom, which I often did not appreciate until much later. His enormous support cannot be underestimated.

Most important, I owe thanks to my family. Linda has supported my writing not only through words and presence, but by assuming the enormous burden of medical internship and residency to free my time for this endeavor. Without her efforts, mine would have been in vain. Rebeka and Gabrielle may not yet understand what is written in these pages, but they did understand its importance to me. They endured as many sacrifices as I did and I hope one day they too will think it worthwhile.

Finally, many different organizations and institutions provided financial support for this project. The Harvard Government Department and the Harvard Faculty of Arts and Sciences provided stipends and fellowship support. I also received generous support through a Newcombe fellowship, a Jacob Javits fellowship from the U.S. Department of Education, and a Josephine de Karmen fellowship. The manuscript was completed during a stimulating year in the unique Program in Ethics and the Professions.

The Ends of Human Life

The Questions of Medical Ethics

Call him Andrew. His face is gaunt and unshaven but peaceful. His eyelids are gently closed. He lies with his skeletal left arm taped to a gauze-covered board and a catheter sewn into his artery. His right hand is flexed, another catheter stuck into a small vein. There is a tube entering his mouth and taped to his nose. Over Andrew's head, his heart's electrical impulses flash across a screen. Every few seconds, like the endless, repetitive steps of marchers, gushes of air resonate from a machine in the corner. Andrew's protruding ribs expand his skin and then slowly descend to their resting level. A few other machines click and gurgle, precisely marking the passage of time.

It is hard to tell from his emaciated appearance, but Andrew is 34 years old. He was diagnosed with AIDS eight months ago. Four months prior to this admission he had been hospitalized for a *Pneumocystis carinii* pneumonia, one of the opportunistic infections associated with AIDS. At that time he was hospitalized for eighteen days, leaving a few days before completing his treatment with antibiotics because he could not tolerate being in the hospital. Otherwise he has never been in a hospital, receiving all his treatments in the clinic. Prior to this admission, Andrew was not known to have other opportunistic infections or neoplasms associated with AIDS. However, over the last two months he has complained of memory problems. Andrew's physician felt he had a mild form of AIDS dementia, but never gave him any formal neurological testing.

This time he arrived at the hospital looking pale with labored breathing and a high fever. The physicians in the emergency room diagnosed another *pneumocystis* infection. For the last seven days Andrew has been in the five-bed intensive care unit (ICU) on intravenous antibiotics and steroids. Yet his clinical condition has only deteriorated; he is hypoxic and semiconscious, rousing to painful stimuli but not initiating any communication or actions.

1

Aware of his fatal condition and counseled by a local support group, Andrew had signed—and two acquaintances had witnessed—a living will which stated the following: "I direct that life-sustaining procedures should be withheld or withdrawn if I have an illness or disease or experience extreme mental deterioration such that there is no reasonable expectation of recovering or regaining a meaningful quality-of-life. The life-sustaining procedures which may be withheld or withdrawn include but are not limited to: Surgery, antibiotics, cardiac resuscitation, respiratory support, artificially administered feedings and fluid." Andrew had not given this living will to his physician, but kept it in his wallet. Nor was there a record that he had granted any particular person power of attorney.

There is some question about his competence when he signed the living will, especially with the suspicion of AIDS dementia. Andrew's lover of two years claims to have discussed the issue with him several times over the past few months; he believes the living will accurately reflects Andrew's wishes. He has urged Andrew's physician to stop his respirator and his suffering.

Andrew's mother, father, and brother have been at the hospital since his admission, maintaining a constant vigil in his room. Their interaction with the hospital staff alternates between cooperation and hostility; they question every new blood sample the technicians draw, every new intravenous infusion the nurses hang, every new sign and symptom the doctors observe. They deny Andrew's lover's version of events, claiming the living will does not reflect Andrew's actual wishes. They are adamant about maintaining Andrew with maximal intervention and immediately curtail any discussion of withdrawing or withholding treatments, or even of making Andrew DNR (Do Not Resuscitate). In vague and elliptical phrasing, they threaten a lawsuit if the respirator or antibiotics are withdrawn.

Dr. Wolf, Andrew's physician, has known him for about a year. He saw Andrew only once before the diagnosis of AIDS for hepatitis. Just after the diagnosis they briefly spoke of Andrew's prognosis with AIDS. Dr. Wolf promised to administer as much medical care outside the hospital as possible and to protect Andrew from a miserable death. During the first hospitalization Andrew's anger and resistance made Dr. Wolf desperate, especially because he thought the chances of coming out alive were less than 20 percent; Andrew survived. After discharge Dr. Wolf took solace in the smile that accompanied Andrew's office visits and seemed to whisper how nice it was to have experienced another week. Yet he remembers the seriousness with which he and Andrew discussed death and his promise to help avoid "a miserable death." He wants to honor that promise.

The ICU medical team is pressing Dr. Wolf for specific guidelines on the aggressiveness of medical care. They want a DNR order because they think Andrew's chances of surviving a cardiac arrest are almost zero. More important, they worry that Andrew's deterioration suggests he is harboring another infection, possibly a fungal pneumonia, in addition to his *pneumocystis*. They want guidance from Dr. Wolf on how aggressive they should be in trying to discover other causes for Andrew's poor response. Should they push for a bronchoscopy? Should they ask the surgeons for an open lung biopsy? Should they simply add new antibiotics without any diagnostic clues? Or should they stop their aggressive care? The ICU physicians are ambivalent about pushing on in part because they think Andrew's prognosis is grim and in part because they think more invasive diagnostic or therapeutic approaches violate his living will. In addition, they are anxious about using an ICU bed, the antibiotics, and other interventions because the ICU is full and, in the last few days, two other critical patients who need intensive care were refused admission because of the bed shortage.[1]

What should Dr. Wolf do? There are questions concerning the physician-patient relationship: Does the living will really represent Andrew's wishes? Was he competent when he filled it out? Is Andrew's lover's interpretation of the living will accurate or the lover's desire? Do Andrew's parents know him better? Or are they pressing for maximal care because they feel some guilt about rejecting him for his homosexuality?

There are also questions concerning the selection of medical interventions: Is death better than Andrew's existence on a respirator? Is Andrew's situation "a miserable death"? What future does Andrew have anyway, even if he survives? Is there "no reasonable expectation of his recovering a meaningful quality-of-life"? Was there such an expectation during the previous admission? Should he be DNR even if the respirator is not withdrawn? Should the hospital ethics committee be consulted? What is the best care for Andrew?

Then there are questions concerning the allocation of health care resources: Should the shortage of ICU beds weigh in Dr. Wolf's deci-

sion about how to care for Andrew? Should the costs of care, exceed-
ing $2,000 per day, influence Dr. Wolf's decisions? Does it make a
difference that Andrew has no health insurance and does not qualify
for Medicaid coverage? Should the hospital, which had a deficit last
year in large measure because of its uncompensated care for AIDS
patients, assume Andrew's expenses? Should Dr. Wolf consider the
hospital's financial status, especially since he admits many other AIDS
patients who also receive uncompensated care? How much medical
care is Andrew entitled to? Has his current care in some way gone over
the limit? What about other patients who need ICU care? How critically ill are they? What are their chances for a meaningful quality-of-
life? Should their prospects be balanced against Andrew's? If Dr. Wolf
should not consider these patients, should the hospital ethics committee?

These are some of the questions confronting Dr. Wolf and the other
physicians caring for Andrew. They do not arise from any unethical
or questionable practices; they are the kind of moral dilemmas that
confront even the most conscientious physicians. Nor are they unique
to caring for AIDS patients; such questions recur in the care of critically ill newborns, incompetent patients, terminally ill cancer patients, patients with other incurable diseases, and indeed, in the medical care of every person. Furthermore, these are not the only medical
ethical questions confronting physicians.[2] There are questions involving the confidentiality of patient information, the ethics of subjecting
humans to experimental treatments, the ethics of transplanting genes
or brain tissue, the proper practice of informed consent, and many
others.

Inescapably, Dr. Wolf's questions lead beyond medicine; they are
"mortal questions"[3] because they intersect with the eternal human experiences of death, parenthood, personal identity, justice, freedom.
Even if the answers we give these medical ethical questions will not
affect the actual health care we receive or the health care decisions we
might have to make, how we confront and resolve them will both
reflect and affect our understanding of ourselves as human beings, of
the good life, of social justice, of the proper way to care for the disabled, debilitated, and dying. Medical ethics is a measure of our own
moral vision; these questions force us to articulate our ideals and values, our ethical self-understanding, and to assess their worthiness.

Over last two or three decades, such medical ethical questions seem to have been converted from a peripheral concern of physicians to a preoccupation affecting almost every clinical decision. Indeed, they have ceased to be mere professional issues and have become matters of great public concern, prompting frequent news stories on television and in newspapers. And the professional and public response has been swift and sweeping. According to the Association of American Medical Schools, in 1972 only eleven medical schools had courses on medical ethics; by 1986 all medical schools required some kind of course in medical ethics or medical humanities for graduation. Further, between 1983 and 1985 the proportion of hospitals having ethics committees more than doubled to a total of 60 percent.[4] Still other hospitals have created ethics consultants or instituted ethics rounds in which particularly difficult cases or ethical issues are examined.

Over the last decade or so there have been many national commissions devoted to medical ethical issues, including one to establish ethical guidelines for research on humans[5] and also the Presidential Commission for the Study of Ethical Problems in Medicine and Biomedical and Behavioral Research, which issued reports on a wide range of subjects including defining death, genetic engineering, terminating life-sustaining care, informed consent, and allocating medical care resources.[6] Individual states have also created their own commissions to make recommendations on various medical ethical issues such as the allocation of resources for organ transplantation.[7] And recently Congress has enacted legislation forming the Congressional Biomedical Ethics Board to advise it on medical ethical issues such as surrogate motherhood. Finally, all this attention to medical ethical questions has spawned a new academic discipline, so-called bioethics, with all the requisite paraphernalia of medical school professorships, conventions, specialty journals, and books.

While all this attention, both from inside and outside the medical profession, has produced more public awareness and discussion of medical ethical issues, it has not created any widespread consensus. Despite limited agreement on procedures and formal language, there seems to be endless irresolution concerning the substance of these medical ethical issues. For instance, while almost everyone agrees that all citizens should be guaranteed an "adequate level of health care," there is simply no agreement on any substantive criteria for defining this or a list of what it actually comes to (see Chapter 4).

Indeed, the most striking characteristic of discussions of medical ethical questions is their persistent irresolution. It is not just that Dr. Wolf's questions are hard and require tentative and subtle answers; rather, it seems as if they simply lack rational answers altogether. The ethical framework in which these medical ethical discussions and debates occur seems to ensure no agreement. To put it another way: within the last two decades or so, medical ethical *questions* have become irresolvable medical ethical *dilemmas.* As one physician stated in reflecting on the practice of withholding medical care: "What does one do, then? We have developed no rational way to decide what treatment to give and what to withhold once it has been decided to withhold 'heroics.'"[8] Another commentator has made the point more generally: "Much has been written in the past three decades about medical ethics, but has this spate of scholarship produced any real or compelling consensus among practicing physicians? It seems that although awareness of ethical issues has been increased and committees have proliferated, the lack of consensus is now even more obvious . . . there is no longer even the appearance of an effective consensus in the medical profession."[9] Discordant positions, irresolution, and an exhausted uncertainty seem the only conclusive products of three decades of discussion on medical ethics.

This preoccupation with medical ethical questions that seem to defy resolution prompts three sets of questions about medical ethics that will guide the inquiry of this book.

1. What is the proper approach to medical ethical questions? How should the issues of medical ethics be characterized?
2. Why in contemporary American society do medical ethical questions seem to lack resolution? Why do we seem to lack an ethical framework in which these questions can be rationally discussed?
3. Is there a resolution to medical ethical questions? Can we construct an ethical framework that will permit these questions to be rationally discussed?

In response to the first question I will claim that, like all professions, medicine is committed to moral ideals. In medicine these ideals include the health and well-being of the sick and the relief of suffering. These ideals are not self-defining. Nor is it immediately clear how these ideals should be balanced when they conflict among themselves or with nonmedical ideals. Because the ends of medicine are public declarations of the profession, shaped by public laws and influencing public values, they cannot be specified or balanced through the substantive and regulative principles of moral philosophy. They can be interpreted and balanced only through political philosophy; that is, medical ethical questions can be rationally discussed and resolved only within a framework constituted by political philosophy. It is only by appeal to our shared political conceptions, to our conception of what constitutes justice and the good life, that we can know whether it is just to consider the well-being of other patients when deciding what care to provide to Andrew or whether living on a ventilator prohibits a "meaningful quality-of-life." On this view medical ethics is a subfield of political philosophy. This political conception of medical ethics will be elaborated in Chapter 1.

Second, a political conception of medical ethics suggests that the persistent irresolution of medical ethical questions is a consequence not of medical technology but, rather, of the political philosophy that informs deliberations on medical ethics. In particular, the current irresolution can be traced to the liberal political philosophy that informs our society's laws, policies, and practices.

Liberalism espouses the ideal of neutrality, namely that public institutions, laws, and policies should not promote any particular view of what is worthy or good. But, absent judgments about what is worthy or good, we cannot decide whether a medical intervention promotes a patient's well-being or is deemed harmful; to determine whether continuing Andrew's care is in his best interests or perpetuates suffering requires knowing whether his life has lost a "meaningful quality-of-life" or not. It is not just that different people will have different views on what is worthy or good and that in *practice* achieving consensus on these judgments will be difficult; it is that by prohibiting the polity from espousing particular views of the good life, liberal political philosophy excludes, even in *theory*, a shared framework for resolving such medical ethical questions. Consequently, the recent upsurge in medical ethical issues and their apparent irresolution stem from the appeal to liberalism and its ideal of neutrality for the justification of our political policies and practices. In Chapters 3 and 4 I will examine debates about terminating care and allocating resources, respectively, to show how the claims of liberal political philosophy underlie the irresolution characteristic of current medical ethics.

Third, resolution of these medical ethical dilemmas requires nothing less than an alternative political philosophy, one in which laws and policies can be justified by appeal to conceptions of the good life. In Chapter 5 I will sketch one possible alternative: liberal communitarianism. The ideal of liberal communitarianism is a federation of communities, each dedicated to democratic deliberations. The citizens of these communities are committed to articulating a shared conception of the good life that, in turn, guides the formulation of laws and policies regulating communal life. Such a vision is liberal because the citizens are guaranteed rights necessary for participation in democratic deliberations; it is communitarian because these deliberations aim to articulate a common conception of the good life that informs laws and policies. For such communities to engage in substantive deliberations, they will have to be small. Consequently, they will have to be federated into a nation that also addresses those issues that transcend smaller communities, such as foreign affairs.

In Chapter 6 I will sketch a model showing how the liberal communitarian vision might be practically implemented in the area of medical care. This model proposes thousands of community health programs (CHPs). Each individual would be given a voucher and permitted to join a CHP. Through the democratic deliberations of its members, the CHP would have to define its own conception of the good life and the resultant particular health care policies. For example, a CHP would have to delineate which medical services it would pay for and which services would be left to individual payment. By considering historical precedents and accepted traditions, I will show that this model is both politically practical and justifiable.

The Political Conception
of Medical Ethics

Technology and Medical Ethics

Why in contemporary American society have medical ethical questions become so interminable? To many there is an obvious answer expressed in one word: *technology.* Before the development of biomedical technologies, the argument goes, medical ethical questions did not arise. The advent of modern interventions, of antibiotics and respirators, of dialysis machines and organ transplants, has literally *created* these medical ethical dilemmas. The medical ethical questions that now preoccupy us are the inevitable, if undesirable, fruits of biomedical progress. The bioethicist Ruth Macklin succinctly summarizes this view:

> In an earlier era, when medicine was about as likely to harm patients as to cure them or improve their condition, doctors rarely were confronted with life-and-death decisions . . . scientific and technological advances have produced the remarkable medical capabilities we know today.
>
> These advances have been a mixed blessing. The use of medical technology in all its forms causes undesired side effects and untoward consequences . . . The other price—no doubt unforeseen—is the *creation of ethical dilemmas rarely if ever confronted in the past.* (emphasis added)[1]

This view has been so widely accepted by physicians,[2] health policy experts,[3] lawyers,[4] bioethicists, and the public that it has attained the status of an axiom, what we might call the technological axiom of medical ethics.

When pressed, advocates of this axiom substantiate it by citing two trends. First, they note that almost all the medical ethical issues that now preoccupy us (see Table 1.1) have been created or produced by medical technologies. For instance, accompanying the development

Table 1.1   A typology of medical ethical issues

Medical ethical issues	Examples
The relationship between the physician and the patient	Truth telling Confidentiality Informed consent
The selection of medical interventions	Terminating care "Baby Doe" cases Euthanasia
The allocation of medical resources	Just health care Patient selection criteria for scarce resources
The application of personally transforming technologies	Genetic engineering Brain tissue transplants Psychosurgery

of life-sustaining technologies are the controversies about when to terminate such care and let patients die, and who should make such decisions:

> A newborn with a serious birth defect, or one whose future is clouded by acquired illness, sometimes confronts parents and physicians with a tragic choice . . . Participants in such a drama must choose whether to prolong the infant's life, or whether to act in a way that will shorten its life, whether by passive or active means.
>   Like many other ethical dilemmas in modern medicine, this one is a product of advances in technology.[5]

> We find ourselves, as physicians, in the midst of debate over practices that lengthen or shorten the lives of dying patients. The controversy has been thrust upon us by an ethical dilemma—between preserving life and relieving suffering—that has resulted from technological advance.[6]

> What has brought us to this position of awesome responsibility [in making quality-of-life judgments for patients]? Very simply, the sophistication of modern medicine.[7]

Similarly, accompanying the development of respirators and organ transplants is the debate over the definition of death:

> In the past, for example, there was no need for a physician to consider the concept of death: there was but one death. This has changed with the advent of new techniques that have made it pos-

sible to sustain life, or at least to sustain living matter . . . Doctors everywhere are now facing philosophical problems such as defining personhood and conceptualizing death.[8]

The question [of death] was a simple one when I was a boy. Then, the medical and legal definitions were the same: Death occurred when a person's circulation and respiration ceased permanently. But by the time I was facing death myself in 1973, a great controversy revolved around how to define it. Advances in medical technology had clouded the issue.[9]

The development of technology and simultaneous rise in medical costs force a search for principles to allocate these medical resources: "Medical science, in league with modern technology, has created an array of life-saving treatments that are both elaborate and expensive. The production and utilization of these new 'high' technologies in medicine have resulted in difficult and largely unforeseen problems of allocation."[10] And the development of new technologies to alter reproduction, genetics, and neurological function generates ethical dilemmas about their use: "[A] number of medical and technologic breakthroughs have created new moral dilemmas. There are problems in the care of the newborn and of the dying, in the use of psychotropic and other drugs to influence and change mood and behavior, in the development of an expanded scope of genetic knowledge and applied clinical applications, and in greater dilemmas of equity and distribution in the health care delivery system."[11]

The technological axiom is further substantiated by juxtaposing the histories of biomedical advances and medical ethics. Beginning in the late 1950s, coeval with the development, refinement, and widespread introduction of medical technologies, it is claimed, was the genesis of medical ethics itself. Initially it was theologians who raised medical ethical concerns. In 1954 Joseph Fletcher, a Christian theologian, published the landmark medical ethics text *Morals and Medicine,* which addressed issues from euthanasia to artificial insemination.[12] A few years later Immanuel Jakobovits finished a study of Jewish medical ethics.[13] And in 1958 Pope Pius XII responded to inquiries by an Austrian anesthesiologist about the ethics of maintaining irreversibly brain damaged patients on respirators.[14] During the 1960s and early 1970s medical ethics entered a second phase in which many physicians began noting and exploring medical ethical issues. In 1966 Henry Beecher, a professor at Harvard Medical School, published his study of unethical practices in clinical research.[15] In 1968, prompted by the maintenance of patients with irreversible brain damage on respirators and by the need for harvesting organs for transplantation, the Ad Hoc Committee of the Harvard Medical School reported a revised definition of brain death.[16] Research advances in *in vitro* fertilization brought ethical worries from other physicians.[17] Beginning in the 1970s a third phase arose with the creation of institutes exclusively devoted to the study of medical ethics, such as the Hastings Center, and the development of a cadre of secular, nonmedical commentators, so-called bioethicists, whose profession was the study of medical ethical issues. Since the mid-1970s, the profusion of medical technologies and therapies has made medical ethics a thriving discipline.

Widespread acceptance of the technological axiom has had three important effects on medical ethics. First, since these ethical dilemmas are considered new, created within the last few decades, the history of medical practice is viewed as unilluminating on medical ethical questions. The traditions and norms of the medical profession, elaborated and articulated over many centuries, are almost completely excluded from the consideration of medical ethical questions. In the extreme, the relevance of these traditions is explicitly denied or attacked as illegitimate.[18] Second, the technological axiom engenders the notion that dilemmas created by technology can concomitantly be resolved by additional technology.[19] Finally, and most important, this focus on technology makes medical ethical questions more a matter of medicine than of ethics. Medical ethical problems are viewed as another issue in which ethics is consulted for principles to provide an answer. These dilemmas do not prompt moral self-appraisal, a reexamination of our ethical ideals. The consequence, as Peter Singer has pointed out, is that "the ethics in bioethics [is] treated superficially."[20]

The technological axiom of medical ethics is wrong. Medical ethics is as old as medicine itself. It is an intrinsic part of medical practice. Medical ethical questions are inherent whenever an ailing person seeks out another person, trained in the medical arts, for knowledgeable advice on the best way to cure or ameliorate his ailments. Indeed, beginning with the Hippocratic oath and extending throughout history, physicians have felt the need to craft codes and oaths, in the words of the nineteenth-century physician Austin Flint, as guiding standards "for the sake of reference whenever differences of opinion arise [and to] indicate proper course to those whose moral perceptions may be defective."[21] These codes have not simply addressed issues of etiquette;[22] they have provided substantive advice on almost all of the pressing contemporary medical ethical issues (see Table 1.1), from confidentiality and truth telling to abortion and euthanasia to terminating care and the allocation of scarce resources.

Advancement in biomedical technology does affect medical ethical issues. It can make certain ethical issues more common and add to their complexity; it can shape the setting and clinical circumstances in which these issues arise; and, in some cases, it can provide alternative resolutions to these issues. In addition, advancement in biomedical technology can have a profound *psychological* impact on our expectations of what medicine can do—or at least should be able to do—in the face of illness. But technology has not *created* most of these medical ethical issues. The underlying questions—should we maintain the lives of defective newborns? should we withdraw care from terminally ill patients? how should we select recipients of scarce life-saving resources?—and the ethical considerations raised by these questions are as old as man and medicine. Technology has simply outfitted these eternal questions in new clothes, but it has not altered the fundamental ethical issues beneath the new appearances. In the words of Dr. Kenneth Ryan, the chairman of the National Commission for the Protection of Human Subjects of Biomedical and Behavioral Research: "Although advances in technology have heightened ethical concerns in recent years, the problems of euthanasia, withholding or withdrawing treatment, truth telling, informed consent, and equitable access to health care have long been with us. They were just never on an open public agenda."[23]

If technology has not created these medical ethical issues nor their interminable irresolution, why are they on the "public agenda"? I will suggest that the answer lies not in our scientific advancement but in our public values. Political philosophy is primarily concerned with the proper ends of human activities and what people should and should not do to realize those ends. One of its roles is to help specify the proper ends of medical practice, how competing ends should be balanced, and what physicians should and should not do to realize those ends. It is the failure of the political philosophy that underlies the contemporary deliberations in medical ethics, of liberalism, to provide such guidance that has created the current preoccupation with and irresolution of medical ethical questions.

To substantiate this claim I shall propose a new framework for rationally discussing medical ethical issues in which medical ethics is an integral part of political philosophy. This approach might be called a political conception of medical ethics.

The Ethical Dimension of Professions

Medicine is a profession not merely because it satisfies certain sociological or historical criteria, but also because it has an ethical dimension. To understand the nature of medical ethics, then, it is necessary to define the ethical dimension of a profession.

Two necessary, though not sufficient, ethical characteristics of a profession are (1) that it is dedicated to ethical ideals and (2) that it serves a subject, a client, for whose benefit the ethical ideals are pursued. A profession is partially characterized by its ends, the purposes that define its activities. What distinguishes a profession's ends from those of other occupations, such as carpentry and pastry making, is that they are ethical ends.[24] A profession's ends are recognized as forming an essential part of the human good and are qualitatively distinct from, higher than, other ends; the ends of a profession are higher goods. Presumably this is why, before the modern era, professions were viewed as "divinely sanctioned vocations" and men were called to them.[25] While the profession's ends are goods, and recognized as good, they are not the highest human ends. They are subordinate, serving to realize other final human ends.

A profession's ends are constitutive of the profession; the ends, and their interpretation, define the profession's mission and distinguish it from other activities. When a person chooses to becomes a member of a profession, he accepts—in the sense of affirming—the profession's ends as his own. An individual professional does not choose the ends; he is obligated to pursue those ends as part of choosing to be a member of the profession. Further, the ends of a profession are not comprehensive; a professional will have ends besides the ones constitutive of his profession. Therefore a professional is never exclusively defined by his professional role; he is always more than a professional. Finally, a profession's ends are usually multiple. There is a hierarchy among the ends; some ends are primary, others are secondary. But it is not the case that if conflicts among the ends arise, one end overrides the others in all circumstances. The balance of ends must be examined in each individual case.

A profession is also partially characterized by the subject of its activity, the client. Professions are other-directed; the ends of a profession aim at the good of someone other than the professional himself. This means that service to others comes before the professional's gain, economic or other, from the service. Because the profession aims to realize its ends on behalf of a client, a special professional-client relationship will be created. And because this relationship is formed to realize ethical ends, it will be governed by ethical norms integral to the realization of these ends. Furthermore, the success or the failure of the profession to realize its ends is evaluated from the client's perspective. Thus the professional has two objects of devotion: sustaining the profession's ethical ends in general and realizing them for a particular client's benefit.[26] In some situations, therefore, conflicts between these two objects of devotion may arise; benefiting a particular client might require contravening other ends of the profession. How such conflicts are balanced, whether the client's benefit or the integrity of the profession's ends takes priority, is a fundamental question of professional ethics.[27]

There are several points to note about the client. First, the client can be either singular or plural. In some professions the client is an identifiable individual and the good is realized in terms of that individual. In others, the client is a collection of individuals. In most instances the client comes to the professional voluntarily, looking for advice or assistance which the professional offers. But this voluntary quality is qualified.[28] Usually the client comes in need and recognizes the professional's superior knowledge and competence to advise.[29] In order to realize the ends of the profession, the client will also have to reveal information to and permit an invasion of private space by the professional. These elements create an inherent inequality and a potential for domination within the relationship. But the inequalities based on differences of need, knowledge, and vulnerability are partially redressed because the client can always leave the professional; the relationship is alienable. They are also partially redressed because the ends which regulate the interaction are realized for the client. Hence, the relationship and the professional should be devoted to the client's benefit and wish to avoid any possible abuse of the client.

The Ethical Dimension of Medicine

How do these abstract comments on the ethical dimension of professions generally help to illuminate the particular case of medical ethics?[30] The ends of medicine include (1) restoring the health of sick individuals, (2) relieving suffering, (3) ameliorating ill health when health cannot be achieved, (4) caring for the sick, and (5) promoting the health of the general community.[31] This list is not exhaustive; it delineates essential ends of medicine that can help to clarify the relationship between the ends of medicine and medical ethics. The list indicates that there is no single end of medicine, only ends. While these ends are ethical, part of the human good, they are not the ultimate human ends. We value health in part for itself, but only in small part. More important, we value it because it permits us to pursue other, higher goals. As is often said, "there is more to life than health." Indeed, a life solely devoted to health, devoid of other ends, is deemed vacuous, while a life aimed at realizing other ends, yet deprived of full health or subject to frequent bouts of pain and suffering, is deemed courageous.

The client of the physician is the sick person who becomes the patient. Thus the physician aims to restore the health or relieve the suffering of single individuals, and his primary obligation is to the patients for whom he cares. This corroborates the hierarchy among the ends of medicine. Because the subject of medicine is an individual, the primary ends of medicine are restoring health and relieving suffering of individuals rather than the community's health. The success or failure of the physician is evaluated not by the physician's economic gain or fame, but by the restoration of the patient's health or relief of the patient's suffering.

This brief delineation of the ethical dimension of medicine, of the ends and subject of medicine, illuminates the nature of medical ethics. First, it provides a way of differentiating medicine from related professions such as public health and nursing, thereby partially clarifying the priority among medical ends. While the physician is dedicated to individuals and therefore to restoring health and relieving suffering of individuals, the public health professional's client is the general public and his primary end is promoting the health of the general community.[32] Hence those with medical degrees who are primarily dedicated to the general health are not medical professionals but public health professionals. Because the ends of medicine encompass the promotion of the health of the general community, the medical professional's ends overlap with those of the public health professional; what distinguishes them is the nature of their client and, correlatively, which end is primary.

The distinction between medicine and nursing does not involve the plurality of the client, but rather a difference in the primary end of the profession. Medicine is devoted to health and the relief of suffering of sick patients, while nursing is primarily devoted to caring for the very same patients. Again, this does not mean that caring is not an end of medicine. It is; caring, however, is not the primary end of medicine, but the primary end of nursing.

Second, and more important, this elaboration of the ends of medicine clarifies why medical ethics is constitutive of medicine. The sets of fundamental medical ethical issues delineated in Table 1.1—those relating to the physician–patient relationship, the selection of medical interventions, and the allocation of medical resources—are intrinsic to medical practice, defined as attempts by physicians to restore the health or relieve the suffering of sick patients. Let us consider each of these ethical issues.

The realization of the ends of medicine necessitates a physician-patient relationship. This relationship is marked by three types of inequality: inequalities of need, knowledge, and vulnerability. A person comes to a physician, his existence or his integrity threatened by illness. He comes in need of knowing what he suffers from, its significance and prognosis. He also needs emotional support in this time of fear and fragility. He comes to the physician because the latter has knowledge of and expertise on his illness. Hence the patient must accept much of the physician's advice on trust. For a diagnosis to be made and treatment rendered, the patient will have to expose both his body and intimate factual details to the physician.

These inequalities make the physician-patient relationship liable to abuse. The inequality of need makes the patient liable to cognitive and emotional abuse; the inequality of knowledge makes the patient liable to manipulation for the pursuit of other ends, such as the physician's economic gain or the advancement of research; the inequality of vulnerability makes the patient liable to ridicule, deprivation, and discrimination if his vulnerabilities are publicly exposed. These inequalities inherent in the physician-patient relationship, not technology, create the medical ethical issues related to truth telling, confidentiality, sexual relations, informed consent; they are inescapable in the very practice of medicine. For this reason, medical oaths and codes, since the Hippocratic oath, have found it necessary to address these issues.

Attempts to realize the ends of medicine for the benefit of the patient necessarily create at least two different ethical issues relating to the selection of appropriate medical interventions. One is the issue of ethical means: What means, or interventions, can physicians ethically use to realize a particular end? This question underlies much of the debates surrounding euthanasia and abortion as well as ethical questions about experimental therapies. For instance, can physicians ethically relieve patients' suffering by euthanasia in the rare but real cases in which patients are experiencing unremitting pain despite proper use of narcotics and other pain-relieving interventions? Can physicians ethically assist such patients to commit suicide? Can physicians dispense laetrile to terminal cancer patients or the latest drug rumored to halt HIV infection to AIDS patients without knowing the efficacy or side effects of these drugs? Another is the issue of specifying the ends of medicine. In many circumstances the physician, committed to the ends of medicine, will be uncertain how these ends are to be understood in the treatment of a particular person. This concern underlies much of the debates surrounding the withholding or withdrawing of life-sustaining care. The pediatric surgeon confronted with a Down's-syndrome infant that has an esophageal obstruction will wonder which approach, repairing the obstruction or permitting the infant to die, will relieve suffering. The issues of ethical means and specifying the ends of medicine in particular cases are inherent in the practice of medicine, in the physician's attempt to restore the patient's health or to relieve his suffering. For this reason, throughout history medical debates and ethical commentaries have addressed the issues of abortion and euthanasia and have offered advice on how to approach vexing cases, especially the conflict between prolonging life or terminating care to relieve suffering.[33]

Medicine, like all social activities, operates under conditions of scarcity. There will always be more social needs than resources to satisfy them; there will always be more ailments to treat than physicians or medical supplies to treat them; and there will always be poor people who need medical care but cannot afford it. These conditions of scarc-

ity raise the issues of allocating medical resources and justice, of deciding what proportion of social resources should be spent on medicine
and how much on education or defense, which patients should be
given first priority for care, and who should pay for the care of the
poor. Questions of the just allocation of medical resources are inherent in the very practice of medicine. Physicians have experienced
them—and resolved them—in the triage of soldiers wounded in
battle, in caring for the sick during plagues, and in caring for the poor
at all times.[34]

The delineation of the ethical dimension of medicine as a profession
not only identifies those ethical issues that are inherent in medical
practice, it also provides substantive guidance on these issues. This
guidance is justified not by appeal to historical precedents, medical
customs, legal requirements, contracts between physicians and patients, or abstract moral principles, but rather by appeal to the ethical
norms intrinsic to medicine as a profession dedicated to certain ends,
to attending to sick people for the restoration of their health or the
relief of their suffering. Consider three examples.

For the ends of medicine to be realized for the patient's benefit, it is
necessary that the inequalities of need, knowledge, and vulnerability
be shielded from abuse through the creation of *prima facie* duties for
physicians. There are what we might call negative duties, duties to
refrain from lying, breeches of confidentiality, and sexual relations
with patients, as well as positive duties, duties to keep patients informed and to obtain their consent before instituting interventions.
These negative and positive duties protect the patient from emotional abuse, manipulation, public ridicule, and discrimination. Consequently, they have formed the core of most medical oaths and codes
from the Hippocratic oath to the ethical codes of contemporary medical societies. This historical precedent does not justify the duties, but
only attests to their being constitutive of medicine wherever and
whenever it is practiced.

The question of whether physicians should participate in capital
punishment by lethal injection offers a second example of substantive
guidance from the ends of medicine. Medicine's dedication to the restoration of health and the relief of suffering means that physicians
should not participate *qua* physicians in state executions, where the
lethal injection is not intended for a criminal's health or relief of his

suffering but merely for his death. Hence, the physician may not participate *qua* physician. The physician *qua* physician would justify his objection to executing a person by lethal injection not by questioning the justification of capital punishment but by arguing that he cannot administer medical treatments for an end that contravenes the ends of medicine. Conversely, a physician might be called upon to participate in an execution *qua* citizen, say, in a firing squad. A physician could not refuse this call on the ground that it conflicts with the ends of medicine; he is not being requested to execute *qua* physician. To object, a physician would have to question the justification of capital punishment in general or this execution in particular. The form of the execution and the role it requires of the physician make a difference to understanding the physician's obligations.[35]

This example might be beneficially contrasted with euthanasia. While both involve killing, the reason that prevents a physician from participating in executions by lethal injection does not apply to euthanasia. In some cases of euthanasia, the killing is a means to realize a valid medical end, the relief of suffering. In these rare instances, the physician cannot object to euthanasia on the ground that it inherently contravenes the ends of medicine. Rather, to defend the prohibition against physicians' participation in euthanasia requires a claim that certain means, such as intentional killing, should not be used to achieve the legitimate ends of medicine.

A third example of substantive guidance from the ethical dimension of medicine arises in the question of whether the physician has a *prima facie* obligation to treat AIDS patients and the sick poor. The commitment to healing the sick, whether they are rich or poor, whether they have AIDS or heart disease, is constitutive of medicine; when a person elects to become a physician he assumes this commitment; it is neither chosen nor transferable, but constitutive of medical practice. If a physician finds himself unable to care for such patients, then he needs to question whether medicine should be his chosen profession.[36]

Although the ends of medicine can provide substantive guidance in resolving some important medical ethical questions, in others they prove insufficient. For instance, while patient confidentiality is an accepted *prima facie* duty, it is not absolute. It is well recognized that in some circumstances, with good reasons, patient confidentiality may be violated.[37] What are the "good reasons"? Can a physician who diagnoses a bisexual man as having AIDS inform the patient's wife? Can the physician do so if he happens to be the wife's as well as the man's physician? Confronted by a conflict between confidentiality and promoting a patient's health, how should the physician act?

Inevitably, such questions cannot be resolved by appeal to the ends of medicine; alone, they offer insufficient guidance for resolving all medical ethical questions. Indeed, we can identify three types of ethical problems—collectively designated as the problems of specifying and balancing—that can be properly addressed only by appeal to an ethical framework more comprehensive than the ends of medicine.

First is the problem of *specification:* the ends of medicine are not self-defining but are in need of specification. For instance, the physician treating a car accident victim who is respirator-dependent and quadriplegic needs to know whether turning off the respirator constitutes relieving suffering or not. Cassell suggests that suffering be defined as "the distress associated with events that threaten the intactness of the person." [38] Is the personhood of the quadriplegic patient, permanently attached to a respirator and confined to a wheelchair, intact? Does the patient's dependence on machines perpetually threaten his personal integrity? The physician's quandary can be addressed only by superseding the ends of medicine and contemplating the meaning of personal identity. This and many other medical ethical questions can be addressed only by specifying the ends of medicine. And this, in turn, can be done only by going beyond the ends themselves.

As noted in the case of the bisexual man who has AIDS, there is a second problem relating to *internal balancing:* the ends of medicine will often conflict and will therefore need to be balanced against each other. Resecting a malignant tumor, for instance, may cause impotence. Which end should take priority, restoring health or preventing the suffering associated with impotence? Determining how conflicts between the ends of medicine should be balanced requires going beyond the ends themselves.

Finally, there is the problem of *external balancing:* nonmedical ends of life, such as independence, learning, justice, honesty, may conflict with and need to be balanced against the ends of medicine. Such external balancing clearly requires going beyond the ends of medicine.

How are the ends of medicine to be specified and balanced? To what *beyond* the ends of medicine do we appeal? How do we construct the more comprehensive ethical framework necessary to address these questions? What is the relationship of this framework to the ends of medicine?

Medical Ethics and Political Philosophy

Specifying and balancing ends must be informed by political philosophy. Clearly, balancing the ends of medicine with other nonmedical social ends, such as distributive and criminal justice, is influenced by political philosophy. Issues such as what proportion of social resources should be distributed to health care, what medical services the state should guarantee all citizens, and what patient selection criteria the state should permit or prohibit, reflect the community's values and ideals. Such medical ethical issues are essentially issues of political philosophy.

But we look to political philosophy not just to help address medical ethical questions that relate to the whole health care system, to the distribution of resources, but also to help in the specification and balancing of ends essential to the physician's treatment of individual patients. To know whether it is ethical to turn off the respirator for a quadriplegic patient requires conceptions of personal identity, a worthy human life, murder, and suicide; to know how much information a physician must provide a cancer patient to obtain proper informed consent for an experimental therapy requires conceptions of autonomy, coercion, and the public good and how to balance these values; to know whether to break the AIDS patient's confidentiality and inform his wife requires a framework for weighing the relative importance of competing individual rights as well as the public good. Such ethical conceptions and such a framework for weighing competing values are the domain of political philosophy. And it is only through political philosophy that a coherent ethical framework, one that delineates and organizes these notions into a consistent perspective suitable to guide the specification and balancing of the ends of medicine, can be realized.

Political philosophy is concerned with the collection of communal ends in a polity, articulated, elaborated, and organized into a coherent framework to guide the ethical reasoning of citizens as members of that community on issues of public concern. Political philosophy reflects and embodies shared values, or what is sometimes referred to as the common morality. Usually this is no simple process since these values are often implicit and inchoate; they often conflict; and they are often embedded in communal practices, traditions of argument, and the like. Political philosophy, therefore, is pursued as the articulation, interpretation, and elaboration of these values for public purposes; it aims to offer a way of connecting the ideals into a coherent ethical framework for public deliberation. At its highest, political philosophy can be thought of as common morality idealized.[39]

This coherent framework constitutes an ideal toward which the polity aspires. By articulating and organizing the community's shared ideals, political philosophy provides a standard that citizens will affirm and appeal to as providing justifications for their actions. In this sense, political philosophy offers a framework for ethical reasoning and public deliberation on matters of political concern and social conflict. It links our shared and common values with our points of ethical conflict, attempting to articulate the former to help resolve the latter.[40]

But it should not be thought that this framework is settled and established once and for all. Political philosophy is a dynamic process over time; certain values may be applied more widely, other values may be rejected, still others may be reinterpreted. Indeed, the process of attempting to resolve political or social controversies may force us to reject our underlying values or to revise the weight we give them. Even as the framework of political philosophy guides our communal deliberations, it may be subject to revision. In this way, political philosophy is similar to scientific theories: it is a constant but mutable framework to guide reflection and action.

To make clinical decisions for an individual patient, the practicing physician must specify and balance the ends of medicine. But this process occurs within a framework constructed from ethical conceptions that have been elaborated by political philosophy. Medical ethics is thus a subfield of political philosophy.

This approach is consonant with the practices of some medical ethicists. It is implicit and sometimes explicit in Daniel Callahan's approach to allocating resources and terminating care and in Norman Daniels' method of determining basic medical services, and it possibly underlies the approach adopted by the President's Commission in some of its reports.[41]

This view might be challenged by those who think that, apart from

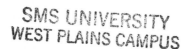

questions relating to the allocation of resources, the specification and balancing of the ends of medicine are not, and should not be, resolved by appeal to a community's shared ideals. Rather, they might maintain, these are private acts, to be performed by the physician in consultation with a patient appealing to religious or personal values, the patient's view of what constitutes a worthy life. Indeed, some might argue that determinations of how the physician and patient relate, whether certain life-sustaining treatments should be terminated or whether patients are able to use certain technologies, should be resolved by appeal to personal moral commitments regardless of communal, political standards.

In response, we need to remember that the ends of medicine and their specification and balancing are neither personal nor those of a single practitioner or patient. They are the ends of a profession to which individual practitioners must adhere; the ends are constitutive of the profession and its practices. As such, the ends and their specification and balancing are public declarations by the community of what the profession stands for. The ends and their specification and balancing regulate the relationship between professionals and members of the community in the particular professional-client relationships; they provide the assumed mutual understanding that serves as a background to this relationship, defining the expectations and responsibilities of each party. These ends define the community's understanding of the purpose of the profession and thereby how the profession is to serve the public good, better the common life, and interrelate with other public activities. For these ends to be declarations that the community can accept—or be persuaded to accept—they must be justified by appeal to the community's shared ethical ideals. Hence they must be justified by appeal to public values that both the professional and the citizen affirm.

Further, a profession serves the community and practices within the community. Its appropriate practices are shaped by the explicit expressions of the community's philosophy, expressed in the criminal and civil law and other regulatory policies. For example, deciding whether to terminate the quadriplegic's respirator for the relief of suffering will depend not just on the patient's personal values but on whether withholding or withdrawing life-sustaining care constitutes murder, assisting suicide, or not; deciding whether to break the AIDS patient's confidentiality will depend not just on the patient's desire for privacy but on communal notions of injury and responsibility, the public standards embodied in tort law. This is not to say that the guiding ethical framework embodied in existing laws and policies will simply dictate resolutions to these ethical questions. Indeed, reflection on these ethical questions may lead to modifications of the community's own ethical ideals and laws. But this means that the framework for deciding these issues is constructed from political, not personal, philosophy.

Even in those areas of medical practice where there may be no laws or public policies to determine how ethical issues should be addressed, the community frequently has an interest in how these issues are resolved. Medical practices can sustain or undermine many social ideals. And therefore, ethical decisions about these practices may not simply be private matters. For instance, decisions such as whether physicians terminate care to infants with Down's syndrome, or artificially fertilize surrogate mothers, or begin purchasing organs for transplantation, both express and forge collective understandings and ideals. These are not merely private choices; they influence how we understand the status and rights of mentally disabled people, the good of children, the value of pregnancy and human organs. While such medical practices may begin as private acts to benefit individual patients, their reverberations affect all of us by changing our understanding of the public good and communal values. Consequently, such decisions implicate the community's values, and their ethics need to be evaluated within political philosophy.

This brings me to the last point: what is considered private and what is considered a public matter subject to political values is itself a public, political decision informed by a conception of the relationship between the polity and the citizen, the public and the private. Consequently, whether certain medical ethical questions are in fact left to personal discretion or practitioner choice, without regulation through laws or policies, is informed by political philosophy and not by any physician's or patient's private ethical dispositions alone. In this way, personal decisions are inherently structured by and embody political conceptions and the method of weighing different values espoused by the community.

To determine what they should do, medical practitioners have to look beyond the ends of medicine and beyond their personal commitment, to political philosophy. If medical ethics is an essential part of medicine, so too must be political philosophy.

Implications of the Political Conception

The claims of the political conception suggest several implications. First, the political conception offers an explanation for a persistent question within professional ethics: How can a profession simultaneously be autonomous and subject to the moral rules of a polity? The political conception accepts that each profession has ends that are unique to the profession. These ends define the purpose of its activities and some of its ethical norms. But no professional ethic can be derived solely from the profession's ends; many ethical questions require that the ends be both specified and balanced by appeal to political philosophy. Thus a profession is partially autonomous, because its unique ends can delineate specific duties and ethical practices. But since these ends are insufficient to address all ethical questions of the profession, there must also be appeal to the shared public ideals. Because all professions must appeal to the same idealized common morality, they are integrated into a whole. Thus we can imagine that each profession has a sphere of its own activity, and these separate spheres are then integrated into a consistent ethical framework through political philosophy. Political philosophy provides a unified framework informing the different subfields of each profession. Another metaphor might illuminate this relationship: each profession can be regarded as a room within a house, with political philosophy providing the foundation and walls that both support each room and define the common areas linking each room into a whole house.

Furthermore, on the political conception, the different professional ethics are part of the dialectical nature of political philosophy. These different professional ethics actively form part of political philosophy. The questions and ethical judgments within the professional realm provide some of the ideals and ethical practices that are elaborated to inform the community's political philosophy. Concomitantly, the resolutions offered by political philosophy to professional ethical questions are tested, supported, and criticized by the particular judgments in actual cases within the practice of the profession. Thus, the sphere of a profession is neither completely autonomous from nor subsumed by political philosophy.

The political conception can be clarified by distinguishing it from three other positions on the relationship between professional ethics and common morality. The first position is the teleological approach to professional ethics articulated by Leon Kass, Edmund Pellegrino, and the advocates of clinical ethics.[42] This view holds that there is a medical ethic intrinsic to medical practice. "The nature and meaning of the medical art" are discovered by examining its end—"health and wholeness"—and the circumstances necessary to realize this end. This end dictates special duties for the physician and guides him in deciding what care to provide patients. The interpretation of the end of medicine and these duties are articulated in medical oaths and codes that physicians should consult for guidance. Within the teleological approach, political philosophy and professional ethics are completely *separable spheres*. On this view the ethical norms of professional conduct can be derived from within the profession based on its intrinsic ends. Thus all professional ethical questions can be answered from within professional ethics. Political philosophy does not affect professional ethics.[43]

This teleological approach to professional ethics must be rejected because, as I have shown, professional ethics, exclusively derived from the ends of the profession, cannot answer all ethical questions arising from professional activities. Ethical issues requiring the specification and balancing of ends are part of professional ethics. And this specification and balancing cannot occur from within the intrinsic professional ethic but require appeal to political philosophy. Thus the realm of professional ethics cannot be completely separable from common morality, as suggested by the teleological approach.

The second position is applied ethics, an approach advocated by bioethicists, especially Beauchamp and Childress, Veatch, Gorovitz, and Engelhardt.[44] Applied ethics denies that there is a medical ethic intrinsic to the practice of medicine. Medical ethics is "derivative . . . justified by reference to more general and fundamental principles and rules. [Thus medical ethics is derived by] applying general moral-action guides to biomedicine . . . Biomedical ethics is thus comparable to political ethics and business ethics . . . [It is] the *application* of general moral principles to an area of human activity" (emphasis in the original).[45] The applied ethics approach conceives of professional ethics as *derived from* common morality. Thus professional ethics is created by the principles of common morality applied to the problems of a profession; there are no intrinsic professional norms; professional ethics is subsumed by common morality.

Applied ethics must be rejected because political philosophy does not completely subsume professional ethics. A profession has autonomous ends and ethical norms that are intrinsic and do not require appeal to the principles of common morality for justification. Further, the applied ethics approach offers no way of balancing conflicting ends because it presents no way of balancing the principles of common morality. Finally, and most important, these principles are not applied to professional ethical issues seriatim to generate the norms of professional ethics. Indeed, the notion of fixed principles applied to problems is erroneous. There is a dialectic in which our reflections on professional ethical issues modify common morality.

The third approach is exemplified by a prominent view of legal ethics.[46] On this view there is a role morality associated with a profession, and this role morality has an uneasy and usually tense relationship with common morality. Political philosophy and professional ethics are separate, connected but conflicting ethical spheres. Professional ethics is role-related and thus intrinsic to the profession and its structure. But the ethical imperatives of this role are always to be tested against the dictates of common morality. Sometimes these two ethical views will overlap, providing very strong justification for an ethical action; frequently the professional ethic will conflict with our shared values. The ethical demands of the profession and political philosophy will thus be in constant tension; they will *conflict but have to be balanced* so that neither has an overriding claim, although each does have a claim.

This view, the balancing approach, is to be rejected because the ethical norms of a profession are not necessarily antagonistic to the dictates of the common morality, requiring a balancing between the two conflicting ethical spheres. There is no inherent tension, but rather a necessity for coherence between professional ethics and political philosophy. Indeed, it is not clear from this approach how this balancing is to be achieved; by appeal to what ethical framework can we justify the balancing, if not to political philosophy? And further, like the teleological approach, this approach fails to recognize that professional ethics cannot resolve the major ethical issues without appeal to common morality. There is a need for coherence between professional ethics and common morality.

Each of these three approaches should be rejected. Professional ethics is not separated from, derived from, or to be balanced against political philosophy. Instead, it is best to see that the intrinsic ends of a profession are incomplete; they need specification and balancing through political philosophy. A complete account of the purposes of the profession—a specification of its ends, a balancing of its internal ends, a balancing of its internal ends with nonprofessional ends—requires political philosophy. Professional ethics can be fully articulated only by references to political values. Professional ethics and political philosophy are not in conflict or at cross-purposes, but professional ethics is insufficient without the values articulated in political philosophy.

This is not to say that there will not be some tensions between professional ethics and political philosophy. There may well be. These tensions may arise from different elaboration of certain conceptions, specification of professional obligations and purposes, and assessments of the weight to give certain values. The political conception, however, denies that these tensions are inherent, arising from a necessary antithesis between professional role and citizen. According to the political conception, the relationship between professional ethics and political philosophy might be characterized by the metaphor of *integration*.

This leads to a second implication of the political conception of medical ethics, relating to what we might call the "division of moral labor."[47] Since each profession has an internal ethic and since, to practice, each profession must come to some understanding of how its various ends should be balanced, each profession will require an interpretation of political philosophy for its professional matters. In other words, for a profession to pursue its activities many professional ethical questions must be resolved. But these can only be resolved by relating political philosophy to the professional activity. Thus integral to each profession will be an interpretation of political philosophy as related to its own professional activities. Consequently, it is incumbent on the profession to address certain ethical questions in a way that it is not for the average citizen. For instance, to delineate patient selection criteria for scarce organ transplants requires balancing the pursuits of health and justice. The transplant team needs to decide whether organs should be allocated randomly on the basis of a lottery or whether they should be given to those who are likely to survive the longest with the transplants. Resolving such dilemmas will require an interpretation of distributive justice. In this way a profession is the initial or primary interpreter of a community's political philosophy within the profession's sphere of activities. The profession's interpretation is the *prima facie* standard that is given deference. This suggests that there is a "division of moral labor." The profession attends to its own professional ethical questions, providing an interpretation of political philosophy for its own ethics. Hence the profession might be viewed as the guardian of its own ethics as well as society's representative doing the primary work on ethical issues relating to the profession.

But the profession's interpretation is not the only, or necessarily the dominant, interpretation of the profession's ethics. Since the professional ethical questions are public questions, any member of the community can provide an alternative interpretation of political philosophy for the professional ethics. In fact, as the professional ethical questions become more important, either by implicating more fundamental communal ideals or by affecting more people, it is likely that community members will scrutinize the profession's interpretation and offer alternative interpretations of political philosophy for professional ethics. The profession's interpretation is given deference but not necessarily precedence. To put it another way, the "division of moral labor" is not rigid; there is job flexibility.

This view explains why professions are permitted to be self-regulating and to articulate their own codes of ethical conduct, but why the polity always retains powers to review professional rules of conduct and ethical codes. Professions are given deference as guardians of their ethic, but not absolute or exclusive rights. Ultimately the appeal is to the community's political philosophy, which can be interpreted by all citizens.

A third implication of the political conception relates to pluralism of professional ethics. Because different communities will espouse different political philosophies, professional ethics will vary among communities. Thus we should expect that different communities with different values and political philosophies will balance health and justice differently. Empirically this will be noted in the different patient selection criteria for scarce medical resources and what medical services are guaranteed citizens as a matter of justice. Similarly, different communities will understand suffering, murder, and the physician's obligation to preserve life in different ways, creating different views on the ethics of terminating the quadriplegic's respirator. And conceptions of personal privacy and confidentiality will differ among communities, producing different standards on the public disclosure of a patient's AIDS diagnosis. The political conception of professional ethics provides a way of doing comparative professional ethics by doing comparative political philosophy.

A final implication of the political conception relates to deprofessionalization. As I have argued, a profession cannot be autonomous in the sense of being self-sufficient. The objectives of the profession's practices depend upon how its ends are specified and balanced internally and externally. Consequently, a profession must be able to articulate and elaborate its ideals in the context set by the community's values and delineate their implications for professional practices and ends. Deprofessionalization occurs when members of a profession are unable to delineate the profession's objectives by appeal to the framework constructed by political philosophy. In such cases the professional cannot justify his, or the profession's, practices. Justification, then, relies on those outside the profession.

This responsibility for ethical interpretation is threatened by professional specialization. As the members of a profession become more specialized, focusing their knowledge and training on technical skills, the attention to the ends of the profession and their relationship to political philosophy atrophies. Professionals then redescribe their ends in narrower, technical terms disconnected from the profession's ethical ends, and these tasks can be practiced independent of the profession's overall end. The consequence is that the specialist ceases to understand and guard his profession's ethics.

In medicine such circumstances might arise when an interventional radiologist is asked to place a feeding tube into a patient in a persistent vegetative state. If the radiologist simply decides whether placing the feeding tube is feasible and fails to consider the ends for which it is being placed and their appropriateness, he has become a mere technician. This trend in medicine has resulted in the rise of professional bioethicists or hospital-based philosophers. Their function has been to interpret political philosophy for the practicing physician and thereby to define the ends and purposes of the physician's practices.

This is deprofessionalization. And, in turn, it fosters both the commercialization of medical activities, since each independent task can be sold for profit, and the abandonment of professional status and standards.

According to the political conception, there is no role for hospital-based philosophers or ethics consultants to address medical ethical dilemmas. Medical ethics is intrinsic to medicine. As each citizen must be a political philosopher, so each physician must be a medical ethicist; to be a physician is to be a medical ethicist because there is no way for a practitioner to determine what should be done without engaging in medical ethics. The aim of medical ethics, then, should not be to create a pool of bioethicists for physicians to consult for the resolution of dilemmas, but to make physicians recognize the intrinsic ethical nature of their practice and to understand the relationship between the ends of medicine and political philosophy. Bioethicists may have a role in this process by helping doctors to become better medical ethicists. But the current role of the professional bioethicists in addressing clinical dilemmas only attests to the deprofessionalization and commercialization of medicine and reveals how far medical ethics has been dissociated from modern medicine.

The Irresolution of Medical Ethical Questions

The political conception of medical ethics can now help to answer the original question of this chapter: Why do contemporary medical ethical questions seem so irresolvable? According to the political conception, medical ethical questions are coeval with medicine. Medical practitioners in every place, at every time, need to address these questions to know how they should care for sick people. What differentiates our era is not the existence of these medical ethical questions, but the sense that they defy resolution, that there is no coherent ethical framework in which to deliberate on them.

To explain this phenomenon, we should focus on the underlying political thought. For it is political philosophy that provides the framework in which these ethical questions are addressed. The political conception of medical ethics suggests that the reason why medical ethical questions seem irresolvable may well inhere not in some defect of medical practice or the advent of biomedical technology or the inherent complexity of moral life, but in our community's political philosophy. In particular, liberal political philosophy informs much of the current moral thought. One of its basic tenets is the principle of neutrality, the notion that the laws and policies of the country should not be based on any particular view of the good life. On this view, there should be no substantive end that is either promoted by or used to justify society's laws and policies. Without an end that informs the ethical framework, it is impossible to determine the ends that medicine should pursue and thus to resolve medical ethical questions. The difficulty presented by liberalism is not merely a practical impossibility arising from the multitude of views espoused in our society. Rather, in liberal political philosophy there is not even a theoretical way of resolving the pressing medical ethical issues.

To defend this view I shall focus on two urgent and controversial medical ethical questions—terminating life-sustaining care to incompetent patients and the just distribution of medical resources—in Chapters 3 and 4, respectively. I shall connect the nature of the controversy surrounding these issues with aspects of the liberal political philosophy that informs much of American public life.

This examination serves three purposes. First, substantiating the claim that these problems remain irresolvable because of certain elements of liberal political philosophy will validate the political conception of medical ethics. Thus the examination of these medical ethical questions tests the validity of the political conception. Second, if the link between these medical ethical issues and political philosophy is valid, then it suggests that the modifications necessary for resolution of these—and other—medical ethical questions are matters of political philosophy. In other words, resolution of medical ethical issues may require revisions in our values and how we understand our political ideals. Finally, as I argued in the previous section, there is a reciprocal, supportive relationship between our ethical judgments and political philosophy. Medical ethical questions and judgments are no less a part of this relationship than political or legal judgments; our judgments on medical ethical issues and the resolutions suggested by our political philosophy must "fit together." In this sense, our medical ethical judgments inform our political philosophy. And thus the study of medical ethical issues becomes political philosophy.

Further, medical ethical issues are a "test" for political philosophy. The adequacy of political philosophy is evaluated by two distinct tests. One is the test of justification. Here the question is: Does the political philosophy cohere with the society's historical traditions, political culture and practices, and shared ethical judgments?[48] Answering this test requires a cultural and historical assessment.

A second test is whether the political philosophy "meets the practical requirements of social life."[49] Here the question is: Does the political philosophy construct an ethical framework in which the practical ethical questions confronting society can be deliberated on and resolved? There are two senses to this question. It might be an inquiry into the probability that government would implement the policies derived from political philosophy. This is a question of *political practicality*. But clearly, the evaluation of a political philosophy cannot depend upon the vagaries of actual power politics. The other sense of this question is one of *philosophical plausibility*. It is a question of whether the political philosophy can, even in *theory*, provide an adequate framework for addressing pressing public issues. In our circumstance the test of philosophical plausibility becomes: Does liberal political philosophy provide an ethical framework for "free agreement, reconciliation through public reason" in matters relating to medical ethics?[50] If the answer is no, then liberalism fails to realize its own objective and may require revision, or even abandonment. Rawls accepts this test and conclusion for his own theory when he writes on the issue of allocating medical resources: "Perhaps the social resources to be devoted to the normal health and medical needs of [normal] citizens can be decided at the legislative stage in light of existing social conditions and reasonable expectations of the frequency of illness and accident . . . If [a solution] cannot be worked out for this case, the idea of primary goods may have to be abandoned."[51]

Historically, political philosophers have not been interested in medical ethics. Although they examine legal questions, especially concerning constitutional law, questions of income inequality, and the like, medical ethical questions have not received much attention. This book should further the concern of political philosophers with medical ethical questions. And such concern may change our practice of political philosophy. Medicine is a teleological activity, aiming to realize substantive ethical ends in practice. Medical ethical questions require addressing the specification of ends and their balancing. Thus, by addressing medical ethical questions, political philosophy will be forced to consider substantive ends and functions and not just procedures and rights.

2

The Nature of Liberal Political Philosophy

Two Forms of Liberalism

I have claimed that political philosophy provides the framework for addressing medical ethical questions and that the persistent irresolution of these questions in American society derives from its liberal political philosophy. What is the nature of this liberal political philosophy?

One of the "constitutive principles of liberalism"[1] is the ideal of neutrality. In modern societies, individuals typically espouse a plurality of conceptions of the meaning, purpose, and value of life, that is, conceptions of the good life. According to the ideal of neutrality, the state should tolerate these different conceptions of the good life and not try to impose a particular view of what is worthy or good. The state is neutral when it does not base its laws on any particular conception of the good life, and thereby permits people to affirm and pursue their own ideas of what is worthy. This liberal ideal of neutrality does not claim that state policies will not have a differential effect on the pursuits of citizens; clearly different policies will generally help some rather than others. Neutrality of effect is impossible, an absurd ideal. Instead, the ideal is for neutrality in justification.[2] "The basic [political] institutions and public policy are [neither] to be designed to favor any particular" conception of the good life nor to be justified by appeal to any particular conception of the good life.[3] On liberal grounds, the state's institutions and policies should create a political framework within which individuals who hold different views can pursue their own conception of the good life. Dworkin succinctly summarizes the ideal of neutrality: "[Liberalism] supposes [as its constitutive political morality] that political decisions must be, so far as possible, independent of any particular conception of the good life, or of what gives value to life. Since the citizens of a society differ in their conceptions, the government does not treat them as equals if it prefers one conception to another."[4]

There are different ways of understanding and justifying this neutrality, and therefore different forms of liberalism. One of the dominant forms is *moral liberalism*, which justifies neutrality by appeal to individual autonomy.[5] The highest human good, according to moral liberalism, is for individuals to fashion their own lives by their own lights. An individual can be autonomous only when he actually exercises his own capacities of choice, judgment, and the like. Autonomy, and the full flourishing of the individual, require that the state let individuals exercise these capacities themselves, without interference. The limits on government action and the content of government policies—an extensive set of individual rights and opportunities—are necessary to ensure that individuals realize the ideal of autonomy. Where government policies are necessary, the justification should be to enhance each individual's ability to choose and create her own life. In education policy, for instance, the objective should be to ensure that children have sufficient knowledge and exposure to choose and create their own lives. The moral liberal believes:

> The content of children's right to education will depend upon what is adequate for living a full life within their society—for being capable of choosing among available conceptions of the good and of participating intelligently in democratic politics if they so choose . . . [Consequently moral liberals] rank children's rights to education above their rights to religious freedom since [moral liberals] believe that this restriction of their present liberty is necessary to create the conditions for future enjoyment of religious and other freedoms. Without education, liberal freedoms lose a great deal, even if not all, of their value.[6]

Similarly, the moral liberal endorses state support of art because it will enhance the opportunity of individuals to create their own lives.[7]

Historically, moral liberalism has been a dominant strand both in philosophy, including Kant and Mill, and in American culture.[8] However, it has been attacked as being not really, or not sufficiently, liberal. Moral liberalism guarantees governmental neutrality and extensive individual freedom from state interference, but it does so to promote a single conception of the good life. Since the principle of individual autonomy is used to justify state laws and policies, moral liberalism permits the state to promote a single conception of the good life to all citizens, regardless of their individual values. In moral liberalism, therefore, there is no neutrality of justification because governmental neutrality is justified by appeal to a view of the highest human good: autonomy.

An alternative has been proposed: *political liberalism.*[9] Articulated by Rawls, Dworkin, and others, this liberalism informs contemporary American political and legal thought. And the fundamental conceptions of political liberalism—its notions of pluralism, autonomy, equality, and its framework for relating these ethical conceptions— have implicitly and explicity influenced medical ethics.[10] My purpose is not to provide a detailed interpretation of political liberalism; but neither is it sufficient simply to review Rawls's two principles of justice to reveal the importance of political liberalism for medical ethics.[11] To understand how such principles are to be interpreted, to what social goods they apply, requires some appreciation for the complexity of the theory. Indeed, it is only through understanding the basic conceptions of political liberalism and the framework they create that their effect on medical ethics can be illustrated.

The Tenets of Political Liberalism

Political liberalism can be understood as being constructed from seven tenets. The first three define the practical and philosophical background for political liberalism, indeed for any political philosophy; the remaining four are the constitutive tenets characteristic of political liberalism.[12]

1. *The Circumstances of Justice.* Two facts of social life form the *practical* background to considerations of justice: scarcity of resources and pluralism of beliefs. Scarcity means that there will always be more demand than supply of resources, which requires a theory delineating social cooperation and the distribution of resources. Pluralism is the historical fact that in modern society people "hold opposing religious and philosophical beliefs, and affirm not only diverse moral and political doctrines, but also conflicting ways of evaluating arguments and evidence when they try to reconcile these oppositions."[13] In modern society there is no agreed-upon view of the good life to guide enactment of laws and policies.

2. *The Justification of Justice.* Because of pluralism, political philosophy cannot be justified by appeal to any transcendental religion or

philosophy. Instead, political philosophy is the articulation, elaboration, and formulation of ethical ideals implicit or latent in existing institutions, traditions, and practices. This theory is then revised by comparison with shared ethical judgments—for instance, that racial and religious discrimination is wrong—and traditional theories. The ultimate aim is to achieve both a coherence between the theory and individual ethical judgments and generalized agreement on the particular philosophy. On this view, the justification of a political philosophy rests on all things—ethical convictions, traditions, practices, and the philosophy—"fitting together" into a consistent whole.[14] Thus, political philosophy is a structure without foundations that is justified by a dynamic "reflective equilibrium" in which there is mutual support—and potential for revision—between particular ethical judgments, ethical ideals, and general principles. This implies that we cannot simply apply principles to cases; "the study of our substantive moral" judgments informs general principles, indeed may lead to their revision or rejection. It also means that political philosophy "starts from within a certain political tradition" and is informed by the values of that tradition.[15]

3. *The Objectives of Justice.* The purpose of political philosophy is practical; it provides a shared ethical "framework for deliberation" that citizens appeal to in assessing the justice of social institutions, laws, and policies.[16] Most important, a political philosophy's framework serves to guide the assessment and restructuring of the "basic structure" of society, that is, "the way in which the major social institutions distribute fundamental rights and duties and determine the division of advantages from social cooperation."[17] These institutions—including the constitution, the legal system, property, economic institutions, educational institutions, and the like—receive primary attention because they define the background into which we are born and in which we create and pursue our lives; this background has a pervasive effect on our lives and their possibilities from birth.

I now move from the general tenets that apply to all political philosophies to the specific claims distinctive of political liberalism.

4. *The Ideal of Neutrality.* According to political liberalism, the only way to accept pluralism while avoiding "the autocratic use of state power" is to espouse neutrality. Excluding from politics the diverse conceptions of a good life found in a modern, pluralistic society is the only way to secure political agreement and resolve social problems.

But while pluralism precludes agreement on a detailed conception of the good life, it does not preclude the sharing of some values and principles by people with diverse conceptions of the good. Thus we can all agree that religious or racial discrimination is wrong. These shared values can provide the "kernel of an overlapping consensus" from which the basic framework of political philosophy is elaborated. Neutrality is preserved because the political philosophy is justified by appeal to values shared by different conceptions of the good life and not by appeal to any particular detailed conception of the good life.

5. *The Conception of the Person.* The entire framework and particular principles of political liberalism depend upon its conception of a person.[18] A person has two moral powers or capacities: "A sense of justice is the capacity to understand, to apply, and to act from the public conception of justice which characterizes the fair terms of social cooperation. The capacity for a conception of the good is the capacity to form, to revise, and rationally to pursue a conception of one's rational advantage or good."[19] By possessing these two moral powers, citizens are *equal* and entitled to the benefits of social cooperation. Citizens are *free* in the sense that they can choose their own good and take responsibility for it, but the particular ends they choose do not affect their political standing, rights, opportunities, or privileges. In other words, our political freedom inheres in the ability to stand apart from our conception of the good. Our political rights do not depend upon our choice of final ends; we are free from politically punitive actions resulting from our choice of religion, political views, careers, or spouses, and from any changes, minor or radical, that we make in these choices during our lives.

6. *The Conception of Justice.* The principles of justice indicate how to distribute goods. To clarify Rawls's now famous two principles of justice, I shall restate them as three principles:

a. Each person has an equal right to the most extensive scheme of equal basic liberties compatible with a similar scheme for all.
b. Offices and positions must be open to all under conditions of fair equality of opportunity.
c. Inequalities of wealth and income must be to the greatest advantage of the least advantaged members of society.

In essence, the first principle is one of strict equality—all citizens get the same rights; the second is one of fair equality of opportunity, ensuring that those who possess the same talents, abilities, and drive should have the same prospects of success regardless of their starting point in the social hierarchy or their family's income;[20] and the third is Rawls's well-known difference principle requiring the distribution of incomes to ensure that the worst-off people are maximally benefited. These principles are "lexically ordered" so that the first one must be fully satisfied before the succeeding ones are applied.

7. *The Conception of the Good.* The primary goods are the things to be distributed by the three principles of justice. Each person, regardless of his particular conception of the good life, affirms the liberal conception of a person. Therefore, each person recognizes that people should exercise their two moral powers as well as have a chance to pursue their own particular conception of the good life. The primary goods are those things "generally necessary as social conditions and all-purpose means to enable human beings to realize and exercise their moral powers and to pursue their final ends."[21] These primary goods, then, are deemed good by every person and define a common standard of what each citizen needs that is derived from the conception of a person but independent of any particular conception of the good life. The five primary goods are as follows:

   a. First, the basic liberties as given by a list, for example: freedom of thought and liberty of conscience, freedom of association, and the freedom defined by the liberty and integrity of the person, as well as the rule of law, and finally the political liberties;
   b. Second, freedom of movement and choice of occupations against a background of diverse opportunities;
   c. Third, powers and prerogatives of offices and positions of responsibility, particularly those in the main political and economic institutions;
   d. Fourth, income and wealth; and
   e. Finally, the social bases of self-respect.[22]

Once the conception of a person, the principles of justice, and the primary goods have been defined, their integral relationship to each other, their mutual dependence, should be clear.[23]

   This summary of the seven tenets of political liberalism will help to clarify why liberal political philosophy produces the persistent irresolution surrounding medical ethical issues in contemporary America. Simultaneously, this examination will provide a test of the *philosophi-*

cal plausibility of political liberalism. The study of the issues of terminating care and allocating medical resources will show how the liberal ideal of neutrality, the prohibition against justifying state laws and policies by appeal to a conception of the good life, precludes, even in theory, any resolution to these medical ethical issues.

3

Terminating Medical Care for Incompetent Patients

On the evening of April 15, 1975, a few friends gathered for a party. Inexplicably one of the group, a 21-year-old woman, stopped breathing. Some of her friends tried frantically to give her mouth-to-mouth resuscitation; after about fifteen minutes she began breathing. Shortly thereafter she again stopped breathing for about fifteen minutes. The police and an ambulance arrived, began resuscitation, and took the unconscious woman to the hospital. In the emergency room, a doctor found the woman with fixed pupils and unresponsive to deep pain. Unclear about the history and cause of the respiratory arrest, the physicians continued to resuscitate her, placed her on a respirator, and transferred her to the intensive care unit. A blood and urine toxic screen revealed no drug overdose, although quinine and barbiturates were detected in the therapeutic range, with traces of valium and librium. There was no evidence of either trauma or poisoning.

After several days without evident improvement, a neurologist, Dr. Morse, was asked to examine the patient. Her ocular reflexes were normal, but she was unresponsive to pain and had decorticate posturing (flexed arms and extended legs), suggestive of significant damage to higher brain functions but preserved brain stem functions.

Several weeks later, still unresponsive, maintained on the respirator and fed through a naso-gastric tube, the patient was transferred to the intensive care unit at Saint Clare's Hospital. A brain scan, electroencephalogram, lumbar puncture, and angiogram all seemed to confirm that she had extensive brain damage with some preservation of her brain stem function. These tests did not help to establish a cause for the events of April 15. The patient continued to receive around-the-clock care by nurses under Dr. Morse's direction.

Although she remained in an unconscious, vegetative state, this young woman was certainly not brain-dead. In fact, she developed cycles in which she would alternate between states of complete unresponsiveness, "sleep," and "awakened" states in which she demonstrated blinking, chewing motions, and periods of crying. Nevertheless, even during these "awakened" periods she was unaware of any human or inanimate object in her environment. After many weeks, it became obvious that there was no real hope of her ever recovering from this vegetative condition; as some put it, "she can *never* be restored to a cognitive or sapient life." [1] This conclusion was confirmed by the examination of several other neurologists.

What should be done? Should this woman's respirator be stopped? Should her naso-gastric feedings be stopped? How vigilant should Dr. Morse and the nurses be in monitoring and treating this patient's condition? Should they order a special bed to prevent the development of bedsores, which often become infected and require antibiotics? Should they continue to monitor this woman's vital signs, measuring her temperature, blood pressure, and heart rate? What should they do if she develops a fever? How vigorously should they try to diagnose its source? Should they treat the fever "empirically" with antibiotics? Or should they just let her die from the infection? If she begins bleeding, should Dr. Morse and the nurses give her blood transfusions? Should they withhold transfusions, waiting to see if she stops bleeding on her own? Fundamentally, all these questions reduce to one: What medical care should this patient receive?

On July 31, 1975, after three and a half months of anguish and prayer, followed by extensive discussion of these questions with their priest and the Saint Clare's Hospital Catholic chaplain, the patient's family wrote Dr. Morse the following note: "We authorize and direct Doctor Morse to discontinue all extraordinary measures, including the use of a respirator for our daughter, Karen Quinlan . . . [W]e hereby RELEASE from any and all liability the above named physician, associates and assistants of his choice, Saint Clare's Hospital and its agents and employees." [2] Uncertain how to respond, Dr. Morse investigated similar medical case histories and concluded that "to terminate the respirator would be a substantial deviation from medical tradition, that it involved ascertaining 'quality-of-life,' and that he would not do so." The local prosecutor and the New Jersey attorney general also threatened criminal proceedings if the respirator was turned off. Karen's father went to court to try to enforce the family's request. Justice Muir ruled against the family, arguing:

There is a higher standard, a higher duty, that encompasses the uniqueness of human life, the integrity of the medical profession and the attitude of society toward the physician. A patient is placed, or places himself, in the care of a physician with the expectation that he (the physician) will do everything in his power, everything that is known to modern medicine, to protect the patient's life . . . Society has come to request and expect this higher duty . . . The nature, extent and duration of care by societal standards is the responsibility of a physician.[3]

The case was appealed, and the New Jersey Supreme Court was forced to decide the question of what constituted appropriate medical care for Karen Quinlan.

The question is deceptively simple. In "normal" cases the objectives of medical interventions seem clear and obvious to all, needing no explication or articulated justification. Instead, such a question usually refers to the physician's technical judgment about the appropriate means to an obvious end. For instance, if a child has an ear infection, the question about what medical care he should receive refers to which antibiotic treatment should be used. Similarly, if an adult has obstructed coronary arteries, the question refers to a choice between a pharmacologic regimen, a catheter-guided balloon dilatation of the artery (percutaneous translumenal coronary angioplasty, or PTCA), or a surgical bypass operation based on rates of success, long-term mortality, and the like.

The force of the *Quinlan* case lies in the fact that these presumed, unarticulated objectives of medical interventions are obscured. Physicians cannot just treat Karen's inability to breathe by asking about the best means to obvious ends. In her case, the ends of medical interventions cease to be obvious and stand in need of clarification and specification. Karen Quinlan's doctors and nurses can decide what care to provide her—whether to continue her respirator or not, whether to continue her naso-gastric feedings or not, whether to treat her next fever or not—only after the ends of medicine have been specified, only after they answer the question: What should be the ultimate objectives of medical interventions for a patient such as Karen?

Since 1976 and the *Quinlan* case, there have been more than seventy-five terminating care cases argued before state supreme courts, lower federal courts, and even one before the U.S. Supreme Court. *Quinlan* and the succeeding cases have clarified three fundamental issues relating to terminating care. First, they have made clear that the decision to terminate care is not exclusively a private matter. At a minimum, society, through the courts or legislatures, must decide whether patients have a right to terminate care; who should exercise this right for incompetent patients such as Karen Quinlan; what procedures and safeguards should exist for the exercise of the right; how conflicts between family and physicians, if they should arise, should be adjudicated; who can challenge a terminating care decision and for what reasons; what care incompetent patients without families should receive; and the like. In addition, as the *Quinlan* case made clear, the decision to terminate care implicates criminal and civil laws, raising questions of murder, criminal abuse, discrimination, and so forth.[4] Decisions about terminating care must also cohere with other social judgments. If Karen Quinlan should be treated, then facilities must be provided for such care and medical insurance should be required to pay. Conversely, if terminating care is deemed acceptable, then physicians and the public need to adjust their understanding of the standards of medical practice and, as Justice Muir noted, of society's moral standards and expectations. Indeed, this understanding will shape the types of interventions patients are given in an emergency and the alternative treatment plans presented to patients. Another state supreme court summarized the inescapable public nature of terminating care decisions in the following way: "Here, the presence of the State is manifested by its capability of imposing criminal sanctions on the hospital and its staff, by its licensing of physicians, by the required involvement of the judiciary in the guardianship appointment process, and by the State's *parens patriae* responsibility to supervise the affairs of incompetents. Taken together, these factors show a sufficient nexus between the State and the prohibitions against withholding or discontinuance of life-sustaining treatment."[5]

Second, it is now clear that the facts of all terminating care cases are distinguishable along three dimensions: (1) the patient's level of mental competence, (2) the patient's general physical condition, and (3) the types of medical interventions being considered (see Tables 3.1–3.3).[6] Karen Quinlan was a "hard case," at one extreme of these three dimensions: a hopelessly ill patient in persistent vegetative state requiring a respirator, artificial feedings, and constant nursing care. But the decisions required in her case—clarifying, specifying, and balancing the ultimate ends of medicine—apply to cases with almost every permutation of these three dimensions. Indeed, part of the force of the *Quinlan* case inheres in making physicians and others recall that in many "normal" or routine medical circumstances the ends of medicine are *not* at all obvious, but rather in need of clarification and specification. For instance, patients with laryngeal cancer frequently face a situation in which surgical removal of their larynx can prolong life but compromise their ability to speak. Should the end of medicine be to prolong life with limited functions or to preserve certain human functions with a foreshortened life span?[7] Similar conflicts arise in the care of a diabetic woman with a gangrenous foot. A below-the-knee amputation would cure the infection and prolong the patient's life; without the amputation she would almost certainly die from complica-

Table 3.1   Patient's level of mental competence

Category	Definition	Examples
Coma or persistent vegetative state	Unconscious patients with no awareness of external stimuli, including pain, or internal needs	Quinlan
Primitive	Conscious patients with minimal awareness of the environment	Patients with severe dementia
Receptive	Conscious patients who are aware of much of the environment but cannot initiate constructive action	Patients with strokes left partially paralyzed and aphasic
Interactive	Conscious patients who can initiate constructive interaction but at a fairly simple level	Patients with mild Alzheimer's disease
Reversibly incompetent	Transiently incompetent patients who are expected to become fully conscious and competent	Adults under anesthesia
Fully competent	Fully conscious and competent adults	Normal adults

Table 3.2 Patient's general physical condition

Category	Definition	Examples
Terminally ill	Patients with incurable diseases that will result in death within a short time regardless of medical interventions	Cancer, AIDS, Lou Gehrig's disease
Hopelessly ill	Patients with diseases or disabilities that make them debilitated, requiring constant or frequent medical or nursing care, without a fatal disease process	Quinlan
Chronically ill	Patients with diseases requiring regular medications or medical care but without being debilitated	Chronic renal failure, diabetes
Healthy	Patients without chronic medical problems, debilitating disabilities, or terminal disease process	Normal adults

Table 3.3 Patient's level of medical interventions

Category	Definition	Examples
Emergency care	Care required immediately to sustain life	Resuscitation
Intensive care	Care requiring constant physician and nurse monitoring	Care for acute myocardial infarction
Acute medical care	Care requiring hospitalization and routine physician and nurse monitoring	Chemotherapy, surgery
Chronic medical care	Care requiring frequent medical treatments without hospitalization	Dialysis
General nursing care	Care requiring nursing interventions without treatment of disease processes	Pain control, G-tube feedings

tions of the infection. Should the end of medicine be to prolong her life but leave her wheelchair-bound, or to let her die with her body intact, having never known disability?[8]

One of the more common situations confronting physicians involves demented patients, with diverse functional capacities, who live in nursing homes and acquire pneumonias or other infections. Routine antibiotics will usually cure the infection and return the patient to the previous, albeit limited, existence. Conversely, pneumonia may be seen, in Osler's words, as the aged person's "friend," permitting a relatively quick, painless death without a progressive loss of function and independence culminating in a pitiful, lingering end.[9] Should the aim of medicine be to prolong the limited lives of these patients or to permit them to die of easily treatable infections? By calling into question the seemingly obvious, cases such as Karen Quinlan's make physicians and the public realize that in these and other routine situations we can decide what care to provide—what treatment plans to consider—only after we have determined what should be the aims of medical interventions.

Finally, the *Quinlan* case not only made physicians aware of the need to articulate explicitly their objectives in rendering routine medical care, it also provided a guiding framework for addressing the issue of terminating care. The New Jersey justices constructed their decision to permit the termination of Karen's respirator around three basic questions: Is there a right to terminate care? Who should act as the decision maker? What criteria should justify the termination of medical care? The court answered these questions by arguing that Karen Quinlan had a constitutional right of privacy and therefore a right to refuse medical care, and that Karen's father should act as her guardian and exercise her right of privacy. Although the court did not specifically delineate criteria to guide the termination of care, it did suggest that the respirator was extraordinary care. In May 1976 Karen's respirator was disconnected. Unexpectedly, she continued breathing on her own and was maintained with artificial nutrition and hydration through a naso-gastric tube. Finally, in June 1985, Karen Quinlan contracted a pneumonia that was not treated with antibiotics, and she died.

This framework and the court's reasoning provided a paradigm guiding most subsequent legal decisions and ethical commentaries on terminating medical care. And in the wake of the *Quinlan* decision there has been a greater willingness to terminate medical care for patients; physicians and society now contemplate and permit the withholding or withdrawal of almost any medical intervention, from respirators to antibiotics to artificial nutrition, for patients in almost any type of condition. And yet, despite this greater acceptance of terminating care, the issue is still surrounded by as much controversy as existed in the conflict over discontinuing Karen Quinlan's respirator. The number of legal battles over terminating care has been accelerating rather than diminishing; the range of cases has expanded, involving more patients with more varied mental and physical conditions. In highly publicized cases, patients considered to have severe, irreversible mental deficits have inexplicably recovered significant function, and other patients, granted the right to terminate their life-sustaining care, have retracted their long-considered desire for termination. These situations raise qualms about irreversible mistakes in such decisions.[10] And physicians, called upon to advise patients and families and to institute medical interventions, feel the absence of guiding standards:

> What does one do, then? We have developed no rational way to decide what treatment to give and what to withhold once it has been decided to withhold "heroics." . . . The problem is simply too difficult for me as a single human being to face in a conscious way. How do I consciously decide to let this person die when everything in my being says that life has the ultimate value? How can I make a decision about the quality of this life? How can I know what the patient would want? . . . Since I am operating in a vacuum and have no reliable criteria on which to base a decision, my choice is ultimately guided by my feelings, prejudices, and mood more than by my reason.[11]

While the legal cases since *Quinlan* have clarified many important points relating to terminating care, they have not answered the fundamental question: What should be the ultimate objectives of medical care? Indeed, the years since 1976 have only highlighted the failure of the framework devised by the *Quinlan* court to guide us in addressing this question. This failure is not accidental, but, as I shall show, is an inherent consequence of the liberal political philosophy that informs the framework guiding medical ethics. Consequently the controversy prompted by the *Quinlan* case has not abated, but persists with no prospect for resolution.

To support this claim I will examine each element of the guiding framework proposed by the New Jersey Supreme Court in *Quinlan* and subsequently adopted as the paradigm for addressing the question of terminating care. I hope to demonstrate that certain tenets of liberalism preclude devising and justifying a shared standard for terminating care, and that to make such decisions people often invoke an illusory consensus or illiberal principles.[12]

The Right to Refuse Medical Care

A fundamental aspect of the New Jersey Supreme Court's framework for addressing terminating care decisions is the recognition of Karen's right to refuse medical care and thereby her right to have the respirator terminated. Recognizing this right is probably the most enduring legacy of the *Quinlan* decision. Where does this right come from? How is it justified?

One of the fundamental moral attributes of a person is the capacity for self-determination or autonomy, the capacity to form, to pursue, and to revise a conception of the good life. A primary reason for the guarantee of basic rights is to ensure that individuals have the possibility to form and pursue their own conceptions of the good life: "The basic liberties (freedom of thought and liberty of conscience etc.) are the background institutions necessary for the development and exercise of the capacity to decide upon and revise, and rationally to pursue, a conception of the good."[13]

The United States constitution explicitly guarantees many of these liberties, such as the right to freedom of speech and the right to free exercise of religion, but there is no explicit constitutional right to self-determination, no "right to be a *human* being; no definition of a person; and indeed, no express provisions guaranteeing to persons the right to carry on their lives protected from the 'vicissitudes of the political process' by a zone of privacy or a right of personhood."[14] Instead judges have had to elaborate the rights necessary for the exercise of self-determination. One way this has been done has been to recognize a constitutional right of privacy not explicitly enumerated in the Bill of Rights. In the 1965 case *Griswold* v. *Connecticut,* which concerned the right of a married couple to obtain contraceptive information and contraceptives from Planned Parenthood, the Supreme Court argued that the Bill of Rights does not articulate every right enjoyed by free citizens. Some fundamental rights, left unspecified, are integral to the exercise of the other specified rights. These unspecified individual rights, which include the right of privacy, are no less rights and no less fundamental: "Specific guarantees in the Bill of Rights have penumbras, formed by emanations from those guarantees that help give them life and substance . . . We deal with a right of privacy older than the Bill of Rights." [15]

A second way in which the right of self-determination has been secured is as a common law right. Using reasoning almost identical to the Supreme Court's in *Griswold,* other courts have argued that the right of privacy ensures the possibility of individual autonomy and freedom. "Under a free government at least, the free citizen's first and greatest right which underlies all others [is] the right to the inviolability of his person, in other words his right to himself." [16]

Whether by the constitutional right of privacy or a common law right of personal inviolability, our society tries to secure a person's right to form and pursue a conception of the good life. Applied to the realm of medical care, this right of personal privacy becomes a right "to determine what should be done with [one's] own body." [17] People will espouse different ends. Different types of medical treatments—even rejecting medical care altogether—will comport better with the different particular ends espoused. Medical treatments are, like other goods, to be chosen based on how they foster the specific final ends the individual aspires to. Thus, the general rights of privacy, liberty, and self-determination inform the more specific right of informed consent and the right to refuse medical treatments in medical practice. The President's Commission summarized this relationship between self-determination and the right to select or refuse life-sustaining care: "Respect for the self-determination of competent patients is of special importance in decisions to forego life-sustaining treatment because different people will have markedly different needs and concerns during the final period of their lives; living a little longer will be of distinctly different value to them . . . the primacy of a patient's interests in self-determination and in honoring the patient's own view of well-being warrant leaving with the patient the final authority to decide." [18] Similarly, in the landmark *Saikewicz* case the Massachusetts Supreme Judicial Court explicitly delineated this relationship between self-determination, the right to privacy, and the right to refuse medical care:

Of even broader import, but arising from the same regard for human dignity and self-determination, is the unwritten constitutional right of privacy found in the penumbra of specific guaranties of the Bill of Rights. As this constitutional guaranty reaches out to protect the freedom of a woman to terminate pregnancy under certain conditions, so it encompasses the right of a patient to preserve his or her right of privacy against unwanted infringements of bodily integrity in appropriate circumstances . . . The constitutional right to privacy, as we conceive it, is an expression of the sanctity of individual free choice and self-determination as fundamental constituents of life. The value of life as so perceived is lessened not be a decision to refuse treatment, but by the failure to allow a competent human being the right of choice.[19]

Following the *Quinlan* decision, the right of privacy and therefore the right to refuse medical treatment have been affirmed by "every [state] court examining the issue"[20] and recognized for (1) competent patients, (2) incompetent patients who were previously competent and left explicit written or verbal instructions regarding their care if they became incompetent, (3) incompetent patients who left no statements regarding their care, and (4) incompetent patients who have never been competent.[21] In the words of a recent landmark decision: "All patients, competent or incompetent, with some limited cognitive ability or in a persistent vegetative state, terminally ill or not terminally ill, are entitled to choose whether or not they want life-sustaining medical treatment."[22]

In the recent *Cruzan* decision eight of the U.S. Supreme Court Justices agreed that individuals have a constitutional right to refuse medical care. However, their justification of this right diverged from previous analysis. A majority of the Court shunned justifying the right to refuse medical care by appeal to more general considerations of self-determination. The Court was also loath to rely on constitutional penumbras or common law to derive this right. Instead, Justice Rehnquist, writing for the majority, acknowledged the right to refuse medical care as an elaboration of the Fourteenth Amendment's provision "that no State shall 'deprive any person of life, liberty, or property without due process of law.'"[23] In this way the Court affirmed a person's right to refuse care and strengthened its legal standing as a constitutional right by relying on an explicit provision of the constitution while avoiding more contentious ethical issues regarding self-determination.

It is fairly clear how recognizing the right to refuse medical care can resolve the problem of terminating care for competent patients and incompetent patients who have previously expressed their wishes. In the case of incompetent patients who *did* express their views before they became incompetent, in a living will or the Medical Directive for example, respecting their choices can be coherently understood as respecting their right to privacy or liberty interest. In such situations, what is really being respected is their previous capacity to choose conceptions of the good life.[24] Indeed, this is the reason we usually respect a dead person's wishes on the disposition of his body or the disbursement of his estate. The case is similar for incompetent patients who are more interactive and capable of forming, expressing, and, maybe, pursuing, if not full conceptions of the good life, then at least their desires. For instance, we might find a coherent sense to granting a person with Down's syndrome who has near-normal intelligence the rights of privacy based on self-determination.

But can incompetent patients for whom we have no explicit statement of their views on medical care have a right to refuse medical care? In the *Cruzan* case Justice Brennan, writing for the minority, claimed: "Nor does the fact that Nancy Cruzan is now incompetent deprive her of her fundamental rights."[25] The rationale for extending this right to incompetent patients was articulated by the Massachusetts Supreme Judicial Court: "We think that principles of equality and respect for all individuals require the conclusion that a choice exists . . . we recognize a general right in all persons to refuse medical treatment in appropriate circumstances. The recognition of that right must extend to the case of an incompetent, as well as a competent, patient because the value of human dignity extends to both."[26] Many within the medical and legal professions have endorsed this view.[27] The President's Commission, appealing to "basic values" instead of rights, argues that "the two values that guide decision-making for competent patients—promoting patient welfare and respecting patient self-determination—should also guide decision-making for incapacitated patients."[28]

Yet recognizing the irreversibly incompetent patient's right to refuse care seems illogical, if not incoherent. This right exists to ensure that individuals can exercise and realize their capacity for self-determination; it is justified by appeal to a conception of the person as free, as having the capacity to choose, to reform, and to pursue his own conception of a meaningful life. Choosing a life plan or even pursuing a desire is precisely what patients such as Karen Quinlan cannot do, or more accurately, lack—and will forever lack—the capacity to do. Incompetent patients irreversibly lack the capacity to make any choices whatsoever, let alone choices about ultimate ends and how medical interventions might affect those ends. To recognize a *right* to refuse medical treatments for incompetent patients precisely when they lack the capacities that justify such a right seems incoherent.[29]

This incoherence is compounded when we juxtapose the right and its use. The justification for terminating life-sustaining care to incompetent patients is their incompetence, the fact that, in the words of the New Jersey Supreme Court, they can "never be restored to a cognitive or sapient life." In other words, courts recognize an incompetent patient's right to refuse medical care, even though the patient cannot make any choices or be self-determining, and then find it ethically justifiable to terminate care and let the patient die precisely because the patient irreversibly lacks the capacity to make choices. This twisted logic was first articulated in the *Quinlan* decision and has been replicated in almost every terminating care decision since: "The evidence in this case convinces us that the focal point of decision should be the prognosis as to the reasonable possibility of return to cognitive and sapient life, as distinguished from the forced continuance of that biological vegetative existence to which Karen seems to be doomed . . . [if] there is no reasonable possibility of Karen's ever emerging from her present comatose condition to a cognitive, sapient state, the present life-support system may be withdrawn."[30] Hence there seems to be a complex—and ironic—contradiction in attributing the right to privacy and the right to refuse medical care to incompetent patients: courts recognize a right of incompetent patients to "refuse" medical treatment in order to terminate their medical treatment precisely because they lack the capacities to exercise such a right.

While they ultimately recognized the right of irreversibly incompetent patients to refuse medical care, the majority of the U.S. Supreme Court clearly recognized and were troubled by this incoherence. Justice Rehnquist wrote that granting incompetent patients a right to refuse medical care "begs the question" because they cannot possibly exercise the right. He further called it a "hypothetical right to refuse treatment" and then placed the term "right" in quotation marks to indicate hesitancy about granting such a right to irreversibly incompetent patients.[31]

Why have courts, physicians, and many others propagated this il-logical position? One source of the impulse to extend these rights to incompetent patients, even at the risk of intelligibility, may be the need to find a legal justification for an ethical position. While many people believe it is ethically justifiable to terminate medical care to incompetent patients, the legal grounds for such a position would be lacking without the recognition of an incompetent patient's right to refuse medical care. Thus to permit realization of the ethical position, the U.S. Supreme Court and others are willing to gloss over the legal rights issue.

Another rationale for recognizing the irreversibly incompetent patient's right to refuse medical care might arise from the peculiarity of using the concept of rights for the realization of more general ethical conceptions. Embedded within the justification offered by the Mas-sachusetts court for extending the right to refuse medical treatment to incompetent patients is the implication that recognizing this right is the way, in the area of medical care, to recognize human dignity; with-out such a right, incompetent patients would lack human dignity, and we would lack a means of recognizing their dignity. "[T]he law pro-tects the 'dignity and equality' of incompetent patients by attempting to honor, in some measure, their right to self determination." [32]

This seems a strange claim. Certainly it would seem possible to recognize human dignity, to respect persons, without necessarily in-troducing the concept of rights. [33] Otherwise we come to the unten-able conclusion that any polity without rights does not respect the dignity of persons, or that the possibility of human dignity depends upon the discovery of rights. Relying on the language and logic of rights in this circumstance to express dignity only confuses us. What precisely does the incompetent patient's *human* dignity consist in? It certainly does not inhere in self-determination. This of course is not to say that incompetent patients should not be respected; it is only to argue that it is incoherent to claim that we are showing our respect and reverence for them by granting them rights to self-determination that ultimately only justify terminating their life-sustaining treat-ments. In any case, there seems to be a profound confusion underly-ing the attribution of rights to incompetent patients when they lack the capacities that justify these rights.

Yet a third rationale for recognizing the incompetent patient's right to refuse medical care is the wish to escape the awesome issue of ter-minating medical care entirely. Recognizing the right of incompetent

patients to refuse medical care transforms the primary ethical question
from: What care should be provided incompetent patients? into another question: How should the right to refuse medical care be exercised? Although there are several distinct ways of answering this question that require substantive ethical decisions, it is almost always
rendered into an easier procedural question: "Since, by definition,
an incompetent patient is unable to exercise his or her own self-
determination by making decisions regarding treatment, this right
must be exercised on behalf of the incompetent patient by someone
else."[34] Thus, by recognizing the incompetent's right to refuse medical care, the ethical issue of terminating care has become a question of
determining "Who decides?" In this way judges and ethical commentators have escaped the need to make—and justify—substantive ethical decisions about the life and death of patients and can fulfill their
duty by simply identifying another party to assume responsibility for
such decisions.

"Who decides?" is the second aspect of the framework offered by
the *Quinlan* decision. In the view of many, it is the fundamental ethical
question of terminating care decisions, and much of the contemporary public debate surrounds the merits and demerits of potential
decision-makers.

The Insignificance of Who Decides

Assuming incompetent patients have a right to refuse medical care,
who should exercise this right for them? The *Quinlan* court recognized Karen's father as the appropriate surrogate decision-maker, although he could decide to terminate care only after a hospital "ethics"
committee confirmed that the patient had no chance of regaining a
cognitive and sapient life. This is the dominant position; many physicians, physician organizations, courts, and commentators share this
view, contending that the family is the best surrogate decision-maker
for an incompetent patient because the family knows the patient best
and is most concerned for the patient's welfare, and the law respects
the family as a privileged association.[35]

But, unlike many of the *Quinlan* court's other rulings, many disagree with this position and each of the arguments for it. In many
cases what is considered "the family" is strained. The closest relatives
may be nieces or nephews who live far away in other states and may

not have seen the patient recently, let alone discussed issues of terminating care with him.[36] Further, while there is not a great deal of empirical data on how well family members know each other's views on terminating care issues, there are at least two empirical studies of the subject suggesting that family members are *not* familiar with the wishes of patients regarding terminating care. Spouses of elderly patients, many of whom had been married for more than forty years, were no better than chance at predicting the patient's wishes on resuscitation, let alone on antibiotics and artificial nutrition, if that patient suddenly had a stroke.[37] Not only might individual family members inaccurately predict a patient's wishes, there are often disagreements among family members about what types of treatment the patient would have wanted.[38]

In addition, critics of the family as the incompetent patient's decision-maker note that in many instances the family, even if it knows the patient's wishes, disagrees and knowingly overrides them. Indeed, some of the more important legal cases have pitted family members against the patient. In *Lane* v. *Candura,* for instance, a daughter sued to have her mother declared incompetent so the daughter could force her mother to have an amputation for a gangrenous leg—this, despite the fact that the mother was competent and clearly opposed the amputation, accepting her own death at 77 years of age.[39] In another remarkable situation, a woman repeatedly refused a brain biopsy to determine the nature of a mass. When she became temporarily incompetent, her husband, who disagreed with her wish, authorized the brain biopsy.[40] Not only might family members disagree with the patient's wishes, there can be conflicts of interest between the patient and the family. Such conflicts have been clearly demonstrated in "Baby Doe" cases, but they also arise in the care of the elderly or incompetent.[41] Incompetent patients may create oppressive financial, emotional, and time burdens; costs for home nursing care or a nursing home may be draining vital family resources; the family may find caring for or visits to the patient physically and emotionally exhausting.[42] That these conflicts may distort the family's choices of care is clear; what is less clear is how often and whether we can detect these conflicts and protect against them.

Finally, others object that no one, including a patient's closest family members, can exercise a patient's right of privacy. It is argued that by the very nature of a right of privacy, no one but the person himself can exercise that right. Hence, no family can have the right to let one of its members die from lack of treatment without explicit authorization from the patient.[43]

Others propose that choices about terminating care to incompetent patients be left to physicians.[44] Several courts have agreed, suggesting that, at least in the cases where medical care will not cure or relieve the illnesses of a terminal patient, the physician should decide when "further treatment will be of no reasonable benefit to the patient."[45] But there are those who object to this, arguing that while physicians' technical knowledge requires that they determine patient diagnosis and prognosis, decisions about whether to terminate treatment are ethical judgments about the worth and quality of life in which physicians have no special expertise or authority.[46]

Still others urge that the courts make the decisions about terminating care for incompetent patients.[47] In *Saikewicz*,[48] one of the first legal cases involving an incompetent patient decided after *Quinlan,* the Massachusetts Supreme Judicial Court seemed to reject the notion of "entrusting the decision whether to continue artificial life support to the patient's guardian, family, attending doctors, and hospital 'ethics committee.'" The court felt that such "difficult and awesome" decisions should be subject to the "detached but passionate investigation and decision" characteristic of courts. Subsequently, the Massachusetts court has qualified this strong stand and reaffirmed the importance of family and physicians in such decisions,[49] although it still maintains that courts or a guardian should decide for incompetent patients who have no family.[50] Frequently, other courts have eschewed judicial intervention, arguing that prior judicial approval is unnecessary for the withdrawal of care.[51] In New Jersey, the supreme court recently sought to avoid routine judicial review, but required that decisions to terminate care to incompetent patients in nursing homes be reviewed by an ombudsman.[52]

But the point is not that the question "Who decides?" seems fraught with controversy, and every potential answer objectionable. For even if the incompetent patient's right to refuse medical care could be given some coherent sense, and even if there could be agreement on the best party to exercise that right for the incompetent patient, the problem of what medical treatments should be provided to incompetent patients would remain unaddressed.

To decide what care should be provided to incompetent patients requires deciding what the objectives of medical care should be. And whoever ends up exercising the incompetent patient's right to refuse medical care must still answer these questions. Some substantive ethical principles must be invoked—and justified—for these answers. There can be no substantive answer to the medical ethical question of terminating care from mere procedural forms of knowing who decides; substantive judgments require substantive principles that cannot be derived from "Who decides?" Inevitably, there can be no alternative to developing a framework for deciding what care to provide patients. "Although we as a society may decide to lodge the authority for making such [terminating care] decisions in private hands, *someone* must decide and, in so doing, appeal to standards of right and wrong. The issue is not whether we will employ substantive standards; rather, the question is *which* standards will guide us" (emphasis in the original).[53]

But if the family or the physician is the incompetent's decision-maker, it might be thought, then there need not be any public standards; the decision-maker can simply answer these ethical questions by whatever criteria she chooses. No decision-maker can have unlimited discretion to make just *any* decision for the incompetent patient; Karen's father could not do anything he wanted. We recognize some decisions as unethical. And not any reason for a decision will do. We recognize some justifications, for otherwise acceptable actions, as unethical. Consequently, it will be necessary to have substantive criteria delimiting the range of ethically justifiable decisions—and reasons for those decisions—made for the incompetent patient. And these criteria will have to be public criteria, criteria that physicians and others share and can appeal to in evaluating the ethics of a surrogate's judgment.

Thus, the real issue is less who decides than what is decided and why. Beneath the procedural determination of who decides, there still must be an answer to the substantive question of what care incompetent patients should receive. The hope that rights and procedures for selecting "Who decides?" can "save us from the agony and absurdity of making ultimate judgments of worth"[54] is a hope against hope. No matter how many ways we try to avoid developing a public framework for deciding what care to provide incompetent patients, no matter how many layers of rights and procedures we devise, no matter how many times we delegate the decision to others, ultimately there is no way to conceal or evade the substantive ethical decision. As one legal scholar has written, in a warning that physicians, medical ethicists, and lawyers dealing with medical issues should heed: "Process [is a] mischievous idea because [it] covers up these substantive decisions with procedural piety, and pretends they have not been made."[55]

So what ethical framework should guide us in determining what care should be given to incompetent patients?

The Relativity of Extraordinary Care

In the *Quinlan* case, the New Jersey Supreme Court was so trusting of Joseph Quinlan's character and love for his daughter and so certain "that if Karen were herself miraculously lucid for an interval" she would turn off her own respirator, they never delineated a framework for actually addressing the decision to withdraw the respirator. While the opinion mentions the ordinary/extraordinary care distinction in passing, no substantive guidelines are offered or defended. The court recognized this oversight and attempted to remedy it in the subsequent decisions of *Conroy* and *Jobes*. In the years since *Quinlan* three ethical frameworks have been advanced to show how the substantive decisions for incompetent patients might be approached: ordinary/ extraordinary care, substituted judgment, and best interests. I will consider each of these in turn.

The Nature of the Ordinary/Extraordinary Care Standard

The ordinary/extraordinary care standard originated in sixteenth-century debates among Catholic theologians over the question of whether or not individuals were obligated to follow a doctor's orders, in particular the degree to which a person had to alter his circumstances because doctors felt it was necessary to preserve his life.[56] The contemporary formulation is best expressed by Gerald Kelly: "*Ordinary* means of preserving life are all medicine, treatments, and operations, which offer a reasonable hope of benefit for the patient and which can be obtained and used without excessive expense, pain, or other inconvenience . . . [*Extraordinary* means are] all medicine, treatments, and operations, which cannot be obtained without excessive expense, pain, or other inconvenience, or which, if used, would not offer a reasonable hope of benefit."[57]

Despite the fact that the ordinary/extraordinary care standard was initially articulated by Catholic theologians, it has been adopted by many secular commentators and has found its way into ethical discussions concerning care for the incompetent. In the years since this distinction entered secular medical ethical discussions, commentators have tried to refine it, to specify more clearly the considerations that would be ethically relevant in terminating care decisions. The result has been at least eight such "clarifying" dichotomies: common/unusual, simple/complex, routine/heroic, medically indicated/not medically indicated,[58] reasonable/unreasonable,[59] beneficial/burdensome,[60] proportionate/disproportionate,[61] and obligatory/optional.[62]

The common/unusual distinction suggests that what is extraordinary is the statistically rare treatment; the simple/complex distinction implies a "technological" separation between a "low" technology intervention and a "high" technology intervention; the routine/heroic distinction also contains an element of the technological but combined with some measure of the degree of intervention, efforts expended by the medical staff, and, possibly, expense; the medically indicated/not medically indicated distinction relies on the existence of strict clinical criteria for an intervention, independent of the patient's mental condition; the next three dichotomies—reasonable/unreasonable, beneficial/burdensome, and proportionate/disproportionate—rely on some measure of benefit to the patient; and finally, the obligatory/optional distinction seems to be less a clarification than a conclusion about types of treatment which the ordinary/extraordinary dichotomy was originally intended to make.

Objections to the Ordinary/Extraordinary Care Standard

As articulated by Kelly and others, this distinction—and its progeny—will not help in providing substantive principles because it is parasitic on other more fundamental ethical judgments which are neither articulated nor justified. Embedded in the ordinary/extraordinary dichotomy seem to be two implicit ethical standards. First are judgments about what factors are appropriate in distinguishing ordinary and extraordinary care. Identifying which factors should be considered is not a factual decision, but an ethical one which needs to be justified.[63] Kelly identifies expense, pain, inconvenience, and hope of benefit as ethically relevant factors to be considered. But what makes these the key factors distinguishing ordinary from extraordinary care? By appeal to what are they justified? Clearly, evaluating the "extraordinariness" of care based on its expense is a moral judgment. It is certainly not a widely shared belief that expense should be part of the consideration in determining whether incompetent patients are treated or not. Indeed, at least in the United States, it is widely argued that the cost of care should *not* be a factor in deciding whether to provide treatment to incompetent patients. Including expense as a consideration discriminates against the poor and uninsured, who could not afford such care.[64] And this is why I have initially proceeded without including considerations of justice. Furthermore, it may be that other factors are relevant to this distinction. Why has Kelly excluded emotional burden on the patient's family, which some commentators think is relevant?[65] Why has he excluded bodily integrity or independence? Neither Kelly nor anyone else offers a justification for this particular list. Ultimately, the factors used to distinguish ordinary and extraordinary care are neither inclusive nor justified.

But there is a second, and more substantial, way in which this distinction is insufficient. These factors are not self-defining. What is excessive expense or excessive pain? How do we define pain or suffering or hope? Using the ordinary/extraordinary care dichotomy relies on a criterion defining when expense and pain are excessive that is never delineated.

This is especially true of the factor "a reasonable hope of benefit." According to this dichotomy, we should provide care which offers a reasonable hope of benefit, but not care which provides no reasonable hope of benefit. But what constitutes "reasonable"? Can we say that to some, such as cancer victims, a 5 percent chance of cure is reasonable, but to others only a 30 percent or a 50 percent chance of cure is reasonable? But if a standard of reasonableness exists, it is left unarticulated and unjustified.

The most important point, however, is that these criticisms extend to the notion of benefit. According to liberal political philosophy, there is no single human good true for all people; pluralism implies differing views of what is ultimately worthy and valuable. Hence there is no single standard of benefit. For some people existing at the receptive level of mental incompetence is worthwhile, and any medical treatment which permits this offers "a reasonable hope of benefit." For others medical treatments which sustain them in this condition, but offer no chance of improved mental functioning, will "not offer a reasonable hope of benefit." To distinguish treatments as either ordinary or extraordinary requires a prior ethical judgment about what should constitute a benefit. And this is never explicated by the advocates of the ordinary/extraordinary dichotomy. Or to put it another way, to identify one treatment as ordinary and another as extraordinary *assumes* an ethical framework for determining what should constitute a benefit and what should not. But this framework is left implicit and obscure in the ordinary/extraordinary care dichotomy.

Thus the ordinary/extraordinary care distinction appears to provide a guiding ethical standard for determining what care incompetent patients should receive, but actually it is "more of an expression of the conclusion than a justification for it;"[66] the distinction "begs the question" by appearing to provide a guiding standard but relying on implicit ethical judgments of what is beneficial and what is not. Practical disagreements over using this dichotomy will mirror disagreements about the more basic ethical judgments regarding benefits and burdens.

And in reality this has occurred. This unjustified dichotomy has produced "an unfortunate array of alternative meanings"[67] and widespread disagreement among people as to what constitutes ordinary and extraordinary care in any particular circumstance of terminating care. To some people "ordinary measures are food, fluids, oxygen, antibiotics and pain killers."[68] To others any medical intervention for an incompetent patient is extraordinary. The President's Commission cites an interesting case involving a 76-year-old man dying of amyotrophic lateral sclerosis (Lou Gehrig's disease). The attending physician argued that "I deal with respirators every day of my life. To me, this is not heroic. This is standard procedure." Conversely, the judge, who was called upon to decide about terminating the respirator, declared it to be an "extraordinary life-preserving means."[69] And recently disagreements over this distinction have moved from respirators to encompass food and fluids. In the *Conroy* case, a nurse thought that a naso-gastric feeding tube "should not be removed since in her view it was not an extraordinary treatment." The attending physician, however, "considered naso-gastric feeding an extraordinary, or optional, medical treatment."[70]

The theoretical and practical problems with this distinction have forced many courts and commentators to conclude that this dichotomy has "too many conflicting meanings" to be useful in resolving the question of what medical treatments to provide incompetent patients.[71] Despite this ambiguity, the ordinary/extraordinary distinction persists in both court decisions and discussions of physicians and families.[72]

The Impossibility of Substituted Judgments

The Nature of the Substituted Judgment Standard

With the recognition of the inadequacy of the ordinary/extraordinary distinction, many have adapted the substituted judgment standard to the issue of terminating medical care to incompetent patients. This standard was originally developed 150 years ago in England to inform guardians about how they might administer and dispose of an incompetent person's property.[73]

According to this standard, the determination of what medical care the incompetent should receive is made by imagining what the incompetent person himself would choose. Substituted judgment is a sort of thought-experiment: the incompetent patient's decision-maker tries to imagine a counterfactual situation in which the incompetent person suddenly is lucid and then to delineate the decision that "would be made by the incompetent person, if that person were competent."[74] The aim is "to reach the decision [about medical treatments] that the incapacitated person would make if he or she were able to choose"[75] by "ascertain[ing] the incompetent person's actual interests and preferences . . . wants and needs . . . values and desires."[76] In the words of one justice, the surrogate "dons 'the mental mantle of the incompetent' and substitutes itself as nearly as possible for the individual in the decision-making process."[77] In legal terminology such a decision is "subjective" because the decision-maker tries to choose as the incompetent patient would.

To some degree the New Jersey Supreme Court adopted this position when it argued that if Karen Quinlan miraculously became conscious for a moment to choose what care she would want, they were confident she would have agreed to terminate the respirator.[78] Substituted judgment has received its most detailed endorsement, however, from the Massachusetts Supreme Judicial Court, which first articulated it in *Saikewicz*.[79] It has reaffirmed the standard in cases involving the medical care of adults who have been incompetent since birth;[80] cases involving the medical care of adults who have become incompetent from disease processes;[81] and cases involving minor children who are mentally normal but incompetent by age.[82] But it is not only the Massachusetts Supreme Judicial Court which has endorsed this standard. The President's Commission argues that "decisionmaking for incapacitated patients should be guided by the principle of substituted judgment."[83] Courts in many other states have also endorsed this view. For instance, the New Jersey Supreme Court, nine years after *Quinlan,* argued that "the goal of decisionmaking for incompetent patients should be to determine and effectuate, insofar as possible, the decision that the patient would have made if competent."[84] And in 1987, this court went on to state: "The 'substituted judgment' approach to decisionmaking for patients in the persistent vegetative state is our ideal."[85] Similarly, a Florida appellate court even applied this standard to a child in a vegetative state, arguing: "It is proper for the court to exercise its substituted judgment even absent evidence of intention of the incompetent person."[86] Legal and ethical scholars have also endorsed this standard.[87]

To a significant degree, the widespread endorsement of this standard stems from its aspiration to actualize the incompetent patient's self-determination, to make the incompetent patient's right to refuse medical care coherent by making the patient himself the one "who decides." As the Massachusetts Supreme Judicial Court wrote in the *Saikewicz* case: "The 'substituted judgment' standard which we have described commends itself simply because of its straightforward respect for the integrity and autonomy of the individual."[88] The substituted judgment standard can "protect and implement the individual's personal rights and integrity."[89] By attributing the actual decision of whether to terminate medical care to the incompetent patient himself, this standard seems to obviate the need for invoking substantive ethical standards articulated by others.

Objections to the Substituted Judgment Standard

How could we know what an incompetent would do if he or she were competent? In the case where the incompetent patient had been competent and indicated his or her wishes explicitly, as in a living will or the Medical Directive, then we need no imagination or thought-experiment or elaborate legal standard to guide us. The patient has already given us specific guidance. Indeed, in such cases there is no substitution of judgment, just the execution of the incompetent person's preferences made while competent.[90] In such cases "substitute judgment" is a misnomer.

These, however, are not the "hard cases." The cases in which we need ethical guidance are precisely those where the incompetent patient has never been competent or, if the patient was competent, never made an explicit declaration about what medical care he would want. Can the substituted judgment framework provide guidance in such cases?

In the case of patients who were never competent—that is, children or adults who have always been incompetent—the standard is simply unjustifiable. Trying to imagine whether a person who has never had the capacity to make ultimate decisions would *want* certain medical treatments, especially life-sustaining treatments, is simply impossible. There is no factual foundation on which to extrapolate what such a patient's preferences would be. It is like the guesswork needed to predict what job a 4-year-old will choose when she becomes an adult. A dissenting justice on the Massachusetts Supreme Judicial Court minced no words in his condemnation of this standard: "The court today has decided that the probate judge has the power to divine the wishes of a severely mentally retarded woman who 'currently functions at the level of a four year old' as to whether she should permit herself to be rendered forever incapable of conceiving and bearing a child. To say the least, this is an impossible task . . . The very condition of incompetence makes the doctrine of substituted judgment a cruel charade."[91]

Other commentators have called substituted judgment a "form of guesswork, suffused by the decision maker's biases."[92] And it is hard to see how it can be anything else. Such a counterfactual seems meaningless: "Thus it is unrealistic to attempt to determine whether [Mr. Storar, a 52-year-old man who has been retarded since birth and has a mental age of 18 months] would want to continue potentially life prolonging treatment if he were competent. As one of the experts testified at the hearing, that would be similar to asking whether 'if it snowed all summer would it then be winter?'"[93] Indeed, even while endorsing this standard, the President's Commission has argued that the substituted judgment standard cannot possibly be used for individuals who have been incompetent since birth, because there are no grounds for ascertaining the views of such patients.

What the substituted judgment standard offers is not a judgment as seen through the mental eye of the incompetent, but a pretense to do such. As one commentator put it, substituted judgment is a "fiction that obscures what actually transpires when a decision is made whether to withhold medical treatment for an incompetent."[94] This standard hides what really occurs: the court or the surrogate decides for the incompetent, in the name of the incompetent, under the guise of recognizing the incompetent's dignity, integrity, and autonomy. In other words, the incompetent patient's decision-maker is exercising his power over the patient, not the patient's power.[95]

But what about using substituted judgment in the more common situation of incompetent patients who were once competent? For such patients it might be possible "that intimate knowledge of a friend or relative allows the formulation of a reliable opinion about how the patient would react to the situation, even if that person had never previously experienced or expressed views upon such a situation. The theory of substituted judgment is that if we know someone well enough—her ideals, values, attitudes, philosophy of life—we can figure out how she would have reacted to a new situation."[96] As noted previously, this ideal is easily violated because the interests of those exercising the incompetent's rights may conflict with the interests of the incompetent. In such situations the process of substituted judgment becomes an exercise of power over the incompetent patient in the name of exercising the patient's power. As an example, consider the actual process of substituted judgment in the case of Earle Spring, in which a Massachusetts court delineates the eight grounds on which it concludes that the incompetent patient himself would not have wanted dialysis treatment:

> (1) the fact that he had led an active, robust, independent life; (2) the fact that he has fallen into a pitiable state of physical dependence and mental incapacity; (3) the fact that no improvement can be expected in his physical or mental condition, but only further deterioration; (4) the fact that dialysis treatments exact a significant toll in terms of frequency and duration of treatments and uncomfortable side effects; (5) the fact that the ward has no understanding of the nature and the purpose of his treatments and cannot cooperate and does not reliably acquiesce in their administration; (6) the fact that his wife

and son, with whom the ward had and has a very close relationship, feel that it would be his wish not to continue with dialysis in the present circumstances; (7) the fact that it is their wish that dialysis not be administered; and (8) the fact that the attending physician recommends against continuation of dialysis treatments in these circumstances.[97]

Where is the voice of Earle Spring? Do we know from his robust life prior to his incompetence that he would not have wanted dialysis? Do we know that he would think his state "pitiable"? Do we know that he would consider dialysis such a significant imposition, especially when many competent patients are willing to endure it? And what do we know of Earle Spring's view from the fact that his wife and son want the dialysis discontinued? Instead of discovering Earle Spring's perspective, this list of "the facts" reveals the view of the judges and the family, who find his state pitiable and intolerable.

In evaluating this use of the substituted judgment standard, it should be realized that the patient's state was in fact not so bad. Prior to asking the court to terminate the dialysis, Earle Spring's family consented to the treatments for over a year. If substituted judgment by the family previously suggested that Earle Spring wanted dialysis, what made them reevaluate their understanding of his conception of life? Over the year, the only circumstance which changed did not have to do with Earle Spring's condition; he did not become more incompetent or more violent. Rather, his wife's circumstances changed: over the year she suffered a stroke. Is the judgment to discontinue dialysis that of Earle Spring or that of his family and the court, who find his violent behavior offensive and draining on the family and therefore are willing to find his state "pitiable"?

Unjustifiable use of the substituted judgment standard does not mean that it is unjustifiable, only that it is liable to abuse. If substituted judgment is to be used as a standard for decision making, then substantive procedural safeguards will be needed to ensure that the patient's wishes and not the family's desires will be implemented. Even in the ideal, can substituted judgment ever be more than "guesswork" in which the decision-maker can express no more than "concerns and sympathy . . . in divining th[e incompetent] person's unknown wishes?"[98]

Empirical studies, as noted previously, suggest that even spouses of many decades, as well as doctors and nurses, cannot accurately imagine what kinds of medical care a patient would want.[99] Even under the best of circumstances—when there is no guilt, no distracting personal interests of the decision-maker, and no other distorting passions— using substituted judgment is suffused with guesswork.[100] Furthermore, the chance of realizing this ideal is dependent in important ways upon the interpretative abilities of the incompetent's particular decision-maker. An empathic, perceptive, and insightful person may be able to predict accurately another person's preferences. But not all of us are fortunate enough to have such spouses or close family members, let alone doctors and nurses. And it does not seem quite right to leave life-and-death decisions to the widely varying capacities of incompetent patients' surrogates without any safeguards or standards by which such decisions might be checked.

More important, is the ideal justifiable? Can we ever "know someone well enough—her ideals, values, attitudes, philosophy of life"— to predict what she would want? The problem is not the philosophical one of knowing other minds. Instead, the problem here is how this ideal relates to the liberal conception of a person. Underlying the ideal of substituted judgment is what we might call the conception of a person with character. The person is constituted by ideals, values, and a philosophy of life, which are open to interpretation to disclose the person's identity. It is by articulating this identity that we can imagine how that person would decide questions of terminating care. Conversely, on the liberal view, no importance can be attached to a person's expressed ideals and conception of the good life. Persons are said to stand apart from their conceptions of the good life because the moral powers include the capacity to *revise* our conception of the good life, indeed even to convert radically when confronted by novel situations such as life-and-death choices. The liberal conception of the person conflicts with the conception of a person who takes constitutive attachments as defining of identity.[101] And in liberal political philosophy it is unjustifiable to base policies on a view of persons which attributes to them a constitutive identity. To do so would be to introduce a particular conception of nonpublic identity to establish a public policy. In this way even the ideal of substituted judgment seems unjustifiable on liberal grounds. To invoke it in order to realize the right to refuse medical care seems to contradict the liberal political philosophy which justifies that right.

That our moral convictions seem to draw us toward the conception of persons with character suggests that the liberal conception of the person, fundamental to liberal political philosophy, may not cohere with our considered judgments. And this in turn suggests that certain fundamental aspects of liberal political philosophy may need to be reconsidered. At the moment I can do no more than mention this point.

It may be worth wondering why, with all its practical and theoretical defects, the substituted judgment standard persists, maintaining undaunted support, especially among lawyers and judges.[102] One motivation, it would seem, arises from the need to realize the incompetent patient's right of privacy and right to refuse treatment.[103] For if these are rights of incompetent persons, then they—not other people—must be able to exercise them. The substituted judgment makes it appear that the incompetent person is invoking his right. But if this is mere appearance, a false appearance, then again there is doubt about the validity of "recognizing" the incompetent's right of privacy. A second motivation for continuing to invoke the substituted judgment standard despite its flaws derives from the hope of avoiding situations in which someone articulates ethical standards *for* the incompetent person. The substituted judgment standard enables the court to evade the issue of articulating and defending a decision of what would be best for the incompetent patient by making it appear that the patient is actually elaborating the standard. But if the substituted judgment standard is groundless and meaningless, then deciding what is best for incompetent patients appears to be the only substantive standard left. And the possibility of having a resolution to the dilemma of what medical care incompetent patients should receive rests on the clarity and defensibility of the best interests standard.

The Indeterminacy of Best Interests

To determine what medical care incompetent patients should receive, it is necessary to determine what should be the aim of medical care. I have investigated two ethical standards that have been invoked to answer this question—the ordinary/extraordinary distinction and the substituted judgment standard—and found each deficient. In order to answer this question, there seems no way to avoid having some explicit conception of what is best for an incompetent patient. It is for this reason that I turn to the best interests standard.

The Nature of the Best Interests Standard

According to the best interests standard, the incompetent patient's surrogate decision-maker should choose those medical interventions that will most benefit the patient. The surrogate must evaluate the "benefits to be gained versus the burdens caused" by the prospective medical treatments, and choose those treatments in which the benefits maximally outweigh the burdens and thereby best promote the patient's welfare.[104] In some situations, the incompetent patient's decision-maker may deem no treatments as best for the patient.

This standard can be contrasted with substituted judgment as follows: substituted judgment is "subjective" because it relies on what the patient wants or might choose in the hypothetical situation that he should become competent; the best interests standard is supposed to be "objective" in the legal sense that it relies on some "objective test based on a notion of what most reasonable individuals in society would be likely to do in the same or similar circumstances."[105] Substituted judgment tries to "divine" the patient's mind, while the best interests position relies on an external standard of benefits and burdens, aiming to do what is best for the patient, protecting him from unwise and foolish decisions.

Using the two different standards can lead to different results in the same case. For instance, in the *Saikewicz* case an interactive incompetent patient, who could communicate his wishes by gestures and grunts, developed acute myeloblastic monocytic leukemia (AMML), and the Massachusetts Supreme Judicial Court was forced to decide whether he should receive chemotherapy. The judges noted that most competent people elect to receive the chemotherapy for Joseph Saikewicz's type of leukemia. This places a great burden on the court to demonstrate why it would be in this patient's best interest to forgo treatment when the vast majority of people who were competent to decide actually elected treatment as being in their best interests; in contrast, justifying the refusal of this treatment based on the substituted judgment standard is easier since we can readily imagine good reasons why any particular individual would reject cancer chemotherapy even if the majority opted for it. As one commentator has written: "Probably the primary reason for adopting the 'substituted judgment' standard over the 'best interests' test in both cases was that very good arguments can be mustered to demonstrate that continued treatment was actually in the best interests of both Karen Quinlan and Joseph Saikewicz." [106] Thus when some commentators suggest that "the substance of such a [substituted] judgment, of course, must be the best interests of the incompetent" [107] or when the courts claim "the substituted judgment doctrine is consistent with the 'best interests of the child' test," [108] there is some degree of misunderstanding, confusion, or obfuscation.

Recently the best interests standard has received considerable attention for two reasons. First, the recognition that the substituted judgment standard has theoretical and practical difficulties in precisely the instances which require substantive ethical judgments has forced courts to consider it. [109] Second, the President's Commission endorsed the best interests standard, and several prominent state courts adopted it in cases that condoned the termination of artificial nutrition and hydration to incompetent patients. [110] Other courts have endorsed the best interests standard when the patient has been incompetent since birth. [111] And this standard has been advocated as the best one to use in deciding what care to provide children. [112]

While it has only recently gained prominence in legal cases and while its proponents imply that it is new, the best interests standard is neither novel nor radical. Since the inception of medicine, the physician has always been dedicated to providing medical treatments that benefit his patient. This standard is merely a formal, legal articulation of the physician's traditional objective. "There is a long tradition in medicine that the physician's first and most important commitment should be to serve the well-being of the patient." [113] Indeed, according to the Hippocratic oath the physician swears "into whatever houses I may enter, I will come for the benefit of the sick." The notion of doing what will benefit the patient is not new but old, as old as medicine itself. What is new in the best interests standard must be found in how these interests are conceived.

Using the best interests standard has two consequences. First, any attempt to decide what is best for an incompetent patient will inherently involve quality-of-life determinations. "Quality-of-life" is among the most abused terms in medical ethics; it contains at least two distinct meanings that are often unrecognized, obscured, or confused. Sometimes people use the term "quality-of-life" to mean a social judgment about a person's *comparative* worth. For instance, we might decide not to provide care to the elderly because they are "worth" less in the sense that they do not have as long to live or are not as economically productive as young people. This comparative sense is associated with, for instance, Nazi claims that the Jews or gypsies were not quite human beings or not worth as much as Aryans. Conversely, quality-of-life can mean a *personal,* noncomparative, judgment about the worth of alternative conditions or situations. Personal quality-of-life judgments are both necessary and common, as when a person decides whether pursuing a certain career, say being a physician, is better than an alternative, or when a man decides between pursuing a career single-mindedly or splitting his time between parenting and a career.

While comparative quality-of-life judgments can be excluded from the best interests standard, personal quality-of-life judgments cannot. To decide whether or not a treatment is beneficial requires judging whether the life with the treatment is of higher quality than without the treatment. There is no way of determining what is best for a person without also having some standard of what will count as best in the patient's own context. And this, by any other name, is a *personal* quality-of-life judgment. Thus, if we are to use the best interests standard, we must recognize the need for personal quality-of-life judgments.[114]

But using the best interests standard for incompetent patients presents a twist on such quality-of-life judgments that is probably the source of all the confusion and abuse of the concept. In the case of an incompetent patient it is not the patient himself, but society, who evaluates the quality-of-life of alternative circumstances. Because the patient is incompetent, society must decide what life situation will be most worthy for the patient. This is not a comparative quality-of-life judgment, in the sense that society is not evaluating the incompetent person's worth compared to other people; rather it is a social judgment about personal quality-of-life, that is, about what type of life an individual should consider valuable or of suitable quality. Thus we might say that in using the best interests standard for incompetent patients, there will need to be a social judgment about a personal quality-of-life which does not entail a social judgment about the comparative worth of that person.

If the best interests standard is to be used to determine what care incompetent patients should receive, then we need some specification of what constitutes a benefit and a burden. In other words, directing us to weigh benefits and burdens is helpful only if we know what is to count as a benefit or as a burden. Hence to use this standard, we require what the President's Commission called some "objective, societally shared criteria"[115] or what others label a "broad social understanding" of benefits and burdens.[116] Lacking such a socially shared criterion, the best interests standard would become vacuous—a good maxim that provides little enlightenment. Is there such an objective, socially shared criterion?

Objections to the Best Interests Standard

Contemporary proponents of the best interests standard are fairly vague on the criteria of benefits and burdens used. Often, the best interests standard is advocated without a specification of what should constitute a benefit or a burden, as if these were natural or self-defining categories. Occasionally, the determination is given as a general formula for calculating when an intervention is in a patient's best interest. One applied ethicist offered the following "algorithm" to express the considerations that should guide the incompetent's decision-maker who uses the best interests standard:

$$\frac{\text{strength of duty}}{\text{of beneficence}} = \frac{\substack{\text{chance of} \\ \text{success}} \times \substack{\text{quality} \\ \text{of life}} \times \substack{\text{length} \\ \text{of life}}}{\text{cost}}$$

Unfortunately the key operative term, "quality of life," is left unspecified and is designated neither a unit of measure nor a qualitative assessment.[117] Indeed, the entire equation seems a mechanical view of assessing benefits without any sensitivity to how people actually conceive of them.

Probably the most explicit and sophisticated attempt to specify a criterion for determining benefits and burdens is found in the *Conroy* case. This case involved an 84-year-old bedridden, demented woman whose mental capacity was primitive. She was being fed by a nasogastric tube, and her nephew requested removal of the tube. In its decision, the New Jersey Supreme Court outlined a "pure-objective test" to determine whether it would be beneficial to withhold artificial nutrition from such an incompetent patient who had never expressed her opinion on life-sustaining treatments. According to this objective test, medical care can be terminated only if "the net burdens of the patient's life with the treatment clearly and markedly outweigh the benefits that the patient derives from life so that the recurring, unavoidable, and severe pain of the patient's life with the treatment would render the life-sustaining treatment inhumane."[118] Pain, and pain alone, is the standard of benefits and burdens. And on this basis, the majority ruled that Ms. Conroy, a patient with little awareness of her environment and multiple physical ailments, should *not* have her naso-gastric feedings stopped. This standard has been endorsed by others who maintain that besides medical prognosis, terminating care decisions require "assessments of the value of life," and these assessments, in turn, are "concerned about the amount of pain and suffering that continued life portends."[119]

But is this an objective and socially shared criterion? In evaluating this standard it is important to distinguish between pain as an experience and pain as a moral value. Clearly pain as an experience is subjective, influenced by a person's psychological and neurological state, cultural heritage, sociological situation, and the like.[120] But the experience of pain is not our interest; rather, we need to know if unremitting and severe pain is an objective moral value for determining what is of benefit or burdensome.

Pain is not a socially shared criterion of benefit or burden. Pain may be an objective moral value in the sense that we all recognize the claim of removing or ameliorating pain. But this does not mean that it is the *sole* or *most important* value in determining benefits and burdens. We are not all Benthamite hedonists, even in a demented, terminal condition. In a strong dissent, one of the judges of the *Conroy* court argued that this hedonist standard of pain is not a shared criterion of benefits and burdens. It is only one factor, and many if not most people will consider other things important:

> In my opinion the Court's objective test too narrowly defines the interests of people like Miss Conroy . . . "Pain" thus eclipses a whole cluster of other human values that have a proper place in the subtle weighing that will ultimately determine how life should end . . . Thus some people abhor dependence on others as much, or more, than they fear pain. Other individuals value personal privacy or dignity, and prize independence from others when their personal

needs and bodily functions are involved. Finally, the ideal of bodily
integrity may become more important than simply prolonging life
at its most rudimentary.[121]

Not only does the actual fact of dissent suggest that pain is not a
shared criterion, but Judge Handler also suggests what other individuals might consider valuable that is not included in the use of pain as
the sole criterion for determining benefits and burdens.

As a practical matter, the advocates of the best interests standard
have not yet offered an objective or socially shared criterion of benefits
and burdens. But failure in these attempts does not show that there is
no objective or socially shared standard; more clever advocates of the
best interests standard might suggest other specifications of benefits
and burdens to provide the best interests with content. We must consider a further question: In a liberal polity, is it even *theoretically* possible to provide these criteria of benefits and burdens that might inform the best interests standard?

Determining what is a benefit and what is a burden is inextricably
linked to a particular conception of the good life. We can only tell if
some situation or thing is valuable or harmful by relating it to a more
encompassing conception of what is meaningful and worthy. The
possibility of using the best interests standard becomes a question of
whether there is an objective, socially shared conception of the good
life. For only with such a conception of the good life could there be an
objective, socially shared standard of benefits and burdens.

In a liberal polity, is there a conception of the good life which could
inform the best interests standard? This question has two aspects: one
is a philosophical question of whether there is an objective conception
of the good life, and the other is a sociological question of whether
there is a shared conception of the good life. The advocates of political
liberalism avoid the first question.[122] Deciding whether there is an objectively best way to live is a controversial philosophical issue. Liberals
such as Rawls claim that answers to such issues should be avoided,
neither denied nor affirmed, in the formulation of public principles
and policies. Such issues as whether there is a best way to live cannot—and need not—be addressed for the resolution of such public
matters. Instead, liberals rely on "the fact of pluralism," the fact that
different people will espouse incommensurable conceptions of the
good life. This means that in a liberal society different people will

evaluate the same situation differently. As a result, in the public realm, the liberal view assumes there is no socially shared conception of the good life or of benefits and burdens: "[G]iven the circumstances of justice in which citizens have conflicting conceptions of the good, there cannot be any practical agreement on how to compare happiness as defined, say, by success in carrying out plans of life, nor, even less, any practical agreement on how to evaluate the intrinsic value of these plans." [123]

None of this is new to physicians. It is precisely this view that justifies the practice of informed consent in contemporary society. American society recognizes the individual's right to consent to or to refuse medical interventions because determining whether a particular treatment will be of benefit is an individual choice which depends upon the individual's particular conception of the good life, particular beliefs, aspirations, responsibilities, family ties, ultimate ends, and so forth. [124] To return to the example of laryngeal cancer, two patients being treated by the same physician at the same hospital may opt for very different treatments. One may value his speech more and accept a shorter life, while the other may value longevity over having the ability to speak. Similarly, given two patients at risk for having a genetically defective infant, one may opt for amniocentesis with possible abortion and the other may refuse to test for any defects, accepting the risk of having a defective child. There is no agreed-upon standard of what is best; it all depends upon what is considered valuable and what is not. Because of this, and because the state aims to be neutral in such choices, the choice among medical treatments must be left to the individual; and the right of informed consent is meant to ensure this respect for individual choice. The President's Commission put it this way: "[D]ecisions about the treatments that best promote a patient's health and well-being must be based on the particular patient's values and goals; no uniform, objective determination can be adequate—whether defined by society or by health professionals." [125]

What is true for competent patients who can give informed consent is also true for incompetent ones. Every judgment about what level of medical care to provide, every determination of which treatments are beneficial and which ones are burdensome, presupposes a particular conception of the good life. "The fact of pluralism" means that there is no such thing as a socially shared view of *the* best interests of the incompetent patient. In a liberal society, there is no "uniform, objective determination" of what "best promotes a patient's" interests. Within liberal political philosophy, formulating objective, socially shared criteria to determine what medical care is beneficial and what care is harmful to guide application of the best interests standard is impossible. Or as one of the New Jersey Supreme Court judges put it: "A 'best interests' standard assumes a consensus that is not there regarding when discontinuation of treatment is in a patient's best interests."[126]

These points suggest that the contemporary debate on terminating care to incompetent patients is a debate among people advocating divergent conceptions of the good life for informing the determination of the best interests standard. In other words, the liberal position about the diverse conceptions of the good life finds expression in the multiplicity of views expressed in the debate about appropriate care for incompetent patients. Hence we can substantiate the claim that in a liberal society there is no criterion of benefits and burdens which can inform the best interests standard by considering the diverse conceptions of the good life advocated in the public debate and how they inform different treatments for incompetent patients.

Prominent positions within the public debate might be categorized into six different conceptions of the good life. This list is not comprehensive, but it does represent some of the most frequently discussed positions. It should, however, be noted that many advocates do not conceive of their positions as philosophical conceptions of the good life and have not developed their conceptions very far. Thus in some cases it will be necessary to reconstruct and fill out the details of a position. Even if the reconstruction presented here does not precisely fit any particular individual commentator's avowed position, it should serve as a clarification of those often undeveloped positions. Finally, the list will proceed from those advocating the most active medical interventions to those who consider more selective treatment acceptable.

1. *The Physical Conception.* This is the classic sanctity-of-life position, sometimes called vitalism. Most basically, it holds that life itself is sacred or, in less religious language, of supreme value. The life of a being born from human parents, no matter how deformed or debilitated, should be preserved and maintained using available medical interventions. Any considerations of cognitive abilities, level of consciousness, possibilities of independent living, age, or attendant physical complications should not be entertained in evaluating which ther-

apies should be instituted. The possibility of extending life is the objective. And the extension of life is to be measured not in years or months, but from moment to moment. On this view the continuation of physical existence, metabolism, the absolute basic bodily functions, is the human good. This alone is needed to justify our actions. One writer succinctly summarizes this position in considering "the profoundly retarded, non-ambulatory, blind, deaf infant who will spend his few years in the back ward cribs of a state institution" and argues: "One who has never known the pleasures of mental operation, ambulation, and social interaction surely does not suffer from their loss as much as one who has. While no one who has known these capacities may prefer death to a life without them, we have no assurance that the handicapped person, with no point of comparison, would agree. Life, and life alone, whatever its limitations, might be of sufficient worth to him." [127] (I exclude from consideration under this physical conception those who advocate that "everything be done" except when the care "merely prolongs dying" or is "futile." These qualifications, while they may be wise and justifiable, already dilute the force of this position by admitting some circumstances in which care can be withdrawn. They also bring in the ambiguity of drawing the lines of when a patient is dying and judging when care is futile. In this sense they clearly involve significant ethical judgments about the quality-of-life.)

In contemporary America, we associate this position with Protestant fundamentalism. [128] Yet the most articulate defense of such a position is probably found among some Orthodox Jews. [129] The advocates of this physical conception of the good, however, need not be religious at all. Indeed, this position, or one very similar, has been advanced by law professors, [130] some physicians, [131] and some liberal journalists. [132] It may even be the position invoked by the New York Supreme Court in the Storar decision[133] and possibly underlies the Department of Health and Human Services' "Baby Doe" rules. [134] Regardless of who precisely espouses this conception, it clearly has an important place within the debate about withholding care, if only to mark what is considered the most consistent position that requires no contentious distinctions among those who are to receive and those who will not receive medical treatment. In some ways it is the "natural" position against which another position is to be critically evaluated.

2. *The Hedonistic Conception.* On this conception of the good, the

basic end of life is the avoidance of pain. This, of course, is the old Benthamite view of persons as loci of sensations, where the objective of life is maximizing pleasure while minimizing pain. Applied to the area of medical care, it leads to the simple rule that "the only possible justification for withholding treatment is pain."[135] Or to capture the original flavor of the hedonistic calculus: "I suggest that we are justified in claiming that death would be better for the infant only if it is reasonable to believe that the negative experiences—the physical pain and psychological suffering that would occur in continued living— would outweigh the positive experiences and pleasures that would occur."[136] We should not forget John Stuart Mill's observation on this Benthamite logic, which notes the inevitable reduction of all human suffering to physical pain.[137] As noted previously, the advocates of this position are many, including the New Jersey Supreme Court.

3. *The Relational Conception.* On this conception the important good of human life is an affective, relational one: the potentiality to enter into human relationships. In the *locus classicus* of this position, Richard McCormick writes that "life is a value to be preserved only insofar as it contains some potentiality for human relationships."[138] The type of human relationships envisioned is not modeled on the Aristotelian conception of friendship but on basic emotional interactions. A infant's life can have "meaning as long as there is hope that the infant will, in relative comfort, be able to experience our caring and love. For when this happens both we and the child are sharing in that 'greater more important good.'"[139] In this conception of the human good the capacity "to give and receive love" and affection, to interact and communicate emotionally, is the fundamental good which makes life worth living. It is important to understand that this good need not require the sophistication of verbal responses, but only the bond of love. The receptions and responses of an infant are the model. And "without these qualities, no distinctly human good can be achieved."[140]

While this conception of the good has Christian overtones, it has attracted many secular advocates as well, partially because it explicitly recognizes what the other conceptions fail to and what appears, intuitively, "to be highly relevant from a moral point of view"—that the value of life exists only in relation to other higher, human goods.[141]

4. *The Autonomous Conception.* This conception derives from the individualist notion that the essential characteristic of human beings is

their ability to conceive and to pursue a conception of their own good. On this view the common purpose of human life is for individuals to construct their own lives, to discover what ultimate ends they value and attempt to realize these goals. The good is the good of self-determination and thus entails a certain independence, which is more mental than physical. The essential capacities are those related to thinking and judging, having the ability to decide what aims and objectives one wants to pursue, being capable of determining what particular acts will achieve the chosen ends, and pursuing them. Philosophically, this is the expression of the ideal of moral liberalism as found in the philosophy of Kant, Mill, and others.

Usually autonomy is seen to be relevant only when a patient is competent, and thus capable of making decisions about his own medical care, and is thought to be irrelevant in guiding decisions about what care to provide incompetent patients.[142] On this view, the so-called moral principles of autonomy and beneficence are inextricably connected. This position has implicitly informed some important positions on withholding medical care, especially within the medical profession. This conception of the good underlies Osler's position as well as the recent advocacy of terminating naso-gastric feedings and minimizing medical interventions for mildly demented—the "pleasantly senile"—patients by several prominent physicians.[143] And when the President's Commission discusses the best interests standard, it suggests that an important criterion should be "the possibility of developing or regaining the capacity for self-determination."[144] This standard seems to underlie some court decisions which do not explicitly employ the language of autonomy or self-determination but do allude to such a conception. In the *Dinnerstein* case, for example, the court sanctioned giving a vegetative patient with heart disease a "Do Not Resuscitate" status because a possible resuscitation would not return the patient "towards a normal, functioning, integrated existence."[145] And the same court, in the case of a minor, mandated chemotherapy because it would give the patient an opportunity "for growth into [a] free and independent individual."[146]

5. *The Economic Conception.* On this conception, the critical good is the ability to engage in socially meaningful work, the capacity to hold a job, to be economically self-sufficient, and to live independently. This conception is fairly obvious and easily quantifiable. Rarely is it offered as an explicit conception of the good, although it is found in

Britain. For example, in discussing the results of a study on treating spina bifida cases, John Lorber considers the most favorable outcomes under the heading "possible breadwinners." These are the children who could "earn their own living in competitive employment and be self-supporting with a secure, independent place in society."[147] And similarly, the criteria for allocating kidney dialysis in Britain rely heavily on age, therefore potential productive years saved, and also exclude any patients with complicating disabilities, including physical handicaps and any mental illness or defects.[148]

6. *The Utilitarian Conception.* Within this view the overall measure of good is in terms of "happiness" or "well-being," which is practically reducible to the absence of pain and suffering. But this conception of the good differs from the previous five, especially the hedonistic conception, because in contrast to the others, the good is not related to specific individual persons. The good is impersonal, or, better, a social good; what matters is an aggregate good, not how each individual realizes her particular goods. This is expressed by the view that people are "replaceable." If they, and related others, such as their family, experience more pain and suffering, making the aggregate happiness lower, than if they were "replaced" by another human being, then it would be justifiable to let them die. An illustration by one of the proponents of this view might clarify the position: "It is also plausible to suppose that the prospects of a happy life are better for a normal child than for a haemophiliac. When the death of a defective infant will lead to the birth of another infant with better prospects of a happy life, the total amount of happiness will be greater if the defective infant is killed. The loss of happy life for the first infant is outweighed by the gain of a happier life for the second. Therefore, if killing the haemophiliac infant has no adverse effect on others, it would, according to the total view, be right to kill him. The total view treats infants as replaceable."[149] It is from the perspective of this "total view" that happiness, the good, is to be evaluated. Hence the view that individuals are "replaceable" for the realization of the maximum happiness of everyone aggregated into a "total" social picture.

This is a view particularly associated with utilitarian philosophers such as Peter Singer, Michael Tooley, and Jonathan Glover.[150] These commentators go to great lengths to explain why such a conception of the good leads to withholding or withdrawing care from infants and possibly the permanently incompetent, but not from normal individuals, by elaborating "intrinsic" qualities of the person that make his continued living valuable enough to be secured by a "right to life." Persons are seen to be human beings who, at a minimum, have desires about the future and are self-conscious. Killing people, then, is wrong first because it has the disastrous side-effect that no one will be happy because people will always worry about being killed, and second because we actually have this desire to live which should not be frustrated. Hence the need for "a right to life" as a way to secure our desire to continue living and the possibility of being happy, a way to ensure maximization of the aggregate good. Killing the incompetent should not make normal people fear for their own lives, nor will it frustrate the incompetent's nonexistent desires to keep living. Hence there is no need to give incompetent patients a right to life to maximize the aggregate good. Indeed, as discussed above, their death usually would be better for the overall happiness. The specification of the essential elements of personhood and the attendant right to life, therefore, are best seen as ways of altering the calculation of the aggregate good. They make "normal" people seem irreplaceable not because they are intrinsically valuable individuals, but because killing them would lower the aggregate good.[151]

It is important to recognize that the claim here is not that an individual's happiness or best interests depend upon the interests and practices of other people, but that the relevant conception of the good is not individualized but aggregated, viewed from the "total" perspective. Seeing the good as aggregated makes the individual's particular good irrelevant except as a contribution to the whole, and the individual himself completely replaceable.

No doubt the summaries of these six conceptions of the good are too brief and schematic. And no doubt the proponents of each position might legitimately complain that the capsulization has somewhat distorted their view. Moreover, there are other conceptions of the good life that are not considered. But this is not intended as a comprehensive review of all possible conceptions of the good. Rather, it is an attempt to demonstrate that there are many different ways of considering what is good for a person, even from a single person's own perspective. Each of these conceptions is not without its difficulties, but each conception can serve to define the ultimate ends and attachments of a human life and can ground practicable criteria for determining whether or not an incompetent patient will benefit from particular medical care. In this sense, each conception could serve as the basis of a surrogate's choice for an incompetent patient. But these different conceptions will necessarily produce different and, what is more important, conflicting judgments about what kind of care will be for the patient's benefit. It is not a matter of which personal perspective we adopt, whether the perspective of the patient or that of a normal adult or of the reasonable man. The issue is rather which conception of the good life we adopt. No matter from which personal perspective we approach the issue, we still need a standard for what will be good.

These different conceptions of the good life would prescribe different medical care as being beneficial for patients. For instance, if we consider Karen Quinlan, a hopelessly ill patient in a persistent vegetative state, both the physical and the hedonistic conceptions of the good would urge that it is in her best interests to be kept alive by all manner of medical care. From one perspective, she is alive and her life is valuable even if vegetative. From the other perspective, she is not suffering and certainly has no unremitting severe pain. Significantly, we can imagine that from her perspective she might easily espouse either of these conceptions of the good and determinations of her best interests. Conversely, the affective and autonomous conceptions of the good would suggest that her best interests are not served by continued care, even antibiotics and naso-gastric feedings. She cannot relate to other people in any way, let alone make any decisions about her life. We can easily imagine that these conceptions of the good life might be hers. Obviously, on either the economic or the utilitarian conception, treatment should be abandoned.

Similarly, if we determine the best interests of Ms. Conroy, an 84-year-old woman confined to bed who suffered from organic brain syndrome, by applying the physical and hedonistic conceptions of the good, she should receive all types of medical care. Indeed in commentary on this case, it has rarely been noted that when the New Jersey Supreme Court outlined its objective standard for withdrawing treatment based on "recurring, unavoidable and severe pain," it concluded that the patient's care should *not* be terminated because she was not experiencing such pain.[152] According to the relational conception, her artificial nutrition and hydration probably should be continued since she is minimally conscious and seems to sense emotion at a very minimal level.[153] According to the other three conceptions, her best interests would certainly be served by withdrawal. Again it is important to emphasize that the decision about Ms. Conroy's care does not depend upon adopting her perspective, since her perspective does not define any particular conception of what is beneficial. Best interests depend not on which personal perspective is adopted, but on which standard of the good life is adopted.

This detailed investigation into the best interests standard suggests that any attempt to find either an objective or a socially shared criterion of benefits and burdens within liberal society will be unsuccessful. In a liberal polity there will be no agreed-upon standard and hence no way of publicly defining *the* best interests of a patient.

There might be one final attempt to articulate an objective, socially shared criterion of benefit. This attempt would go back to the liberal conception of a person articulated in Chapter 2. In this conception, a person is conceived as having two moral powers, a sense of justice and the capacity for a conception of the good life. Thus individuals must have the capacity to form, to pursue, and rationally to revise a vision of the ultimate good and purposes of life. Now it might be argued that this conception of the person should provide the grounds on which we determine what care to provide incompetent patients in a liberal society. After all, it is by appeal to this conception of the person that the principles of justice are justified. Using this conception, it might be thought that when a person becomes so incompetent that he irreversibly lacks the capacity to formulate or pursue a conception of the good life, he ceases to be an equal citizen, and at that point there is no reason to continue to provide him with medical care. Hence it would be justified to terminate medical interventions to Quinlan and Conroy, and to all patients whose level of incompetence extended from coma to the receptive type (see Table 3.1).

In response two things should be noted. While it may be claimed that this conception of the person is the shared conception that should inform public principles and policies, it is certainly not shared when it comes to terminating care. Indeed, the strong standard, justifying the withholding of care from patients whose mental deficits range from coma to receptive, is not one that all agree to. As this survey of the various positions in the current debate over terminating care suggests, there are several prominent positions that oppose this standard. The New Jersey Supreme Court, among others, has espoused the hedonistic conception; several prominent bioethicists espouse the relational conception; and there are religious people who espouse the physical conception. This conception of the person applied to a standard of benefit is in no way a shared view. If anything, this suggests that the conception of a person is not as widely shared as might be supposed. Indeed, the fact that this position is not widely shared in relation to incompetent persons might suggest that it is not the "intuitive idea" of the person which informs our political culture—or that this intuitive idea needs refining and qualifying.[154]

But what is more important, adopting this position, using the conception of a person which informs liberal political philosophy, to delineate criteria of benefit in defining the best interests standard would be to violate the liberal ideal of neutrality. Using this conception to define a standard of benefit would be to make autonomous individuality the standard of good as applied to incompetent patients, and thus to adopt the autonomous conception of the good life outlined previously as the one informing public laws and policies. In other words, to set the standard of benefit by whether an individual had irreversibly lost the capacity to formulate or pursue a conception of the good life would be to justify a public policy by appeal to a particular conception of the good life which is not shared. To do so would provide a solution to the problem of medical care for incompetent patients. Yet such a solution would violate the liberal tenet of neutrality. It would impose the ideal of autonomy on other citizens; it would make liberalism another "sectarian doctrine." Thus a solution to the problem of medical care for the incompetent is theoretically possible. But any such solution cannot be consistent with the tenets of liberal political philosophy. In other words, the tenets of liberalism undermine the possibility of using the best interests standard.

I have argued that using the best interests standard to decide what care would be most beneficial to an incompetent patient would require either an objective or a socially shared standard of benefits and burdens; otherwise it would be an indeterminate standard. But we have seen that the advocates of this standard have not provided such a criterion for determining benefits and burdens. Furthermore, I argued that every standard of benefits relies on a conception of the good life. But "the fact of pluralism" suggests that there will be a multiplicity of these conceptions and therefore a multiplicity of standards of benefits and burdens; there will not be a shared conception of the good life by which to determine what best promotes a patient's health and well-being. This point was emphasized by my survey of six different conceptions of the good life, which suggested different treatments for different patients. Thus, given the liberal affirmation of "the fact of pluralism," a socially shared standard is impossible. Finally, trying to invoke any particular conception of the good life, for example the autonomous conception, to provide a standard of benefits for the best interests standard would be inconsistent with the liberal ideal of neutrality.

Thus the most severe problems in utilizing the best interests standard arise not from practical difficulties, such as disagreements over the patient's diagnosis or prognosis, but from philosophical inconsistency between the standard itself and the tenets of liberal political philosophy. There is no way to use the best interests standard and fulfill the liberal ideal of neutrality. The best interests standard is untenable in a liberal polity. The choice is between affirming this standard and affirming the tenets of liberalism; these positions cannot be espoused simultaneously.

Illiberal Resolutions to the Problem of Terminating Care

The arguments of this chapter suggest that within liberal political philosophy there is no framework for deciding what care to provide incompetent patients. The ordinary/extraordinary dichotomy relies on implicit determinations of what would benefit the patient; the substituted judgment standard seems an attractive fiction, imposing the judgment of the surrogate on the incompetent patient; and the best interests standard lacks a socially shared standard of benefits and burdens to guide its use. This presents a problem: In a liberal polity, how is the issue of terminating care to incompetents in fact resolved? The answer is by appeal to illiberal solutions. Our society has not forsaken the best interests standard, but, without acknowledgment, it violates the tenets of liberalism. In the interpretation, application, and justification of standards used to guide terminating care decisions, we can discover implicit and sometimes explicit use of illiberal principles. I shall outline four common approaches.

The first solution, already encountered in the *Conroy* objective test, is to suggest that pain, or sometimes pain and suffering, constitute objective standards of benefit and burdens for incompetent patients. Clearly, when judges invoke this hedonistic conception of the good life to determine what care incompetent patients receive, this conflicts with the liberal ideal of neutrality.

The second, and probably most common, solution is to make the decision private by leaving it to the incompetent patient's family. In previous sections I have already noted many of the attractions as well as the difficulties of this solution. But there is another consideration worth mentioning: having the state support the family's power over its members, by granting the family final authority to decide what care the patient receives, conflicts with the tenets of liberalism. The President's Commission suggests five reasons to leave terminating care decisions to the family:

1. The family is generally most concerned abut the good of the patient.
2. The family will also usually be most knowledgeable about the patient's goals, preferences, and values.
3. The family deserves recognition as an important social unit that ought to be treated, within limits, as a responsible decision-maker in matters that intimately affect its members.
4. Especially in a society in which many other traditional forms of community have eroded, participation in a family is often an important dimension of personal fulfillment.
5. Since a protected sphere of privacy and autonomy is required for the flourishing of this interpersonal union, institutions and the state should be reluctant to intrude.[155]

I have already noted that the first two reasons offered by the President's Commission are suspect. But the last three reasons for leaving terminating care decisions to the family are in overt contradiction to liberal tenets. In a liberal polity, it is not the state's role to support traditional institutions because they are either traditional or the only bastions of community left. In a liberal state, providing support for either traditions or communities because their preservation is deemed especially important violates the ideal of neutrality. Furthermore, the fact that many people find the family "an important dimension of personal fulfillment" does not mean that the state can establish a policy of always deferring to the family without violating the ideal of neutrality. For this would impose a view of how individuals should view their familial relations which may not be a shared element of everyone's conception of the good life. That the idealized model of the family as a nurturing union does not extend to all families has become glaringly obvious in the course of the AIDS crisis. Conflicts with family members, especially for homosexual victims of AIDS, are common. There can be no presumption that all citizens think the family, as traditionally defined, should be given "recognition as an important social unit."

The point is not that the family should not be deemed important and granted special privileges. Rather, the point is that this position is in conflict with liberalism. If we want to endorse and promote the family as an important unit, which is the best and most appropriate decision-maker for its incompetent members, then the justification for this cannot be found within liberal political philosophy. Through what was once called benign neglect, a liberal polity may permit social unions to flourish, but it cannot support them either with special legal recognition or with financial resources because this would be imposing a conception of the good life on all members of society.[156] To the degree that we find the family an important public institution worthy of political recognition and protection, we deviate from the tenets of liberal political philosophy.

A third solution is the assertion that there exists a social consensus on how incompetent patients should be medically treated. The California Supreme Court expressed this view when it wrote: "When dealing with patients for whom the possibility of full recovery is virtually nonexistent, and who are incapable of expressing their desires, there is also something of a consensus on the standard to be applied."[157] But there is no such consensus on any standard for terminating care. In the previous sections I have delineated the many diverse opinions held within our polity that fuel the current controversy. Indeed, if a consensus existed, the entire issue would have disappeared because there would be a socially shared perspective by which to determine what care to give incompetent patients; there would be no more court cases, no more public debates and controversies. The persistence of the debate, without an apparent shared perspective, belies the existence of a consensus. The assertion of a consensus seems purely imaginary, more a hope than a reality.

The final mechanism adopted to resolve this medical ethical issue is to follow the old maxim "avoid death." Whenever there is doubt about what care to provide a patient, the reaction is to intervene and preserve life, because "there is always time to allow the patient to die with dignity tomorrow—to allow someone to die one day too soon is a mistake that cannot be rectified."[158] As the President's Commission put it, "health care professionals serve patients best by maintaining a presumption in favor of sustaining life."[159] And the New Jersey Supreme Court was explicit in recommending that "when evidence of a person's wishes or physical or mental condition is equivocal, it is best to err, if at all, in favor of preserving life."[160]

There is no doubt that in the years since the *Quinlan* decision courts, physicians, and the public are more willing to set aside the maxim "avoid death" and to sanction the termination of medical interventions in particular circumstances.[161] And yet in most cases, without specific guidelines directing physicians and families to stop care, medical interventions are continued. "Avoiding death" is the assumed position that can be altered only by specific directive. But just as with pain, averting death is an illiberal solution because it presumes a conception of the good life, a judgment that life is worth continuing under any circumstances, at any cost.

These are the real ways in which the care of incompetent patients is decided. They clash with the tenets of liberal political philosophy. Consequently, each resolution is only temporary; each illiberal resolution soon becomes undermined by liberal doubts and attacks. The use of pain or death to determine what care should be given incompetent patients is attacked because other important human values are ignored. Liberal doubts concerning the virtues of the family as surrogate decision-maker make it increasingly difficult to let decisions remain private, without review by the courts or a public agency. Finally, the increasing number of court cases and the persistent public debates deny the reality of any ethical consensus. So the controversy goes on unabated, with no end in sight.

The Ill Effects of Irresolution

Liberal political philosophy undermines each attempt to justify a particular view of how incompetent patients should be treated by making each view appear as one personal perspective among a variety of legitimate value judgments. The consequence is interminable controversy that adversely affects physicians, the public, and liberal philosophy itself.

Despite the persistent unresolved questions, physicians must still care for incompetent patients. The consequence is the physicalization

of medical practice; in short, the care for human disease and derange-
ments of human bodies becomes divorced from care for the entire
human being. Lost is concern for the role of disease in the person's life
plans, the relationship between disability and human fulfillment, the
possibility of life well lived ready for its natural end. The claim here is
not that the irresolution surrounding terminating care of incompetent
patients somehow *creates* the physicalization of medicine. Admittedly,
the growth of biological knowledge and technological advancements
already forcefully propel medicine in this direction. The ethical irresolution, however, encourages and exacerbates this tendency.

In the face of what one physician called "a vacuum [without] reliable criteria on which to base a decision" regarding the withholding
or withdrawing of medical treatments, practitioners still must make
fundamental judgments about what interventions to provide patients.[162] In response to this dilemma, some physicians positively affirm the preservation of life, regardless of a patient's mental capacities,
as the end of medicine. Other physicians try to fulfill the liberal spirit
and find a neutral posture. Often they view preserving life as the correct response. As noted in the previous section, both society and the
medical profession encourage this view.[163] Still other physicians, de-
spairing of finding principled grounds for terminating care, follow
their clinical instincts. And from medical school on, from their men-
tors' and their patients' expectations, their instincts are well trained to
intervene to prolong life. Indeed, physicians are rarely challenged for
intervening but often criticized for "going slow."[164] "Physicians do
not easily accept the conception that it may be best to do less, not
more, for a patient. The decision to pull back is much more difficult
to make than the decision to push ahead with aggressive support."[165]
Whether it is positively affirmed, liberally espoused, or instinctively
assumed, prolonging life becomes the "default" response for physicians facing clinical decisions without clear ethical guidelines on terminating care. As a result, aggressive treatment, without concern for
the "whole" patient—the physicalization of medicine—is the standard of care.

The point here is not to claim that all physicians strive to preserve
life at all costs and that there are no physicians who feel uneasy about
such practices. Many physicians do think it is ethical to withhold care
from incompetent patients, do think prolonging life can be unethical,
and urge their colleagues to use restraint. But these are explicit appeals

against the common practice, and their justification is more personal than public.[166] Liberalism has undermined any attempt by physicians to appeal to a shared framework of the ends of medicine to justify fewer interventions.[167] Without such a framework, aggressive interventions to prolong the physical being rather than caring for the whole being become the natural—and presumed neutral—reaction.

The effect of this ethical irresolution is not limited to physicians, but touches people in many ways. The agony of having loved ones die is multiplied by the indecision surrounding the terminating of medical care. One person described her mother, "who does not know me or other members of the family," as "a corpse we cannot bury."[168] And the father of child kept alive in an intensive care unit only to die after six months writes: "What they never understood was that one *can* care deeply enough about a child like Andrew to want his misery ended. Allowing Andrew to die naturally was what we wanted *for* him, not just to him. I thought often when I did go in to see him about his massive pain. He was sometimes crying then—a nearly soundless, aimless cry of pain, undirected and unlistened to, except, I sometimes thought, by me. As often as I wanted to gather him into my arms I wanted him to be allowed to die. What is the name for that?"[169] Clearly, such situations have prompted the proliferation of court litigation to terminate care. When there is conflict among family members or between family members and the medical team, and there is no shared framework to appeal to, court is where the battle ends. And even in situations where there may be complete agreement for terminating care, the uncertainty over the ethical standards may create hesitation without judicial sanction.[170]

The inability to terminate care can affect people in diverse ways. Families cannot just leave "the corpse they cannot bury" lying in a hospital bed. Sometimes this impulse for an end, the desire to let the dead finally die, can make caring and compassionate people perform monstrous acts. Every so often a brief press report reveals the darkest side of the ethical and hence legal uncertainty that drives this excessive care. We read of a son who held a nurse at gunpoint until his father's life-support system was turned off and his father, a cancer patient who had been in a coma for almost two weeks, died. The son said he had promised his father "not to let him linger." And all during the event he repeated over and over that "he wanted his father to die with dignity."[171] We read of a father who shot his 3-year-old daughter in her hospital crib. Following a head injury, the child had been lying in a hospital bed in a coma for over eight months.[172] We read of a 76-year-old Florida man sentenced to twenty-five years in prison for shooting his wife of fifty-one years who suffered eight years of "excruciating pain and agony" with Alzheimer's disease and osteoporosis.[173] We read of an 89-year-old Texas rancher convicted of murder for shooting his 72-year-old brother who suffered from Alzheimer's disease. The convicted man said: "I regret having to do what I did, but I don't regret doing it. I felt he would have done it himself if he could have."[174] We read of a 36-year-old man trying to disconnect his terminally ill mother from a life-support system in the intensive care unit of a New Jersey hospital.[175]

These people are not crazy; they do not have a history of mental instability; they do not subscribe to any outlandish religions involving sacrificial practices; they are not professional criminals or hired guns; they are not killing to collect fantastic inheritances; they are, at first approximation, normal people. They basically aim to do the right thing for their families and yet find themselves possessed by these agonizing circumstances to kill.

For others the response is just the opposite: paralysis. The moral responsibility for deciding when to terminate care often lies with the family. But with this responsibility comes the added burden that in a liberal society there is no shared ethical framework by which to justify a decision. It is not that people should be able to evade or deny their moral responsibility; nor do we think that such awesome decisions to terminate a human being's medical care should be easy. We would rightly be horrified if people made such decisions without feeling the force of various positions. But there is a difference between making such a decision which can be publicly discussed and justified to others by appeal to shared moral conceptions, and making the same decision in circumstances without common ethical conceptions. In the latter situation the decision loses its ethical quality, seeming to be more a matter of taste and preference and less a position that can be defended and justified. Furthermore, there is a difference between discussing a moral position on terminating care that the polity might effect, and being obligated to decide personally the ethical issues for a loved one. The consequence of focusing all the responsibility on family members while denying them a shared ethical framework for guidance is that many people, while they agree that terminating care is permissible and would want their own care terminated, eschew doing so for their loved ones.[176] Placing such moral responsibility on single individuals without a shared social perspective may be demanding too much of conscientious citizens.

Finally, the irresolution surrounding the issue of terminating care suggests serious difficulties with liberal political philosophy. The issue of terminating medical care is important for political philosophy in part because it indicates a failure of liberalism to fulfill its avowed objective of providing a guiding framework for addressing public ethical questions. The importance of this conclusion, however, extends beyond this single issue to typify a more general problem with liberalism.

We can distinguish two types of public ethical issues based on their content. One type consists of matters of justice that concern the fair distribution of rights, opportunities, and income. The second type involves issues that concern not social distribution to individuals, but the qualitative aspects of collective life. These issues concern what goods are deemed public goods, how public goods should be valued, how shared traditions should be interpreted and perpetuated, how public spaces should be used, how public projects should be executed, and the like. We might label this second type of public issues "matters concerning the quality of common life." Terminating medical care for incompetent patients constitutes a matter concerning the quality of common life.[177]

One way of understanding liberal political philosophy is through its approach to these two types of issues. Liberalism attempts to restrict the public agenda by excluding certain subjects from public debate. Liberalism limits those ethical issues that can be addressed within politics to matters of justice. These distributive matters, it is felt, are fundamental and can be addressed by appeal to neutral principles such as Rawls's principles of justice. (For the moment I will not question the validity of this claim; I leave its evaluation to the next chapter.)

Because matters concerning the quality of common life can be addressed only by appeal to an ethical framework informed by a conception of the good life, liberalism tries to exclude them from the public agenda. But this is not possible.

Matters concerning the quality of common life have traditionally been viewed as public ethical issues to be resolved through political deliberation, although not by appeal to the principles of justice or any other neutral principles. As I argued in this chapter, the issue of terminating medical care for incompetent patients, and similar issues, are public ethical issues; they can only be privatized if the polity itself adheres to coherent standards for all types of interventions touching upon the borderline of life and death. At the very least the polity must decide standards delimiting justifiable termination decisions, and, in some instances, it must itself actually decide upon and justify terminating medical care to individual incompetent patients. Further, such standards and decisions are clearly ethical; they do not involve measures of efficiency or taste or improvements in material life. They entail commitments to what is good and valuable; they involve the interpretation and affirmation of certain ethical ideals. Choosing various alternative policies can radically change a community, making it one in which certain goods are cherished and pursued or one in which certain goods are not valued. And yet the issue of terminating medical care to incompetent patients, and more generally, matters concerning the quality of common life, are not matters of justice. While terminating medical care relates to the right of privacy, through the right to refuse medical care, it cannot be addressed just by appeal to such a right or to any distributive principle. Such a public ethical issue is not exhausted by, but rather transcends, justice. To address the issue, the polity would have to appeal to ethical ideals besides those related to the distribution of rights, opportunities, and income. Indeed, as I have shown, such decisions can be made only by appeal to conceptions of the good life.

Liberalism tries to exclude from political debate those ethical issues that can be resolved only by appeal to conceptions of the good life. But when this cannot be done, when these issues will not remain private and call out for a public solution, the deficiencies of the liberalism become apparent. For in failing to provide a framework for principled deliberation on matters concerning the quality of common life, liberalism undermines its own objective: these issues are public ethical issues and yet liberalism cannot address them.

Just as some moral philosophies attempt to reduce all ethical considerations to moral imperatives, so liberalism tries to reduce all political issues to matters of justice.[178] But our public life encompasses more than justice. Matters concerning the quality of common life are public ethical issues to be addressed by appeal to a shared ethical framework. In limiting political deliberation to matters of justice, liberalism constricts, distorts, and denudes our public lives—and therefore our medical ethics.

4

The Just Distribution of Medical Resources

By considering the issue of deciding what medical care should be provided to incompetent patients, we explored the dilemma created for liberal political philosophy by public deliberation on matters concerning the quality of common life. Every attempt to resolve this issue without invoking a conception of the good life—through the use of individual rights, the ordinary/extraordinary distinction, and the substituted judgment standard—fails. Hence the turn to the idea that decisions about care for incompetent patients should promote the patient's "best interests." But, as we saw, this standard can help only when informed by a conception of the good life. Yet the liberal ideal of neutrality prohibits justifying any law or policy by appeal to a single conception of the good life. It thereby precludes the public affirmation of a single conception of the "best interest." Thus I concluded that the perpetual ethical irresolution surrounding the determination of what medical care incompetent patients should receive has its source not in the practical issues of uncertainty over a patient's prognosis or who should be the patient's surrogate, but in the philosophical tenets of liberalism.

But, it may be thought, matters concerning the quality of common life are not, or should not be, *political* issues; liberal political philosophy is fundamentally a theory of justice, concerned with the fair distribution of rights, opportunities, and income. While liberalism may not provide an adequate ethical framework to guide deliberations on issues relating to terminating medical care for patients, it is argued, its virtues and philosophical plausibility rest on its ability to structure a framework for addressing matters of justice. In this way, liberalism can at least fulfill its objective in the realm of justice.

In this chapter I investigate this claim by asking: Does liberal political philosophy provide a deliberative framework to guide us in creating a just scheme to distribute medical resources? Do the liberal principles of justice permit us to devise a philosophically plausible conception of just health care?[1]

The allocation[2] of medical resources continues to be a topic of intense controversy, suggesting the absence of an ethical resolution. I will show that this public irresolution is a necessary consequence of the very principles of liberal justice. Any scheme of just health care will have to be informed by a conception of the good life. Part of our polity's inability to devise a national health insurance plan, to create a scheme supplying basic medical care for the entire population, and even to agree upon a theoretical construct for the just distribution of medical resources, can be traced to the liberal ideal of neutrality.

Justice and Health Care Policy

In 1971, as part of the debate over national health insurance, Representative Wilbur Mills, the chairman of the powerful House Ways and Means Committee, scheduled hearings on renal dialysis. Shep Glazer, who then was vice-president of the National Association of Patients on Hemodialysis, was scheduled to address the Committee. Minutes before his appearance, his wife connected him to a dialysis machine and he testified before Congress, literally showing the politicians that patients on dialysis could lead normal lives, could continue to work and raise children, if they could be dialyzed.[3]

At that time, Shep Glazer was among the 4,000 Americans with chronic renal failure being kept alive by dialysis. Only those fortunate enough to have major medical insurance policies that covered the cost of treatment, to be enrolled in a Veteran's Administration dialysis program, or to receive community-supported dialysis were being kept alive. In 1971 almost 40 percent of all dialysis was being done in the home at a cost of $5,000 to $7,000 per year after an initial investment of $12,000 to $19,000 for the dialysis machine.[4] Hospital-based or center-based dialysis was much more expensive, costing between $15,000 and $25,000 per year.[5] Further, for more than 50 percent of patients, dialysis was only a temporary measure on the way to kidney transplantation, the preferred, cheaper, and permanent treatment for renal failure.

In his testimony, Shep Glazer told Representative Mills and the House Ways and Means Committee his story and asked them for help.

Let me introduce myself personally. I am 43 years old, married for 20 years, with two children, ages 14 and 10 . . . [I] have a major medical [insurance] policy [which pays for dialysis] but the funds [will] soon be consumed by the expensive treatments. . . I was a salesman until a couple of months ago, until it became necessary for me to supplement my income to pay for the dialysis supplies. I tried to sell a noncompetitive line, was found out, and was fired.

Gentlemen, what should I do? End it all and die? Sell my house for which I worked so hard, and go on welfare? Should I go into the hospital under my hospitalization policy, then I cannot work? Please tell me.

If your kidneys failed tomorrow, wouldn't you want the opportunity to live? Wouldn't you want to see your children grow up?[6]

Shep Glazer forced Wilbur Mills and the Congress to confront some difficult questions: Should he be allowed to die even though the technology existed to save his life? Wouldn't every congressman, indeed every man or woman, want to be dialyzed? Should Congress pay the few thousand dollars per patient required each year to keep alive those unfortunate but productive people who, through no fault of their own, are endowed with nonfunctioning kidneys?

But if Congress paid for Shep Glazer's dialysis, why not for the diabetic's insulin, for the "cardiac cripple's" bypass operation, or for the leukemic's bone marrow transplant? And if Congress should pay for acute medical treatments or medications for chronic diseases, why not long-term nursing home care for the elderly or rehabilitative medical care for those with spinal cord injuries or other disabilities? Should Congress be obligated to pay only for vital life-sustaining medical interventions, not for chronic treatments? Or should Congress pay only for cost-effective care, so that somehow the value of the benefits should outweigh the price of the treatment?

These questions can be reduced to two: If Congress should not pay for all these medical interventions, are there any it should pay for? Are there any medical treatments citizens should be entitled to as a matter of justice?

Congressmen felt the emotional as well as the ethical sway of Shep Glazer's appeal. But they also recognized the force of these inescapable inferences. Senator Hartke argued for dialysis patients: "More than 8,000 Americans will die this year from kidney disease because they cannot afford an artificial kidney machine or a kidney transplant.

These will be needless deaths—deaths which should shock our conscience and shame our sensibilities . . . How do we explain that the difference between life and death is a matter of dollars? How do we explain that those who are wealthy have a greater chance to enjoy a longer life than those who are not?" Senator Bennett retorted: "We have equally serious problems which we have not begun to attack which are not so striking as the kidney problem. There is the problem of hemophiliacs, who must constantly receive blood transfusions if they are to remain alive . . . [The action today] demonstrates that we are picking out one particular sector of the whole health care problem, and because it is dramatic, we are trying to push it ahead of everything else. We can only handle so much."[7]

Yet in October 1972, after a thirty-minute debate in the Senate and after just ten minutes of consideration in a House-Senate conference committee, Congress included in the Social Security Amendments of 1972, H.R.1, an extension of Medicare coverage to pay the health care costs for those individuals suffering from chronic renal failure. Thus was enacted the End-Stage Renal Disease (ESRD) Program to provide federally funded financial coverage for the health care of renal failure patients who needed dialysis and those who could obtain a kidney transplant. Dialysis, alone among medical conditions, was defined as a citizen's need.

Since being instituted by the federal government, the ESRD program has greatly expanded and the patients have changed. In 1974, the first full year of the ESRD program, it cost $228.5 million and served 16,000 patients. By 1985 the program cost over $2.1 billion for almost 85,000 patients, in excess of $24,000 per patient.[8] In 1973 the average age of dialysis patients was under 40, with only 7 percent over 55 years of age.[9] And chronic dialysis really did rehabilitate people: 42 percent were working and only 13 percent were disabled or retired. In little more than a decade, by contrast, over 40 percent of all dialysis patients were 60 years of age or older.[10] In addition, 26 percent of all dialysis patients had diabetes and an additional 25 percent had other compounding medical diseases.[11] The result is that today only 18 percent of patients remain employed after going onto dialysis.[12] Overall, end-stage renal disease patients constitute less than 0.3 percent of the total Medicare population, yet consume 4 to 5 percent of the Medicare budget.[13]

In the view of many, the development of the dialysis program typifies the more general "crisis" in American medical care. The current system—or more accurately, health care agglomeration, since the institutions providing health care are too haphazard and disconnected to be accurately described as a system—is simply failing: costing too much, leaving many without services, while providing others with expensive services of questionable benefit.

Consider the costs of health care: In 1950, medical care was about 4.5 percent of the gross national product (GNP), while in 1987 medical care costs exceeded 11 percent of the GNP. In real terms, medical care expenditures have more than doubled in less than forty years. In actual dollars this means we are now spending more than $550 billion, or more than $2,000 per person, on health care each year. This is the highest amount of any country in the world. The country with the next highest per capita expenditure, Canada, spent only $1,483 per person in 1987.

In 1965, before Medicare, the federal government paid about $3.6 billion for personal health care, about 10 percent of the total national expenditures on health care; in 1977 this increased to $40.9 billion, 27.4 percent of the total; and by 1985 this amount was $112.6 billion, representing 30.3 percent of the total personal health expenditures. As a percentage of the federal budget, health care has risen from 4.4 percent of all federal expenditures in 1965, to 11.3 percent in 1977, to over 13 percent in 1985.

Yet despite these enormous costs the provision of care is woefully inadequate. Consider those without medical insurance: Almost 35 million Americans under age 65 had no health insurance for part of 1984, an increase of 6 million in five years. An additional 20 million Americans under 65 were underinsured. And the Medicaid program, designed to help the poor obtain medical care, is failing. Nationally almost 60 percent of the poor, as defined by federal guidelines, are ineligible for Medicaid health coverage, and only 30 percent of poor children are covered. And these restrictive eligibility rules are being further "tightened . . . to deal with the [Medicaid] funding crisis."[14] But even those with insurance or Medicare recipients are having to pay enormous amounts of their own incomes for medical care. In 1984, for example, the Congressional Budget Office estimated that Medicare beneficiaries with incomes under $5,000 per year spent almost 21 percent of their income for out-of-pocket medical expenses. Nearly one-third of the elderly had incomes below $5,000 per year.[15]

In general even with Medicare the elderly are losing ground: Total out-of-pocket expenses for health are now a larger proportion of living costs for the elderly than *before* Medicare.[16]

Consider the effects on access to care and health: The number of poor patients in need of emergency care transferred from the emergency wards of private community or for-profit hospitals to public hospitals for economic reasons is estimated at over 250,000 annually.[17] In major cities this economic "dumping" of patients without insurance or with Medicaid or Medicare coverage has increased from threefold to sixfold over the last four years. Worse, twenty states report infant mortality increases in poor regions since 1981.[18]

While many people have no insurance and are not receiving needed medical care, many others are receiving extremely expensive "high technology" interventions which, in the opinion of many, have questionable benefits. Consider some interventions: Recently attempts to save very small infants, those weighing less than 750 grams (less than 1 pound 10 ounces), with neonatal intensive care interventions have resulted in the fact that "60 to 80 percent of infants died during the initial hospitalization, and the developmental outcome reflects a handicap rate approaching one third of all survivors." Yet for infants between 500 and 999 grams, the cost per surviving child was in excess of $100,000 in 1978 dollars.[19] A similar phenomenon is occurring with AIDS patients for whom there is no cure, or prospects for a cure, only palliative treatments of secondary infections and tumors. On average, AIDS patients will consume approximately $50,000 in medical care services from the time of diagnosis to death. The Public Health Service estimates that in 1991 medical care for AIDS patients will cost between $10 and $25 billion, accounting for 1.2 to 2.4 percent of the total U.S. health care budget, for fewer than 0.1 percent of the population.[20]

And the future appears worse. Costs continue to rise, nearly 10 percent per year. Many complain that health care costs are an important factor in compromising American industrial competitiveness. Consequently, corporations are trying to force workers to assume an increasing share of their health care costs. The private insurance coverage for many individuals is becoming less comprehensive, leaving individuals to pay for more types of care. And each year the federal and state governments try to contain Medicare and Medicaid costs by reducing eligibility, by requiring increasing co-payments, and by reducing payments to hospitals and physicians.

Table 4.1   Levels of the distribution of medical resources

Distributive Levels	Issues
Political	Determining the proportion of GNP devoted to medicine
Medical	Determining the most important medical services
Patient-centered	Determining the patients who should receive specific medical services

What should be done? What system should we adopt to give us just health care, adequate health care for all people, without consuming a disproportionate share of our social resources?

These are not just policy questions, they are questions of distributive justice. And to answer them we need an ethical framework in which to address distributive issues in health care; we need a theory of justice in health care. For it is only by appealing to a theory of justice that citizens can resolve their uncertainty or the conflicting answers different people provide to these distributive questions. A theory of justice in health care provides the justification for society's health care policies; it provides a framework by which principled resolutions to practical disagreements over the distribution of resources can be found. It is by thinking through the meaning and demands of justice as they relate to health that we become clear about what should be done in particular situations, such as Shep Glazer's request for dialysis. So in this time of crisis, in trying to develop health care policies under extreme budgetary pressures, in trying to guarantee citizens essential medical services despite scarcity of resources, we look to political philosophy to provide, in the words of the President's Commission, "ethical principles that offer practical guidance so that health policymakers in Federal, state, and local governments can act responsibly in an era of fiscal belt tightening without abandoning society's commitment to fair and adequate health care."[21] Can liberal political philosophy answer this request for ethical guidance?

To answer this challenge, we need to focus the problem by defining the specific issue to be addressed by political philosophy. Within health care there are three levels of distribution of resources (see Table 4.1).[22] The first level is the *political* level. At this level the distributive question is: What proportion of social resources should be allocated to medical care? This is a question of comparative urgency among the various demands for social resources, from education and defense to housing and health care. The second level is the *medical* level. At this level the distributive question is: What medical services should be guaranteed to citizens? This is a question of comparative urgency among the various medical services, from dialysis and organ transplantation to prenatal and well-baby care. The third level is the *patient-centered* level. At this level the distributive question is: What considerations should determine the availability of services and patient selection for medical services? This is a question that involves delineating the criteria for selecting among patients to receive medical services. These criteria are both clinical and ethical.

Distinguishing these various levels of distributive choices does not imply that the levels are independent of each other—quite the opposite. Each higher level constrains choices at a lower level. The quantity of social resources devoted to medicine will influence the range of services that can be provided and how restrictive patient selection criteria must be. In Britain, for instance, distributive choices at the medical level devote few resources to dialysis, forcing physicians to develop very strict patient selection criteria.[23] Similarly, decisions at the patient-centered level can affect higher-level distributive choices. Clearly in the United States, Congress's decision to grant equal access to dialysis and kidney transplants to all people has raised the total medical resources devoted to end-stage renal disease. This constrains Medicare funds for other medical services and increases the overall amount of the federal budget devoted to health care.

I shall claim that the fundamental ethical issue in the area of the distribution of health care resources concerns the *medical* level. The essential question is: What medical services are most important and should be defined as needs and therefore guaranteed to all citizens? And the challenge for liberal political philosophy is to provide a framework for delineating those medical services to be considered needs.

This is not the usual approach adopted by those trying to reform the health care system to provide adequate care to all people without excessive cost. Instead, they use the economist's traditional macro/micro typology. Thus, economists and politicians worry about the macro level, devising cost containment schemes and limiting reimbursements to reduce the overall expenditures on health care. Conversely, health policy analysts and physicians have focused on the

micro level, studying unnecessary care, variability in the use of procedures, and clinical outcomes to devise clinical criteria for deciding
what treatments to provide patients and, thereby, to reduce the use
and cost of medical care or to guarantee wider access to care.[24]

But by not recognizing the *medical* level of distribution, those
adopting the macro/micro dichotomy ignore the fundamental distributive questions in health care. For the sake of argument, assume we
could change physicians' practice habits and eliminate the 10 to 25
percent of unnecessary medical services overnight. "Even if all useless
care were gradually eliminated, we could anticipate only a temporary
respite from rising costs;"[25] in a short time, just two years, we would
again be confronting rising medical costs and the need to contain
them. More important, if we had this "saved" money previously
wasted on unnecessary medical care, what are the basic medical services that should be provided instead? This is a question at the *medical*
level of distribution. Similarly, if the health care budget is capped and
will not receive a larger proportion of social resources, we will be
forced to decide what medical services should receive priority and
what services should be cut. Again, this becomes a question at the
medical level of distribution.

The importance of the medical level of distribution for defining a
just distribution of health care resources can be further grasped by
considering our actual deliberative process for determining what constitutes a fair distribution of health care resources. In reasoning about
justice in health care we work simultaneously from both the political
and the patient-centered directions, trying to establish what might be
thought of as a "reflective equilibrium" on justice in health care. The
place where the requirements of justice at these two levels meet, and
their differences are resolved, is the medical level. In this way the medical level is the distributive level in which the different demands on
justice are balanced and the requirements of justice specified.

To be specific: Our deliberations on the requirements for justice in
health care begin by considering how resources and services should be
distributed at the patient-centered level. There is a strong intuition
that medical services should be distributed equally among those in
need of the services, or at least that all citizens should be given equal
access to the medical services. This principle of equal access specifies
a fundamental requirement for distribution at the patient-centered
level. It is not necessary to analyze this claim now except to state that

it does seem to be one of the settled intuitions about the just distribution of medical resources.

Concomitantly, we also begin thinking about the distribution of resources at the political level. Clearly there are limited resources and moderate scarcity, necessitating the specification of the urgency of various social programs and what proportion of the GNP each type of program should receive. There is, of course, no definitive specification of the precise proportion of the GNP that should be distributed to each program; but there is some way of roughly ranking the competing programs and some sense for a limit on each program before it disrupts the ranking. The different priority rankings of social programs will reflect different views about which programs are important and which are secondary. (Precisely how these priority rankings are made, the ethical ideals they entail, and the way citizens decide between the competing views are very important issues, but something I shall not explore in detail. I can, however, say that many of the criticisms of the way liberal political philosophy specifies essential medical services would seem to apply to the priority ranking of social programs at the political level; see the section on democratic political procedures later in this chapter.)

After an initial specification, the distributions at the political and patient-centered levels must be "balanced." The political limits on social resources devoted to medical care provide a ceiling. The patient-centered principle determines how the available medical services are to be distributed among those needing them. Then we face the crucial question of justice in health care: What medical services can be provided within the political limit, constrained by the need to satisfy the patient-centered distributive principles? This question is answered by ranking the most urgent medical services, and selecting the most important services that fit within the limit set at the political level when they are distributed according to the principles set at the patient-centered level.

Once the priority ranking of medical services is specified, there may well be another "balancing." Having seen what medical services will be provided to citizens within the resource limit set at the political level, we may choose to increase this limit if, on reflection, these services seem inadequate. And we may go back and forth, adjusting the resource limits and guaranteed services. In this way an equilibrium is established between the distributive determinations at the various levels. The just distribution among resources at the political level is balanced against the services that can be guaranteed at the medical level within the patient-centered distributive criteria. The aim is to make the distributions at all levels satisfy the claims of justice.

These considerations suggest that no scheme of medical services can simply be open-ended; every just scheme must specify and justify a ranking of medical services to remain within the limit on total resources devoted to medical care at the political level. Without such a ranking, the demands for medical care would overwhelm other social programs. In this way, an open-ended health care scheme that adhered to no limit on the social resources to be devoted to medical care would not only be impractical, but, for this very reason, would be unjust in denying resources to other worthy social programs. Consequently, every theory of justice in health care must provide a principled way of ranking the importance of medical services.

This explains the importance of distinguishing the medical level of distribution. It also explains the claim that the most important distributive level for a theory of justice is the medical level. By specifying the relative urgency of the various medical services, we can ensure that citizens will be provided the most important medical interventions according to the distributive principles set at the patient-centered level within the just limits defined at the political level. Only by having this ranking of medical services can justice be achieved in medical care. Hence, providing a principled way of ranking the urgency of medical services is the primary objective for a theory of justice in health care.

In the view of many people, we are facing a "health care crisis." The problems outlined earlier have explosive potential and threaten to ignite the entire system. One way of averting this crisis would be to conceive of a just health care system and the just distribution of health care resources. The question I shall pursue in the remaining sections of this chapter is the following: Can liberal political philosophy offer a suitable conception of justice in health care to help us solve these practical problems? In particular, can liberal political philosophy provide a principled ranking of important medical services?

The Inadequacy of the Right to Equal Access

The Nature of Equal Access

Over the last ninety years or so, the call for a just health care system in the United States has been given a common answer: the principle of equal access. A just health care system requires that each person should have a right of equal access to medical care, or as it is sometimes put, that each person has a "right to an equitable share of total health care resources." [26]

The motivation for this principle is fairly clear: decisions about where to build hospitals, who should be admitted to a hospital, whom doctors should examine and treat, and the like, should be based on ill health and the need for medical services. While phrased in positive terms, the essence of this conception of justice in medical care is a negative claim, a claim that personal characteristics, such as race, gender, geographic location, political power, education, wealth, marital status, religion, or social status, should *not* count in determining what medical care a person has access to or actually receives. In the United States, with a privately financed health care system in which individuals directly pay about 28 percent of all health care bills and the majority have privately funded health insurance, usually through employer-based programs, the most tangible meaning of this right to equal access is that a person's ability to pay should not determine whether or not that person's medical needs are met.

This conception of justice in health care has broad support. We find it in the call for "a democratization of medical service" [27] by a 1918 Ohio Commission on health care, and again in a 1952 report by the President's Commission on the Health Needs of the Nation proclaiming: "Access to the means for the attainment and preservation of health is a basic human right . . . The same high quality of health services should be available to all people equally." [28] This seems to be the idea people have in mind when they urge recognition of a right to health care. It also motivated the adoption of major health care legislation, including Medicare, and it continues to inspire the perennial endeavors to enact national health insurance, despite the long history of defeat for such programs, and more modest reforms of the system. [29]

This call for equal access to medical services is more than political rhetoric or, rather, it is persuasive political rhetoric because it strikes a deep resonance within American culture. In part, it articulates for medical care one of our guiding ideals of justice, the principle of equal opportunity.

While agreement on a right to equal access to medical care is important, it also seems importantly deceptive. In its strongest version, the right of equal access to medical care requires that, if dialysis is available to any citizen, then every other renal failure patient should have an equal opportunity to receive dialysis.[30] But it does not by itself suggest whether dialysis should be provided at all. Equality of access applies only to the *patient-centered* level of distribution, but is silent at the *medical* and *political* levels. As one commentator has written, equal access "is always access *to something,* but to what?"[31] Should citizens have access to dialysis? Or heart transplants? Or any treatment that will be of benefit? Or just life-saving medical care? Or just primary care, emergency care, and routine hospitalization? This principle of equal access is an inadequate conception of justice in the distribution of health care resources because it fails to provide a principled justification for determining *what* medical care services citizens should receive.

The defenders of the equal access principle might respond by arguing that there is a natural and implicit way of defining what medical services should be provided, namely *medical need.* There is a standard of normal human functioning, what one doctor has called a picture of "the well-working of the [human] organism as a whole," and medical needs are needs for services to remedy deviations from this ideal of well-functioning wholeness.[32] As one philosopher writes: "A person needs, from the standpoint of health care, whatever is both necessary and feasible to enable him or her to approach natural human functioning as closely as possible."[33]

Biomedical science offers a fairly clear way of identifying the range of natural human functions that constitute a healthy organism and the range of deviations labeled diseases. Furthermore, this conception of medical need is not just a theoretical definition, but also one that actually guides current medical practices. As members of the Institute of Medicine wrote: "During the last several decades most of what we do as health professionals has shifted from a simple focus on the prevention of death to efforts to restore individuals who are physically or mentally below par to their maximal potential function within the larger society. We have moved . . . to deal primarily with technologies and treatments aimed at improving the capacities of individuals within their lifespan to assume more fully their work and family roles."[34] Another physician put the argument about function into perspective: "Control of illness and improvement of function are the principal objective of medical care . . . Age adjusted death rates have declined over the past 50 years, the purpose of what the doctor does is less the maintenance of life and increasingly the improvement of functional effectiveness . . . The quality of care must be measured by its effect upon functional impairment caused by disease."[35]

Thus, the advocates of the principle of equal access might contend that they have provided an adequate conception of justice in health care. At the *patient-centered* level distribution is based on equal access, while at the *medical* level the required services are delineated by medical need determined by medical practices for the remedy of impairments to normal functions of a human organism. Thus what we might call the refined principle of equal access is as follows: People have a right to needed health care to maintain their normal functioning and to cure or ameliorate their deviations from normal human functions, so far as possible. Or as one bioethicist has stated the idea: "People have a right to needed health care to provide an opportunity for a level of health equal as far as possible to the health of other people."[36] This refined principle seems to motivate many health policy proposals, including a recent suggestion by experts at the Rand Corporation: "At the very least, essential services include all effective diagnostic and therapeutic services—that is, services that benefit the patient when provided by the typical provider . . . Thus, what we mean by essential services is really two-fold. One is medical services of proven efficacy . . . [and second] the timely provision of experimental services in controlled settings where [efficacious treatments do not exist]."[37]

Objections to the Right to Equal Access

Some may object to the refined principle of equal access, arguing that there is no objective determination of normal human functioning; all judgments of deviation are relative, depending upon the environment in which they occur and the social values of the judges; the classification of diseases and deviations from normal human functioning cannot be objective or natural because these determinations are "historically and culturally conditioned."[38]

Whatever the validity of this claim, the more basic problem with adopting the equal access principle informed by the biological notion of medical needs as our conception of justice in health care is its voraciousness. The refined principle generates limitless demands at the *political* level of distribution.

The refined equal access principle seems to entitle every citizen to what might be called "Presidential" medical care. While some treatments for "alopecia (baldness), most cosmetic surgery, and personal attendance by a physician–traveling companion for general reasons of health safety" may be excluded, the rest of medical care, almost everything doctors can now do or might do in the future, from dialysis to hip replacements, from *in vitro* fertilization to cancer chemotherapy, from transplantation of any organ or organ parts to genetic therapy, would seem to be guaranteed every citizen.[39] The refined right to equal access seems to guarantee citizens "everything beneficial."[40] Or as one commentator has written, it can be "used to legitimate a claim that there exists a right to have *all* bodily infirmities corrected if scientifically possibly or conceivable (and a correlative duty on the part of society to take all necessary steps toward that end)."[41]

If we combine this ethical mandate to provide patients equal access to every beneficial diagnostic and therapeutic intervention with the technological powers of biomedical science, there would seem to be no limit to needed medical services and, therefore, costs. Physicians could extend preventive screening tests, such as mammography and hypercholesterolemia detection programs, in an effort to discover untreated diseases; they could relax criteria for patient selection and extend current therapies to more patients; and they could try many new, but expensive, treatments for ailments and defects that are now left untreated. As the President's Commission argued, a health care system designed according to equality of access to all beneficial medical care "might swallow up all of society's resources, since there is virtually no end to the funds that could be devoted to possibly beneficial care for diseases and disabilities and to their prevention."[42] An economist and medical ethicist wrote: "The problem with using need [as conceived by physicians] as the basis of an ethical theory of health care distribution is that it opens the door to unlimited spending on this one good, to the potential exclusion of many other individual and social goods."[43] Thus the entitlements created by the refined right of equal access to medical care would seem insatiable and the costs astronomical.[44] And despite its persuasive political appeal, this consequence of the refined right of equal access has made many reluctant to implement it as health policy, whether through a national health insurance scheme or any other "equal access" reform.

This consequence is not just a practical but also a philosophical objection. Any conception of justice that justifies unlimited demands on social resources is *ipso facto* unacceptable. We look to a theory of justice to guide us in distributing scarce resources, in justifying selecting among competing social demands, not to remove all limits to these demands. Any distributive principle that legitimates unlimited demands either must be abandoned or must be supplemented by other principles. This has been implicitly recognized by an advocate of the refined right of equal access, who grudgingly acknowledges that such a conception will have to be qualified by "efficiency and aggregate utility." At times we are not told how these factors should be balanced,[45] while at other times it is suggested—but never justified—that aggregate utility "be balanced against justice, with each having an equal force."[46] Ultimately, the issue is not how we should weigh equality of access to all beneficial medical care against utility or efficiency, but that having to restrict the refined right of equal access by utility is a clear admission of its inadequacy as a conception of justice for medical care.

This situation has prompted those who advocate the principle of equal access at the *patient-centered* level of distribution to abandon the notion of medical need at the *medical* level of distribution. Medical needs characterized by deviations from normal human functioning and wholeness, they argue in a further refinement, are not medical needs for matters of justice. Society neither does nor should find every deviation from normal human functioning worthy of social resources. Attending to some diseases is more urgent than treating others.[47] While society recognizes every deviation from normal human functioning as a medical need, not every medical need is a citizens' need; only the most urgent ones are citizen's needs. Just as society does not ensure individuals all educational instruction available but pays for some minimum education as an essential need, leaving individuals to obtain any additional educational training they desire through their own resources, so too with medicine. Society should not provide access to all medical care that remedies deviations from normal functioning, but only to some basic minimum, "and then it is up to each individual whether he wishes to sacrifice other goods in order to give himself additional forms of" health care.[48] This basic minimum is more limited than all medical care for every deviation from normal human functioning. Thus at the medical level justice requires providing equal access only to services that ameliorate urgent medical needs.

This more limited level of provision has been variously called a "decent minimum,"[49] "minimally decent care,"[50] "basic health services,"[51] "basic health care,"[52] "essential health care."[53] The President's Commission argues for "an adequate level of health care" and defends this more restricted social guarantee by juxtaposing this level of care to the more expansive notion:

> Because an adequate level of care may be less than "all beneficial care" and because it does not require that all needs be satisfied, it acknowledges the need for setting priorities within health care and signals a clear recognition that society's resources are limited and that there are other goods besides health. Thus, interpreting equity as access to adequate care does not generate an open-ended obligation. One of the chief dangers of interpretations of equity that require virtually unlimited resources for health care is that they encourage the view that equitable access is an impossible ideal. Defining equity as an adequate level of care for all avoids an impossible commitment of resources without falling into the opposite error of abandoning the enterprise of seeking to ensure that health care is in fact available for everyone.[54]

But what is this "adequate level of care"? What are the basic health services? How much medical care is a decent minimum? Is Shep Glazer's dialysis part of the basic health services? Is a kidney transplant? Of course, simply calling dialysis part of an "adequate level of care" does not make it so. "An adequate level of health care" is not a self-defining concept. Indeed, the President's Commission admits it is "amorphous" and vague, especially at the lengthy margins. But if such a concept is to play a fundamental role in determining the just distribution of medical care resources at the *medical* level, then we will need a principled way to define this basic level of care, to determine what illnesses are urgent enough to qualify as health care needs for the purposes of justice. Specifying the just distribution at the medical level, specifying what will be deemed a medical need from the political perspective, is the fundamental challenge to any conception of justice.

But how do we do this? Norman Daniels suggests that there are three possible ways to elucidate this concept: (1) a list of the services which are basic, (2) a criterion by which medical services can be classified as essential or not, and (3) a general decision procedure through which we can decide what medical services constitute the basic ones.[55]

In the next three sections of this chapter I shall explore each of these approaches.

Unjustified Lists of Basic Medical Services

The Nature of the Lists

Because the lists provide tangible determinations for budget calculations and reimbursement guidelines, economists and legislators frequently specify the notion of an "adequate level of medical care" by listing the basic medical services. Over the years, many different lists have been suggested.

In its 1952 report, the President's Commission on the Health Needs of the Nation suggested that a national system for financing health services should provide "comprehensive health services" emphasizing coverage for acute but not chronic medical care. The list was composed of "hospital care; the services of physicians and other health personnel in office and home as well as in the hospital; the more expensive drugs and appliances, and limited dental care . . . [but should] not be expected to cover the costs of prolonged hospitalization for such diseases as tuberculosis and mental disease." [56] Twenty years later, to encourage the expansion of HMOs, Congress enacted the Health Maintenance Organization Act of 1973. This specified a list of "basic health services" that HMOs were required to provide for their prepayment fee. This list consisted of:

(A) physician services (including consultant and referral services by a physician);

(B) inpatient and outpatient hospital services;

(C) medically necessary emergency health services;

(D) short-term (not to exceed twenty visits), outpatient evaluative and crisis intervention mental health services;

(E) medical treatment and referral services (including referral services to appropriate ancillary services) for the abuse of or addiction to alcohol and drugs;

(F) diagnostic laboratory and diagnostic and therapeutic radiological services;

(G) home health services; and

(H) preventive health services (including voluntary family planning services, infertility services, preventive dental care for children, and children's eye examinations conducted to determine the need for vision correction).[57]

Subsequently, this particular list has been commonly cited, most notably by the economist Alain Enthoven, in devising "practical" health plans for the nation.[58]

Another health economist, Karen Davis, proposed a list of "comprehensive benefits" that should be provided by a national health insurance program. This list ignored chronic care and care for drug abuse but did include coverage for medications. Such a program, Davis argued, "should cover both in-hospital and ambulatory services, including services of health centers and clinics, prescription drugs, preventive services for children, maternity and family planning services, dental services for children, and at least limited skilled nursing-home and mental health benefits."[59]

Finally, it may be worth examining a list of "basic health care" proposed by a physician. In discussing the future of American health care, Howard Hiatt, a former dean of the Harvard School of Public Health, argues that society should ensure funding for certain basic medical care programs, such as chronic care facilities and prescription drugs. His list includes:

- Emergency medical services arranged geographically to ensure availability for all.
- A system of primary care for all Americans, so that every citizen who wants one has a gatekeeper.
- Acute hospital care, both secondary (for childbirth, for example, and for relatively straightforward problems such as appendicitis and pneumonia, when the latter are too complicated for home management) and tertiary (for more complex problems like heart and brain surgery, and certain kinds of cancer chemotherapy).
- Community care programs for the poor, with special emphasis on the needs of pregnant women, infants, and children.
- Community care programs for the elderly, including home care programs, day care centers, and nursing homes.
- Hospitals, day care centers, and proper custodial facilities for the mentally ill and the mentally handicapped.
- More extensive preventive programs directed at cigarettes, alcohol, diet, and drugs.[60]

These, of course, are not the only lists of medical services which might qualify as "an adequate level of medical care." While other lists have been suggested,[61] these are among the most detailed lists from a variety of respected authorities on health care that have received significant public attention.

Objections to Lists of Basic Medical Services

The lists themselves seem insufficient for defining an adequate level of medical care. First, these lists cannot stand alone to define basic health care because as broad categories they cannot specify the particular services that are actually covered and those interventions that are excluded. The lists alone will not indicate whether dialysis is part of an adequate level of health care. Presumably not all surgical procedures are basic health services. But which operations are? It would seem that appendectomies are basic medical care, but what about cosmetic surgery, hip replacements, or heart transplants? Furthermore, how should we decide if potential new medical innovations such as transplantation of the ovaries or genetic therapies are basic health care?

Simple lists of categories of care are too indeterminate to answer these questions. Consequently, the lists will need to be supplemented. One way is to view the lists as "shorthand" designations for more general criteria that actually define what constitutes basic care. But what are these underlying criteria? How are they justified?

It might be thought that the existing system for determining appropriate levels of medical care is a natural criterion. Without an explicit elaboration of an alternative criterion, these lists seem to rely on the judgment of physicians—and, in some instances, regulatory agencies such as the FDA—to specify the actual medical services deemed appropriate and inappropriate. As the President's Commission argued: "What makes the HMO list into an 'adequate level' specification is its combination with a delivery mechanism that relies on professional judgment to determine appropriate amounts of services on a case-by-case basis."[62]

But why should physicians' determinations of medical need define basic medical services? In the previous section it seemed clear that physician-defined medical need was not a suitable criterion for determining what services society should guarantee citizens. Furthermore, this criterion is itself indeterminate and likely to lead to unlimited demands for resources. For some interventions, appendectomies for instance, this "professional judgment" seems to be settled; for other treatments, such as prostatectomies and hysterectomies, there is no clear agreement on what is appropriate. And in the United States, this disagreement about appropriate interventions inclines physicians to define "more medical care as better medicine."[63] Physicians believe they have "a duty to do all that [they] can for the benefit of [their] individual patients."[64] And in clinical practice, suffused with uncertainty and haunted by the fatal consequences of missing something, this view encourages aggressive diagnostic work-ups, intensive care unit admissions, high surgical rates, and the like. This tendency can be observed in the curious fact that physicians' families utilize significantly more medical services than the average American or even the average upper-middle-class American. It can also be noted in the wide geographic variation of certain medical practices across the country.[65] Hence, if a list of basic services is to be applied by physicians in individual cases, we risk transforming "an adequate level of care" into "all health care that is of any benefit."[66] This would seem to make lists as limitless as the refined principle of equal access.

Some have suggested that the expansive tendencies of these lists and physician-defined criteria of medical need could be contained by restructuring financial incentives or by establishing some monetary upper limit on the use of medical services. Enthoven, for one, recommends combining the HMO list of basic health services elaborated by physician-defined medical need with "substantial copayments . . . and deductibles" to minimize frivolous, unnecessary, and marginal care.[67] But if the use of the list's medical services is to be influenced— more accurately reduced—by financial incentives, then we have adopted a monetary criterion of "an adequate level of care." Yet to use these financial incentives we need to be convinced that they will ensure people access to a decent minimum level of medical care. And clearly to do this, we would already need some idea of what would constitute the decent minimum level of care. So at least initially this procedure of combining lists of services with financial incentives to limit their use seems circular.[68] In any case, we are back to the fundamental point: used alone, the lists do not define an adequate level of health care. If they designate some underlying criterion, then this criterion needs to be defined and justified. But the seemingly natural criterion of physician-determined necessary medical care does not seem workable or justifiable. In the next section I will consider an alternative criterion.

Even if the lists were somehow sufficient to determine those interventions that are part of basic medical care, we would want to know what justifies the lists. Are they simply arbitrary, or is there a reason for what services are included and excluded?

Enthoven concedes that there is nothing "sacred about this particular list of services"; it just happens to be the one used. But using an arbitrary list of medical services to define how much medical care society should guarantee citizens as a matter of justice seems unjustifiable. Certainly, if a renal failure patient were denied dialysis he would rightly feel the victim of a gross injustice, forced to die or impoverish himself just because his ailment happened not to be covered by an arbitrary list of basic health services. And this sense of injustice would prompt him and others to practical political action. As Enthoven observes, arbitrary lists which limit health care will engender enormous political pressure for their elimination.[69]

It might be suggested that the arbitrariness of the lists is only apparent. The purpose of the lists is to establish some consensus on basic medical services that justifies limits on health care. The lists serve as what Scanlon has called a "construct put together for moral argument" representing "the best available standard of justification that is mutually acceptable to people whose preferences diverge."[70] The lists then seem arbitrary because they are merely instrumental. Nevertheless, they might be justified for the purposes of justice because they represent the compromise position on which all can agree; the lists are used because they are agreed on. This instrumental view does seem to be the motive guiding some of the proponents of these lists. Hiatt suggests that his list is to serve as the basis of a "consensus about what is 'basic'" since it is a list "on which perhaps all but extreme partisans might agree."[71] On this view, the response to renal failure patients is that society agreed on a list of basic services and excluded dialysis. The list is not arbitrary but the result of a social agreement.

Suddenly a whole new range of questions emerges. What procedure was used to generate this supposed agreement? Is the procedure itself justifiable? In later sections I will explore the possibility of delineating such a procedure; at the moment it may be sufficient to ask: Does such a consensus exist? A liberal polity accepts and affirms pluralism, the fact that individuals will espouse a variety of incommensurable conceptions of the good life. Pluralism, however, undermines the likelihood of consensus. While shared traditions, "ideals implicit or latent in the public culture," might secure agreement on abstract principles of justice,[72] these do not seem strong enough to forge agreement on concrete lists of medical services. Indeed, incommensurable conceptions of the good life and the consequent conflicts of interest seem likely to preclude any instrumental consensus on the urgency of particular goods or services. In a pluralist society, the existence of such a consensus cannot be taken for granted, hypothesized, or presumed to be permanent. Those who base their lists on a consensus must demonstrate that one actually exists, or can be forged. And the advocates of these lists have yet to do so.

Indeed, the four different lists themselves already offer *prima facie* evidence against any widespread consensus in the United States on basic medical services.[73] While all lists include acute hospital services, the President's Commission and the HMO Act of 1973 specifically exclude both chronic care and significant mental health care. The President's Commission and Davis include medications, appliances such as glasses, and dental care on their list, but these are excluded in the HMO Act and by Hiatt. Similarly, Congress included care for alcohol and drug abuse, which the President's Commission and Davis did not specify on their lists. In financial terms, these disagreements are not insignificant. In 1985, costs for nursing home services were over $35 billion; costs for drugs, eyeglasses, and other medical appliances were another $35 billion; and dental services cost an additional $27 billion.[74]

Additional evidence against a consensus on a basic list of medical services is found in the recent controversy surrounding Oregon's attempts to create a list of basic medical services to guarantee all Medicaid patients. The proposal is to generate a list of the most important medical services that would be funded by the state's Medicaid program. By limiting the funded services, Oregon also hopes to provide Medicaid to more people, including poor single individuals and childless couples. Yet members of Congress and federal health officals are not so willing to accept these rankings of basic medical services.[75]

Enumerating a list of services which some people think deserve priority only gives the appearance of defining the minimum medical care that society should guarantee each individual as a matter of justice. Indeed, when we explore the usefulness of these lists it appears that they rely either on some underlying general criterion or on some procedure for determining "an adequate level of health care." In the next sections I shall scrutinize these possibilities.

The Weakness of the Liberal Opportunity Criterion

The Nature of the Liberal Opportunity Criterion

One attempt to develop a coherent set of criteria for defining basic medical services has been to use the utilitarian criterion of pain and suffering. Pain is often a patient's presenting complaint. And in some cases, such as lower back pain, migraines, or sickle cell crises, eliminating the nagging or sharp pain is all a patient wants and all a physician hopes to achieve. But as a general standard, this utilitarian criterion does not seem to designate accurately those services considered basic. For instance, some people might suffer from their physical appearance even when there is no deformity due to congenital malformation or accident. They suffer because, say, their noses, chins, or wrinkles are not what they want. Yet most specifications of basic medical services exclude cosmetic surgery—as opposed to plastic surgery—even when it does seem to relieve suffering because it does not aim to restore normal functioning or health.[76] Hence, as a general criterion for justifying those medical treatments we think are basic and should be socially guaranteed, pain and suffering seem to specify the wrong services.

A different attempt is offered by Norman Daniels, who extends "Rawls's theory to health care"[77] to justify a criterion for specifying those basic medical services that liberal society should guarantee as a matter of justice. In contrast to previous attempts to apply Rawls's theory to health care, Daniels does not add health care to the list of primary goods distributed by the difference principle.[78] Instead, he articulates and justifies this liberal criterion by considering four questions: (1) What are health care needs? (2) Why are these needs important? (3) What is the nature and extent of the social obligation to provide for these needs? What medical needs are citizens' needs? (4) In practical terms, what health care services is society obligated to provide?

Daniels begins by accepting the conception of health needs as those services needed to maintain, and to restore deviations from, normal human functions. He believes these deviations are "fixed, primarily by nature" and can be objectively identified by physicians.[79] Second, these deviations from normal functioning are important because they compromise opportunities we value. Because people have an interest in forming, pursuing, and revising their conception of the good life, they will also value having the opportunity to choose among the range of possible conceptions of the good life, "the normal opportunity range," and to pursue their own. Ill health—deviations in normal function—compromises this opportunity: "Impairment of normal functioning through disease and disability restricts an individual's opportunity *relative to that portion of the normal range his skills and talents would have made available to him were he healthy*. If an individual's fair share of the normal range is the array of life plans he may reasonably choose, given his talents and skills, then disease and disability shrink his share from what is fair" (emphasis in the original).[80]

This analysis suggests why individuals consider deviations from normal functioning important, but to justify social guarantees, Daniels connects this view to the liberal guarantee of fair equality of opportunity. Rawls's principles of justice sanction socioeconomic inequalities, despite moral equality, on the condition that desirable social positions with powers and benefits are open to all, that these inequalities are, in some sense, earned, and that they further every person's realization of his own good.[81] Social institutions can permit inequality only if they mitigate these morally arbitrary "social contingencies and natural fortune" through inheritance taxes, educational programs, and the like. These are the guarantees of fair equality of opportunity. Equality of opportunity is one of our ideals commonly invoked in political rhetoric, law, and philosophy. Indeed, the level playing field is one of the most commonly invoked images of American public life, and the position it articulates "has been the great agreed-on undebated premise of our politics."[82]

Daniels argues that "the moral *function* of the health care system must be to help guarantee fair equality of opportunity."[83] Health services should ensure individuals a chance to maintain their human functioning and to cure or mitigate their natural disabilities and accidents of fortune, and thereby should guarantee individuals the opportunity to pursue their own conception of the good life. Health care serves a social function analogous to that of basic education, as a mechanism to ensure that morally arbitrary natural and social factors do not prevent individuals from having and exercising their opportunities. The social obligation to pay for basic health services derives from the social requirement to guarantee fair equality of opportunity. We can call Daniels' criterion for basic medical services the *opportunity criterion*.

This opportunity criterion specifies basic medical services as "services needed to maintain, restore, or compensate for the loss of normal species-typical functioning."[84] They include (1) preventive services—programs for public health, vaccination, food and drug protection, nutrition education, and education for healthy life-styles; (2) personal medical and rehabilitative services—services that cure diseases and restore normal functioning, such as antibiotics and appendectomies; (3) chronic medical services—services, such as dialysis, aimed at those diseases that cannot be cured but only ameliorated; and (4) nursing and social services—services for those whose ailments cannot be cured or ameliorated, including Seeing-Eye dogs, Braille education, wheelchairs, and specially designed vans for the paralyzed.[85] Beyond this socially guaranteed tier of basic medical services, Daniels recognizes an "upper tier" of medical services which need not be socially guaranteed because they do not affect opportunity, including treatments for alopecia (baldness), cosmetic surgery, and amenities in care, such as private hospital rooms (when not medically indicated because of infections).[86] These nonessential medical services are left to individuals to purchase with their incomes depending on their preferences and desires.

Objections to the Liberal Opportunity Criterion

Does this liberal opportunity criterion actually differ from the criterion of providing people with access to all beneficial medical care? Or, to put the question another way, is the standard of beneficial care used by physicians the same as care that guarantees opportunity?

As noted previously, most of a physician's practice does not involve life-or-death decisions, and much of the effort of medical research is not directed at life-saving therapies but at permitting individuals to realize their maximal functional capacities. The power of Daniels' analysis inheres in the way it illuminates the moral side of the physician's objectives in practicing medicine, linking medical needs to opportunity and, therefore, to the claims of justice. As such, the criterion Daniels outlines is not so much a critique of the medical care system as a justification for extending what physicians usually do—when financial reimbursement and other distorting incentives do not influence their professional judgment—to all members of society. Daniels has offered us a criterion for determining what medical care constitutes the basic services which justify providing "Presidential" medicine to all.

What types of medical services does the liberal opportunity criterion exclude from the basic level? It rules out amenities such as private hospital rooms and efforts by physicians to improve physical and mental functions beyond the normal range by, for instance, research into "blood-doping" for runners or research on genetics when the aim is to improve mental abilities, such as mathematical or musical talents, beyond the normal range. It probably also rules out some routine medical interventions such as sterilization, tubal ligations and vasectomies, and nontherapeutic abortions, since these procedures actually contravene normal species functioning and thus do not constitute health care needs according to the biological model.[87] But these exclusions from the basic medical services are, to quote Daniels, "minor."

The liberal opportunity criterion mandates that people receive most of what modern medicine has to offer as a guarantee of fair equality of opportunity. It would seem to justify such controversial—and expensive—interventions as intensive care for very low birth weight infants, since 13 to 30 percent can survive to lead a normal life without developmental handicaps. Further, the criterion would also justify many new, expensive technological interventions—*in vitro* fertilization to restore fertility, genetic therapy to repair inherited physical defects such as sickle cell anemia or thalassemia, artificial organs, including dialysis and artificial hearts, and new computer-assisted devices for the deaf and the paralyzed—as basic since all aim to restore people to near-normal functioning. Indeed, there is very little in the way of costly medical services now provided by American medicine, and available in the future with current research, which would *not* be part of Daniels' basic tier of medical services to be guaranteed by justice.[88] It seems that Presidential medical services for all "are needed if fair equality of opportunity is to be guaranteed" to the citizens.

Like rights to equal access and lists of basic medical services, Daniels' opportunity criterion fails to provide an adequate way of identifying basic medical services that should be guaranteed by society as a matter of justice because it seems to make almost every medical intervention "basic." The opportunity criterion identifies basic medical services in a way that contains, in practice if not in words, no principled limit on the demand for medical services. While Daniels only briefly considers the fact that the basic tier of health services may be too vast and costly, he does suggest that the opportunity criterion may need to be supplemented by a procedure for balancing such demands.[89] Two possible procedures are frequently suggested: some hypothetical choice procedure, such as Rawls's original position, and democratic procedures. I will next investigate whether these procedures can provide a principled way of specifying the "truly" basic medical services, the most important medical services that promote fair equality of opportunity.

Hypothetical Choice Procedures and Conceptions of the Good Life

The Liberal Legislator's Choice

Since the publication of Rawls's *A Theory of Justice* with its original position, the basic outlines and justifications of hypothetical choice procedures have become a standard part of ethics. Such procedures contain four elements: (1) a hypothetical person—or group of persons—who (2) try to deliberate on and resolve fundamental ethical questions, (3) consistent with certain principles and (4) deprived of biasing information, that is, behind a "veil of ignorance."[90]

In the present context, we want to know what basic medical services should be guaranteed as a matter of justice. The specific dilemma a hypothetical deliberator confronts is: If all the medical services that promote fair equality of opportunity were part of basic medical care, then the costs of medical care would overwhelm other social programs. Thus, the hypothetical deliberator must rank, "weigh," or "strike a balance between"[91] the various demands for resources to protect fair equality of opportunity, determining the most important medical services that define "an adequate level of medical care" and that society should guarantee to citizens as a matter of justice. The hypothetical deliberator's answer must be consistent with the tenets of liberalism, including the ideal of neutrality and the principle of fair equality of opportunity. And finally, he can know some general information about society, such as general principles of social theory and more particular facts about the types of health problems that exist in society, their frequency, the source of these problems as best as can be known. However, he cannot know any individualizing information, neither his own health status—his age, health, genetic inheritance, or what diseases he would be likely to contract—nor his own life pursuits—his talents, occupation, conception of the good life.[92]

We shall call the hypothetical deliberator who is deciding what should be basic medical care the *liberal legislator.* He is a *legislator* because he deliberates at the legislative stage, trying to devise actual social institutions and policies within the framework of the principles of justice. He is a *liberal* legislator because the laws and policies he devises must satisfy the tenets of liberal political philosophy.

The idea of such a hypothetical choice procedure is very attractive. It is supposed to model our moral convictions. It should reveal which social institutions all reasonable persons would agree to as just when not biased by their own personal interests and desires.[93] Further, by excluding information of an individual's conception of the good life, the hypothetical choice procedure ensures that the principle, law, or policy selected will not be justified by appeal to a particular conception of the good life and will, thereby, be consistent with the tenets of liberalism. Consequently, a process of reasoning through these hypothetical choice procedures has been commonly used in discussions of allocating health care resources.[94]

Such hypothetical choice procedures will help us discover what justice in health care is only if we can go beyond the vague, intuitive suggestions that the liberal legislator should "weigh" or "balance" competing claims for social resources and help us imagine the substance of such deliberations.[95] How might the liberal legislator refine the opportunity criterion? What would he consider the most important or the "truly" basic health care services? What arguments would he use to justify his choice? Exploring the substance of the liberal legislator's deliberations is a test of the *philosophical plausibility* of such hypothetical choice procedures. The issue is, assuming that any of the current health care institutions are changeable, can we sketch a framework for a just health care system consistent with the tenets of liberal political philosophy which can specify the basic medical services that will remain within the limits set at the political level? Will the liberal legislator's deliberations reveal what medical care services are to be considered "truly" basic, requirements of justice, while honoring liberal principles?

Four Possible Health Care Schemes

To simplify, let us imagine that the liberal legislator is confronted by a choice among four proposed schemes of medical services derived from positions that have been articulated in the current debates over the distribution of health care resources. As presented, these schemes are very rough outlines, covering only a few of the many potential medical services, concentrating on life-saving technologies and nursing and home health care services. Nevertheless, they are specific and distinctive enough to illuminate the substance of the liberal legislator's deliberations.

Scheme 1. This is roughly the current system. (1) Life-saving technologies would be used as they currently are, defined by medical need which is judged by physicians; (2) additional support services, such as nursing home care or home health care, would be roughly as they currently exist; (3) research would continue into all types of care, with the emphasis, as in the current system, on high-technology life-saving care, with less stress on palliative medical treatments for chronic diseases.

Scheme 2. This system would eliminate life-saving care for the elderly but provide more palliative care for their chronic diseases.[96] (1) Life-saving technologies would be employed only for those under a fixed age of 70; (2) additional resources would be aimed at enhancing support services and medical care for the chronic disabilities concentrated in those over 70; (3) research would focus on curing and ameliorating diseases of the young and the chronic ailments of the elderly, such as interventions to cure or ameliorate arthritis, hearing impairments, incontinence, and so forth.

Scheme 3. This system would focus medical care on conditions in which there is a real chance for an independent, autonomous life, a chance to pursue projects and plans.[97] (1) Life-saving technologies would be prohibited from those who had no chance for an independent life, such as incompetent patients, neonates under 1,000 grams, certain burn victims, artificial heart transplant recipients, Stage IV heart patients, and the like; (2) only those support services which helped individuals live independently would be provided; custodial and institutional nursing care would not be provided; (3) research would focus on preventive care and on treatments and technologies which would permit people to lead independent lives and realize their projects, such as interventions to ameliorate—or cure—paralysis and treatments, like organ transplantation, that permit a return to a normal, functioning life.

Scheme 4. This system would focus medical care in the most cost-effective manner, not on the basis of particular diseases or disabilities. (1) Life-saving technologies would be permitted only if cost-effective, only if they were inexpensive or distributed on an age-based criterion, saving the lives of people who were young and could lead productive lives, but not if they merely extended the lives of those over, say, 55 or 60 who would not have many productive years left; (2) only cost-effective support services would be provided, emphasizing home health care but not custodial or institutional care; (3) research would focus on cost-effective treatments and technologies, but not on "extraordinarily" expensive interventions, such as computer-assisted methods to help the paralyzed walk and artificial hearts. This scheme is akin to the British National Health Service.

How do these schemes affect the opportunities of patients? Scheme 1 has its most important effect on longevity, enhancing the individual's range of life plans by extending life as well as providing the opportunity to live a long life itself, independent of having the opportunity to pursue a range of more particular projects. But there are curtailments of the range of life plans—opportunity costs—that scheme 1 does not ameliorate. For some, maybe even many, the long life will be accompanied by infirmities and lack of support services that will inhibit pursuing some of those very plans and opportunities. Without extensive home care or social support services, the chance of traveling for pleasure or living independently outside a nursing home, for instance, may not be possible for some of the elderly. Conversely, the more extensive support services available in scheme 2 will enhance the range of life plans per year by securing opportunities to live independently and pursue a broader array of projects. But here the "opportunity cost" will be the likelihood for a shorter life compared to scheme 1 and the concomitant diminished time to pursue projects and opportunities.[98] Scheme 3 will ensure greater opportunities for individuals who can live independently and are able to pursue their projects and plans with some medical interventions. It aims to ensure that individuals have the opportunity to make plans and pursue them, if they are capable. But the "opportunity cost" will fall on those who cannot live independently even with medical interventions; such people will receive less care and might well die sooner or live with fewer support services to ease their infirmities. Scheme 4 will ensure the maximization of opportunities for welfare, providing more care to the young and those able to live productively with the care. The "opportunity cost" would fall on those who suffered from "expensive" diseases. Patients requiring significant resources, patients with incurable diseases requiring frequent medical interventions, and the elderly would probably not receive many medical services.

To summarize these schemes we might say: scheme 1 eliminates the curtailments of opportunities due to a shortened life; scheme 2 eliminates the curtailments of opportunities due to a poor quality-of-life; scheme 3 eliminates the curtailments of opportunities due to dependence; scheme 4 eliminates the curtailments of opportunities due to inexpensive disabilities.

How would these schemes affect patients with different ailments? Shep Glazer would probably not receive dialysis under scheme 4 or, when old, under scheme 2.[99] Andrew, the AIDS patient, would probably not receive extensive medical care under schemes 3 or 4. The elderly would receive life-saving care but not extensive support services under scheme 1, and just the reverse under scheme 2. Intensive care for neonates would be restricted under schemes 3 and 4, but not under schemes 1 and 2. Organ transplantation would be supported under schemes 1, 2, and 3 but not scheme 4; schemes 1 and 3 would find research into improving organ transplants urgent, while schemes 2 and 4 probably would not. Schemes 1 and 4 would not place a high priority on research into expensive technologies that would ameliorate—or possibly cure—handicaps such as blindness, deafness, and paralysis, while schemes 2 and 3 probably would.

Which scheme strikes the balance among competing medical services to produce a just health care system? Which scheme of "truly" basic medical services should the liberal legislator choose when deliberating behind a thin veil of ignorance, trying to satisfy the principles of justice and of liberalism? There seem three possible grounds of reasoning that the liberal legislator might adopt in deliberating about the choice: a technical assessment, a quantitative assessment, or a qualitative assessment.[100]

None of these assessments will be suitable for the liberal legislator. Only by violating the tenets of liberalism can the liberal legislator weigh the demands on resources and justify a selection among these four different schemes of the just health care system.

The Technical Assessment of Health Care Schemes

The liberal legislator might compare the health care schemes on technical matters, considering which scheme is least liable to generate enforcement problems, which is easiest and cheapest to administer, and the like. As twenty-five years of Medicare and Medicaid have taught us, these technical matters are neither trivial nor cheap. But it is hard to imagine why, if the liberal legislator is trying to select the *just* scheme, such issues of administrative efficiency should be the focus of his deliberations. That such technical issues should be the justification for the selection of a scheme of just medical services could only be acceptable "all other things being equal." But to know when "all other things are equal" requires determining that these different schemes are equally just and that there is no ethical basis for selecting among them. And this, in turn, requires some standard of assessment for determining the "truly" basic medical services. This is precisely the standard we are now trying to find, which the technical assessment does not help us with.

The Quantitative Assessment of Health Care Schemes

Daniels suggests that in deliberating among alternative schemes of health care services the liberal legislator should weigh the various schemes and select the one that prevents, cures, and ameliorates those diseases and disabilities "which involve a *greater* curtailment of an individual's share of the normal opportunity range" (emphasis added).[101] In other words, the just scheme should aim to remove the most restricting disabilities, ensuring that individuals can pursue a greater share of the normal conceptions of the good life given their native talents and skills.

The appeal of this quantitative assessment is clear. Although there may be some controversy about the calculation, a numerical calculation for determining the just scheme of medical services obviates the need for complex moral judgments by providing objective data. In this way, the quantitative assessment has strong affinities with utilitarian calculations for justice. But, precisely for this reason, it also seems flawed on three grounds.

Such a quantitative weighing may work in the trivial case of selecting between two health care service schemes that are identical except that one provides some additional services. While similar situations may confront congressmen debating whether to fund a single new medical program, this is not the situation confronting the hypothetical liberal legislator, and not likely to be the situation confronting an actual legislator who is trying to select a just scheme of "truly" basic health care services. The liberal legislator needs to be able to compare more complex alternatives. In particular, he needs to be able to decide whether scheme 1 eliminates the greater curtailment of opportunities to pursue conceptions of the good life by securing longevity or whether scheme 2 permits a greater range of opportunities by securing people a shorter life with a better quality-of-life and broader range of conceptions of the good life per year of life, and so on for schemes 3 and 4. To use Daniels' quantitative weighing criteria in selecting between these schemes, then, the liberal legislator needs a quantitative scale for the range of opportunities by which to compare the schemes. Is there such a scale?

First, defining what constitutes an opportunity is both a normative and a controversial judgment. Opportunities do not come packaged and labeled; they need to be identified and defined. This is especially true when the types of opportunities we are trying to maximize are not opportunities for jobs, but opportunities to choose among the conceptions of the good life available in a society. Indeed, trying to delimit the opportunity to pursue the types of conceptions of the good life that "it is reasonable for persons to choose in a given society" is controversial.[102] After all, who decides what types of opportunities are reasonable to pursue? And on what basis do we justify these opportunities? Consider some examples. It seems reasonable to want to ensure that individuals can take walks in the country; so we would want to secure for paralyzed people the means to ambulate. But does this mean the opportunity to walk themselves, or would we be satisfied with letting them be pushed in a wheelchair? The former is still not possible and would require committing funds for further research, while the latter is fairly easily secured with wheelchairs. Similarly, it seems reasonable to ensure that individuals can hear sounds. But does this mean that we should secure the opportunity to hear conversations, or the opportunity to hear symphony performances without distortion? One objective might be satisfied by fairly inexpensive hearing aides; the other might require cochlear implants at a cost of $12,000 each. Still further, it might be reasonable to secure the opportunity to have children. But does this mean we ensure that couples have the opportunity to adopt children, or is the opportunity we aim to guarantee the experience of conceiving, carrying, and delivering a child? And if it is the latter opportunity that we want to secure, does this mean we need to offer every couple *in vitro* fertilization or whatever fertility interventions are necessary?

Deciding which of these alternative interpretations of opportunity are the ones that should be secured clearly requires ethical judgments. Any choice will be highly controversial. There seems no way even of identifying the relevant opportunities to be compared without invoking some conception of the good life.

Second, conceptions of the good life are not indivisible entities, but complex schemes containing a number of diverse facets that are not readily comparable. There are the vocational as well as avocational components. And within these components there are those that predominantly engage the mental faculties and those that predominantly engage the physical faculties. In addition there are the more familial and domestic facets of conceptions of the good life, as well as the elements of romance and sex or sexual freedom. And there are other components, such as the desire to live long, the desire to live free of financial or physical or emotional dependence on others, the desire to serve others, and the desire to be financially successful or famous. (These may not all be appropriately characterized as desires—the actor may feel them as obligations, religious callings, or whatever—but we need not delve into those matters here if we acknowledge that these are components of life plans.)

Individuals recognize that realizing one facet of a conception of the good life does not mean that the goods which are contained in another facet are also realized.[103] And further, the goods realized in any of these facets are not necessarily comparable to the goods realized in the other facets. Goods are not singular or reducible to a single interchangeable unit. The joys of delivering and raising children are not the joys of listening to orchestral music nor the satisfaction of playing Beethoven piano sonatas nor the thrill of playing for a professional sports team.

In short, the potentialities of life are numerous, the actualities diverse, and the goods incommensurable.

This complexity in conceptions of the good life translates into complexity in opportunities to realize conceptions of the good life. To use Daniels' own phrase, opportunities are nonhomogeneous and incommensurable. The opportunity to pursue athletic skills is not the opportunity to pursue musical endeavors. Consequently, trying to guarantee individuals the opportunity to pursue an array of conceptions of the good life normally available in society requires guaranteeing incommensurable opportunities to pursue many different facets of conceptions of the good life.

None of this is new or revealing; it is just a restatement of the fact that goods differ in kind and conceptions of the good life are incommensurable. Or, to put it another way, while we often speak of opportunity in the singular, in actuality there are only opportunities in the plural. But the fact of complex and incommensurable conceptions of the good life and opportunities to realize conceptions of the good life suggests that there are no discrete quanta by which to measure the greater share of the range of life plans. In most cases it makes no sense to sum up the number of facets of the conception of a good life an individual can pursue, like the number of dishes at a smorgasbord, for comparison with another individual. Conceptions of the good life, or the facets of such conceptions, are qualitatively different and incommensurable; they are not entities we quantify for comparisons.

Similarly, there is no single quantitative scale for the range of life plans. True, we might say that an individual who crushed his hand beyond repair has a reduced range of life plans because the injury will preclude his playing the violin or any number of activities requiring two hands that he might have pursued before his mishap. Also we might maintain that a person with multiple disabilities, such as spina bifida with paralysis and some mental retardation, has a reduced range of life plans compared with a person who is (only!) paralyzed. But the simplicity of these comparisons is deceptive. The comparisons involve one individual's range of plans which completely subsumes the other's; there is no qualitative difference in the range of plans. This is an atypical situation. Usually the complexity of life plans makes the range of life plans open to individuals incomparable on a quantitative scale. This becomes obvious when we consider comparisons between qualitatively different ranges of life plans. Who has a quantitatively greater curtailment of the range of life plans, an individual who is infertile and cannot have children, or an individual who is deaf and cannot listen to Beethoven, or an individual with a crushed hand who cannot play Beethoven, or a paralyzed individual who cannot play sports, or an individual confined to bed with active rheumatoid arthritis who cannot play sports or Beethoven but can listen to Beethoven and bear children? Each disability involves a reduction in the range of life plans compared to individuals who lack these specific disabilities. But the reductions occur in qualitatively different facets of life plans. One individual will be unable to pursue projects involving manual dexterity but will be able to listen to music and have a family; another individual will be unable to have a family but will be able to pursue projects requiring manual dexterity and auditory acuity; and a third individual will be unable to listen to music but will be able to have a family and engage in some activities requiring manual dexterity. And yet because these are so qualitatively different, there seems no precise scale for quantitatively counting up the number of reduced facets of conceptions of the good life for comparison. Indeed, we would be at a loss to say which had a quantitatively *greater* loss in the range of conceptions of the good life, or, equivalently, different people would disagree about which disability constituted a greater loss.[104]

Thus there will be some gross comparisons of the reduced range of conceptions of the good life in some simple cases, but there will be no suitably precise quantitative scale for determining which range of conceptions of the good life is greater. Using a quantitative scale for measuring the limits on the range of conceptions of the good life to weigh which medical services are more urgent will be, in Daniels' own words, a "fairly crude" measure[105]—so crude a measure, in fact, that it cannot even help us in comparing the reduced range of life plans for the one-armed person with those of the infertile or blind person.

Applied to the liberal legislator's relatively simple choice between the four schemes of "truly" basic health services, Daniels' proposed weighing criterion also seems too crude to be helpful. The range of life plans available to individuals in scheme 1 does not subsume those available under schemes 2, 3, and 4, and similarly for the other comparisons; each scheme secures qualitatively different facets of life plans. Intuitively, it seems impossible to say which scheme prevents, cures, or ameliorates the diseases and disabilities which involve a quantitatively greater curtailment of the range of life plans. Without a precise quantitative scale there seems no single way to count up the number of facets of life plans secured by each scheme for the liberal legislator's comparison. Consequently, there seems no precise way for him to figure out which scheme would lead to the prevention, cure, or amelioration of those diseases which produce the greater reduction in the range of life plans.

There is yet a third objection to the quantitative assessment of opportunities. Even if we assume that the previous objections are erroneous and there is some quantitative way to determine which medical service scheme actually ameliorates the diseases that involve a greater curtailment of life plans and gives people the opportunity to pursue a greater share of life plans, a liberal legislator would not want to use this kind of assessment. Such an assessment is analogous to a utilitarian calculation and does not respect individuals.

Assume, for the sake of argument, that the quantitative calculation endorsed scheme 2. Someone like Shep Glazer might well be denied dialysis. The justification offered him would be that providing dialysis to all who needed it would not be part of the medical services of a system aimed at protecting fair equality of opportunity because dialysis does not enhance the range of opportunities to pursue various life plans as much as other medical care services. This, of course, is not to say that dialysis does not permit those with kidney failure to pursue a wide range of life plans. Clearly, by saving their lives, it does. Rather, on a *comparative* basis, dialysis ameliorates a disease which restricts a smaller range of life plans to fewer people than do other medical services. Therefore, it is less urgent and has less of a claim to be socially guaranteed as part of the "truly" basic medical services which protect equality of opportunity. Is such an explanation satisfactory to a citizen in a liberal polity?

The liberal legislator admits that dialysis does enhance the range of life plans available to those people suffering from kidney failure. Hence dialysis does protect equality of opportunity. In justifying the exclusion of dialysis from the "truly" basic medical services, the liberal legislator is aiming to minimize the reduction in curtailments of the opportunities to pursue life plans averaged over all citizens. In this calculation, the opportunities of kidney failure patients are being sacrificed to enhance the opportunities of others in society, without the opportunities of the renal failure patients also being enhanced. Requiring trade-offs of individual opportunities toward devising policies which maximize the overall fair equality of opportunity means that some individuals must sacrifice their opportunity in order to secure or promote the opportunities of others. Those patients denied services which do not lead to the minimal reduction in curtailments of the range of life plans are wronged, asked to die or live more compromised lives, for the greater opportunities of others. As Daniels himself writes: "If social obligations to provide appropriate health care are not met, then individuals are definitely wronged. Injustice is done to them . . . [If] the just design of a health care system requires providing a service from which I could benefit [a service which protects equality of opportunity], then I am wronged if I do not get it." [106]

What is being objected to are the *grounds* for the liberal legislator's weighing of the diverse schemes. The objection is not against weighing the various medical services to specify the most important ones to be guaranteed to all citizens; rather, the objection is raised against the *manner* of weighing, the use of interpersonal comparisons toward minimizing the overall reduction in opportunities to pursue life plans. When the quantitative assessment is used, it does not matter how these opportunities are distributed among citizens, whether a few are deprived of most opportunities while others have their range of opportunities greatly enhanced. What counts is that overall, the greatest number of opportunities is enhanced. This is clearly illustrated by the fact that such calculations put those individuals who suffer from rare diseases, or rare forms of common diseases, at a significant disadvantage because they will always have quantitatively fewer opportunities to be enhanced by medical services. The loss of their opportunities will be compensated for by the greater gain of others. It is precisely this form of reasoning, this form of aggregation and maximization in defining just social institutions, that liberals object to in utilitarianism. [107] And it is just as objectionable when done by a liberal legislator.

To avoid the faults of utilitarianism, the liberal legislator will have to reject Daniels' quantitative assessment and use an alternative way of weighing the various medical care services.

The Qualitative Assessment of Health Care Schemes

The liberal legislator might evaluate health care institutions that protect fair equality of opportunity by a qualitative standard. According to this standard, the liberal legislator weighs or strikes a balance among the various opportunities by determining which opportunities are more important or more worthy of pursuit. He then chooses the scheme of medical services that secures these most important opportunities. Can the liberal legislator make a qualitative assessment among the various opportunities and still satisfy the tenets of liberal political philosophy?

One possibility might be for the liberal legislator to follow the original intent of the principle of fair equality of opportunity and rank those opportunities to enter jobs and careers as most important. But this seems unacceptable. To justify ranking the opportunities to enter jobs and careers over securing other opportunities requires invoking some conception of the good life that deems such ends very important. This ranking is not neutral. Many conceptions of the good life do not rank the opportunity to secure a job as the most important opportunity. For some conceptions of the good life, mere living is a more important opportunity; according to other conceptions of the good life, nonoccupational opportunities, such as having children and raising a family or striving for salvation, are more important than occupations. Further, using occupational opportunities as a criterion would bias health care against the old, who use a significant proportion of health care resources but who are not likely to be in the market for jobs and careers. The elderly value health because it secures the opportunity to pursue avocational interests, hobbies, and friendships, not gainful employment.[108] Making the qualitative assessment that the opportunities to enter jobs are the most important opportunities seems incompatible with liberal principles.[109] Indeed, when one physician introduced into the decision of whether to provide care to infants born with spina bifida the criterion that only those who might be able to obtain a job and become economically independent be given intensive medical intervention, the response was one of widespread outrage.[110] This ranking not only violates the tenets of liberal political philosophy but also seems to conflict with considered moral judgments.

A second possibility for a qualitative assessment of opportunities might be for the liberal legislator to define the most important opportunities by imagining the opportunities most people, or a given average person, value.[111] The liberal legislator might then define the "truly" basic medical services as those necessary to secure these most valued opportunities. Because the veil of ignorance prohibits him from knowing personalized information, the liberal legislator would not know the particular kind of life plans that he—or other people— would pursue. Instead he would have to assume that "most people would make roughly the same assessment of the value of [medical services] against general handicaps, such as blindness or loss of a limb, that affect a wide spectrum of different sorts of lives," [112] or that "there is some consensus in the society on the relevant values—that there is some value that 'everyone sets' on various increments of health protection." [113] Is this assumption valid? Do people make the same assessment of the importance of opportunities and the value of different medical services? Is there an average person's view on the importance of opportunities and medical services?

We can gain insight into this issue by considering common clinical situations confronting patients. Cancer patients sometimes have to choose whether to undergo chemotherapy or radical and deforming surgery for the chance to live an additional year or few years, or whether to forgo such therapies for a shorter but less painful life. Some people with acute myelogenous leukemia (AML) may have to choose whether to undergo conventional chemotherapy with a 30 percent chance of cure or whether to have a bone marrow transplant, which has a 50 percent chance of cure but, for those who are not cured, an 80 to 90 percent chance of dying within six months. Similarly, patients with hypertension may have a choice between equally effective drugs, one of which costs about $120 per month and another which costs about $15 per month, where the latter has more side effects including the possibility of impotence. Of course these patients also have the option of forgoing all treatments and the daily use of drugs, and accepting the risk of a shorter life span. Some non–insulin-dependent diabetic patients have the choice of controlling their blood sugar by restricting their diet or by regularly injecting insulin or by taking an oral hypoglycemic drug every day. Some women who have not been able to become pregnant can forgo having children, forgo having their own genetic children and adopt, or undergo a number of diagnostic tests and try the therapeutic options, including *in vitro* fertilization, for the chance to have their own genetic children.

The choice between the various options can depend upon individual tastes and interests, but it will also reflect considered moral judgments about the worth of the different opportunities secured and forgone, which, in turn, depends upon the person's conception of the good life. In a modern society, different people will deem different medical treatments and therapies more important. To some people the chance for several additional years of life, the chance to complete projects, to develop relationships, and so forth, is not worth the pain and deformity associated with cancer treatments; to others life offers opportunities for which it is worth enduring any amount of pain and deformity. Some people want their own genetic child no matter what and are willing to sacrifice their job or enjoyable marital relationship and to endure repeated operations; to others infertility is a problematic annoyance but not worth trying to alter if one is so afflicted. It all depends upon a person's aims and projects and overall conception of the good life. Because liberal society recognizes that people will espouse a plurality of conceptions of the good life, it recognizes that there is no single choice about what clinical intervention is best. Consequently, a liberal society recognizes the right of informed consent to secure individual self-determination in the arena of health. As the President's Commission wrote: "The Commission argued that decisions about the treatments that best promote a patient's health and well-being must be based on the particular patient's values and goals; no uniform, objective determination can be adequate—whether defined by society or by health professionals." [114]

What is true for the individual patient deciding between competing treatment options is also true for the liberal legislator deciding between competing schemes of health care services. [115] The liberal legislator trying to define health care policies for a liberal polity will accept that reasonable people will affirm different conceptions of the good and will value opportunities differently. And depending on how individuals value these different opportunities, they will find different medical services more or less important. The different evaluations will depend not merely on each individual's personal interests, diseases, actual physical handicaps, and the effectiveness of the remedies available, but also on each individual's conception of the good life. In this way, the different evaluations reflect differences in conceptions of the good life; the multiplicity of conceptions of the good life implies that people will *not* make the same assessment of the importance of different opportunities or, what amounts to the same thing for the liberal legislator, different medical services. Given the expectation of a diverse set of incommensurable conceptions of the good life, then, there is no *prima facie* reason to expect—and every reason not to expect—

that there will be a consensus on a single, uniform "value that 'everyone sets' on various increments of health protection." The plurality of conceptions of the good life means that there will be no average person's view.[116]

The reasonable or average person's choice or the choice most people would make is a fiction, the type of fiction commonly adopted in legal reasoning. But in the eyes of liberals this is a dangerous fiction. For the assumption behind it denies the plurality of conceptions of the good life, one of the basic tenets of liberal political philosophy.

Conceptions of the Good Life in Assessing Health Care Schemes

Rejecting the technical, quantitative, and qualitative bases for weighing different medical services does not mean that a legislator cannot choose among the four health care schemes. Such a choice is possible, but only by appeal to a particular conception of the good life. Only by rejecting liberal principles can a legislator actually determine which scheme of health care services is just.

This point can be more concretely illustrated by returning to the four schemes of medical services being considered by the liberal legislator. We can outline four different conceptions of the good life that justify selecting one of the schemes of medical services but not the other three. And, equally important, there will be no compromise scheme which is mutually acceptable to the diverse conceptions.[117] As in Chapter 3, I will offer only a broad sketch of these conceptions of the good life as ideal types. The point is to show that different conceptions of the good life will justify different schemes of "truly" basic medical services because in these different conceptions the opportunities to pursue certain aspects of life plans that are secured by medical services are valued differently. By invoking one of these conceptions of the good life, a legislator—although not the liberal legislator—could justify implementing one of the four schemes of health care services.

1. *The Physical Conception.* This conception of the good life emphasizes the opportunities of longevity, the ever-present opportunity to have new experiences and role changes, the possibility of continuing relationships, and the chance to watch the maturing of children and the birth of grandchildren or great-grandchildren.[118] This is the conception characterized by Hobbes, who views death as the greatest evil

and finds all motivation grounded in the fear of death. It is also supported by religious views and a less lugubrious secular view of life:

> Given an identifiable individual, countless possibilities for his con-
> tinued existence are imaginable, and we can clearly conceive of what
> it would be for him to go on existing indefinitely. However inevi-
> table it is that this will not come about, its possibility is still that of
> the continuation of a good for him, if life is the good we take it to
> be . . . A man's sense of his own experience . . . does not embody
> this idea of a natural limit. His existence defines for him an essen-
> tially open-ended possible future, containing the usual mixture of
> goods and evils that he has found so tolerable in the past. Having
> been gratuitously introduced to the world by a collection of natural,
> historical, and social accidents, he finds himself the subject of a *life,*
> with an indeterminate and not essentially limited future. Viewed in
> this way, death, no matter how inevitable, is an abrupt cancellation
> of indefinitely extensive possible goods.[119]

This view is very common and seems to underlie our current health
care system—scheme 1—with its emphasis on life-saving treatments,
intensive care units, high-technology artificial organs, and transplantation, rather than preventive health care, palliative medical care, and
other support services.[120]

  2. *The Relational Conception.* The relational or devotional conception of the good life emphasizes intergenerational obligations and the
importance of posterity and cultural perpetuation. On this view, the
young are to receive what we might call the opportunities of hope and
aspiration, the most complete range of opportunities for education
and training, for the development of projects, families, and relationships. The old, on the other hand, are to receive what we might call
the opportunities of wisdom and sagacity, the opportunities created
by acknowledging finitude and by serving the young, willing the traditions to posterity.

> It should be the special role of the elderly to be the moral conserva-
> tors of that which has been and the most active proponents of that
> which will be after they are no longer here. Their indispensable role
> as conservators is what generates what I believe ought to be the *pri-*
> *mary* aspiration of the old, which is to serve the young and the fu-
> ture . . . It is this seemingly paradoxical combination of withdrawal
> to prepare for death and an active, helpful leave-taking which pro-

vides the possibility for meaning and significance [of old age] in a contemporary context.[121]

This view would seem to justify scheme 2, with its age-based criterion for medical services. Within the American polity this view is probably not as widely espoused as the physical conception, but it does have advocates among ethicists and politicians.[122]

3. *The Autonomous Conception.* This conception of the good life emphasizes having the mental capacities to formulate life plans and long-range objectives necessary to the life plan, to evaluate and revise the life plan and objectives, to be a full participant in social and political life, and to have the physical functioning and vigor to realize such plans and objectives. On this conception a person's capacity to formulate conceptions of the good life and fulfill such conceptions, and participation in society, are essential human goods. The opportunities for these activities, what we might call the opportunities for independent living, are most important. This conception is familiar to us, especially as a version of the liberal ideal portrayed by many American writers and, in the philosophical tradition, by Mill. The autonomous conception would seem to justify scheme 3, providing medical services which can ensure independent living for completion of life projects rather than using an age-based distribution criterion. Within the current debate about allocating medical resources, this is probably the view most consistent with Daniels' opportunity criterion and is consistent with the positions advocated by others.[123]

4. *The Utilitarian Conception.* This emphasizes the opportunity for maximizing the aggregate welfare of society as a whole. On this view all outlays, including those for medical interventions, should be evaluated by a cost-benefit approach, where the benefit to be measured is the overall opportunity for individual welfare or well-being, the individual satisfaction of subjective preferences. Such a view is not unfamiliar; it is frequently expressed by economists and government budget analysts, by utilitarian philosophers, and also by many physicians and others who question the use of high-cost medical services for what appear to be small increases in welfare, life expectancy, or quality-of-life.[124] Generally, such a view would endorse scheme 4, restricting any medical intervention which provided improvements in life expectancy or quality-of-life at "extraordinary" expense and restricting costly medical interventions to those recipients in whom im-

provements in welfare would be larger or would enhance opportunities for welfare over more years, that is, the young.[125] This seems to be the view which underlies the allocation of resources under the British National Health Service.[126] In the United States this view underlies the call to restrict dialysis in favor of other services which have a larger improvement in welfare[127] and underlies at least one major American hospital's refusal to initiate a heart transplantation program: "[W]ith the rapid proliferation of expensive medical technology, there is a clear responsibility to evaluate the new procedures in terms of the greatest good for the greatest number . . . To deny many patients the services of the hospital for procedures and care known to improve survival and quality of life in an effort to help a few through the very difficult and resource-consuming procedure of heart transplantation was considered by the trustees to be unjustified at present."[128]

There probably are other schemes of health care services that would be endorsed by different conceptions of the good life. The point, however, is not just to multiply examples. Affirming the plurality of conceptions of the good life means accepting that there is no univocal weighing of these various opportunities. Further, this plurality of conceptions of the good life suggests that there will not be a compromise scheme that people will accept for the purposes of justice. After all, those who espouse the relational conception of the good life, and endorse scheme 2, oppose scheme 1 because it ensures opportunities for a long life, encouraging the elderly to deny death, and because it does not ensure the opportunities created by services which improve people's quality-of-life. Indeed, the proponents of scheme 2 are opposed to continued research and development of life-extending technologies not simply because they are costly, but because they foster and perpetuate the erroneous idea that people need not accept aging and death. Reciprocally, they oppose the denial of death because it perpetuates attempts to develop life-extending technologies to the exclusion of other types of medical treatments.

> Some "modernizers" in the field of aging believe in the possibility of indefinitely extending human life. I take a more traditional view. I say that not only can the nation not afford the notion of extending middle-age vitality indefinitely but also that the very notion is wrong. My idea of an enlightened national policy is that we should shift the emphasis from quantity to quality [of life] . . . The effects

of such a national policy might be a greater emphasis on prevention of disease and staying healthy; on improving routine medical care for the elderly, especially in the area of chronic, crippling, and disabling diseases and long term care; and on slowing down research on life-extending technologies. We have developed an idolatrous enslavement to technology and need to replace it with an emphasis on the quality of life.[129]

Similarly, those who espouse an autonomous conception oppose scheme 1 because it provides services to those who cannot pursue an independent life, while constricting services that might help others to lead such a life. Finally, the utilitarian conception opposes scheme 1 because it wastes scarce resources on medical care for the dying, the old, and the chronically incapacitated. It is not uncommon to hear those who endorse the utilitarian conception wondering why neonatal intensive care units are "wasting" money on saving infants who are likely to have significant handicaps instead of spending it on prenatal care that will help many others. We can go through each scheme of medical services noting why people with different conceptions of the good life will reject it. Again, opposition to the alternative schemes will result not just from differences of subjective preferences or trivial concerns, but from genuine philosophical differences, differences about what is the best way to lead a life. Overall, the diversity of conceptions of the good life provides strong reason to doubt the existence of a voluntary consensus for a compromise scheme which does not coincide with any particular conception but is mutually acceptable to those who espouse any conception of the good life. In particular, it is hard to see that there could be any compromise between the advocates of scheme 1 and schemes 2, 3, and 4.

Now, it might be argued that without a consensus on the "truly" basic medical services, the liberal legislator should designate scheme 3—or something akin to it—as the "truly" basic medical services, justifying this choice by appeal to the autonomous conception of the good life. He would argue that this conception embodies the conception of a person which informs the liberal principles of justice and should therefore be the one which determines how to balance the just demands for resources.

But to invoke the autonomous conception of the good life as the justification for a health care policy would be to make liberalism a comprehensive conception of the good life, and thus to make moral liberalism the basis of political decisions. But this violates the liberal ideal of neutrality. Although the autonomous conception of the good life has "great importance in liberal thought," it "becomes another sectarian doctrine" when used to justify public laws and policies.[130] Furthermore, it is an important fact of the debate about just health care that while a distribution which would be derived from this autonomous conception, such as scheme 3, may have some advocates, it has very few. In addition, there is no reason to suspect that this would be the compromise scheme that would be acceptable to the advocates of the other schemes. This lack of support for the application of the autonomous conception to determining the "truly" basic medical care services suggests that people do not find this conception the one that should guide public deliberations on justice in health care. This brings into question the notion that this conception matches our considered moral convictions on matters of justice.

Conclusion

The liberal legislator's objective is to specify the institutions and policies that promote fair equality of opportunity. Applied to health care, his aim is to define the "truly" basic medical care services, the subset of all medical services that protect opportunities, that society should guarantee its citizens as a matter of justice. He must weigh or balance all the possible ways to protect equality of opportunity while honoring the tenets of liberalism.

In deliberating, the liberal legislator's problem is not the absence of "a wealth of empirical knowledge," the lack of information on "the prevalence of various illnesses and their severity, and the frequency of accidents and their causes."[131] All the empirical knowledge in the world—or even in a fully informed imaginary world—will not tell the liberal legislator which opportunities to pursue various life plans should be protected by the basic medical services. The liberal legislator needs some criterion or standard of assessment for balancing or weighing these opportunities. But we have found each standard of assessment to be flawed or incompatible with the tenets of liberalism. A technical assessment—selecting the scheme of medical services which will be easiest to administer, and so forth—seems irrelevant. A quantitative assessment—selecting those medical services which protect the greatest number of opportunities for the greatest number of citizens—either does not exist or becomes a utilitarian standard. A qualitative assessment—selecting those medical services that protect the most important or worthy opportunities—violates the liberal ideal of neutrality. There seems no way for the liberal legislator to weigh the various schemes in a manner consistent with liberal principles.

The hypothetical choice procedure leaves the liberal legislator without a standard of assessment by which to weigh the various opportunities to be secured by each scheme of health care services and thus without a way to justify selecting one health scheme over another. Indeed, without such a standard there really seem to be no grounds for deliberation. For there would seem to be no basis on which the legislator could compare and evaluate the justice of the alternative schemes. Consequently, the liberal legislator's deliberations seem ominously quiet.[132] This is not to say that no deliberations are possible. It is possible to choose among the four proposed health care schemes, but only by appeal to a particular conception of the good life.

Thus the fundamental problem of such hypothetical choice procedures is not *practical* but *philosophical*. It arises from the way in which the liberal ideal of neutrality precludes weighing the diverse and incommensurable opportunities enhanced and forgone by different schemes of basic medical services. This procedure cannot help us to determine what basic medical services society should guarantee its citizens as a matter of justice and what services it should leave to personal preference. As a result, it does not help us to determine what a just health care system is.

The Last Hope: Democratic Political Procedures

The Turn to Democratic Political Procedures

After the failure of the hypothetical choice procedure, there remains one further possibility for providing a plausible articulation of basic medical services consistent with liberal tenets: democratic political procedures.[133] There are two distinct motives for endorsing such procedures. One is philosophical skepticism. From the perspective of the skeptics, the failure of lists, a criterion, or a hypothetical choice procedure to specify basic medical care suggests that such a question is not amenable to philosophical analysis; it seems beyond or outside of philosophy. Dissatisfied with the vague guidance provided by theories of justice on allocating resources to patients, many physicians are drawn to this skepticism. Political theorists have linked this view with the endorsement of democratic procedures: "I suspect that *no philosophical argument* can provide us with a cogent principle by which we can draw a line within the enormous group of goods that can improve health or extend life prospects of individuals . . . The remaining question of establishing a precise level of priorities among heath care and other goods is appropriately left to democratic decision-making" (emphasis added).[134]

Thus the skeptics urge us to accept democratic political procedures in determining justice in health care not because democracy embodies a political ideal and fosters essential human activities, but as an instrumental solution. On the skeptical view, democracy is not an end in itself but merely a necessary means, the guarantor of closure; democratic political procedures are introduced as the philosopher's equivalent of Sylvester McMonkey McBean's Fix-It Up Machine.[135]

The skeptical justification of democratic political procedures is unsatisfactory. First, while there may be *no* philosophical arguments consistent with liberalism for defining the basic medical services, I outlined at least four philosophical conceptions of the good life that offer cogent justifications for different schemes of basic health care services. This means that the failure of philosophical principles for justifying choices among health services is not inherent but a consequence of liberal principles. More important, skepticism is a highly controversial philosophical position not affirmed by all. To use it as the justification for democratic procedures is certainly inconsistent with the tenets of liberal political philosophy.[136]

A second motivation for turning to democratic procedures rests on the indeterminacy of the principles of justice. On this view, fulfilling the principle of fair equality of opportunity is a threshold test of justice. Any and all schemes of basic medical services that promote fair equality of opportunity pass the threshold and are designated "equally just." Selecting among these different "equally just" possibilities, then, is not a matter of justice, but a matter for democratic political procedures. Thus democratic political procedures are affirmed not out of skepticism, but as a method of resolving indeterminacy in the principles of justice, of selecting among "equally just" laws and policies. In the words of Rawls, democratic procedures are the final stage of "an attempt to find the best policy as defined by the principles of justice."

> [J]ust laws and policies are those that would be enacted at the legislative stage. Of course, this test is often indeterminate: it is not always clear which of several constitutions or economic and social arrangements, would be chosen. But when this is so, justice is to that extent likewise indeterminate. Institutions within the permitted range are equally just, meaning that they could be chosen; they are compatible with all the constraints of the theory . . . This indeterminacy in the theory of justice is not in itself a defect. It is what we should expect. Justice as fairness will prove a worthwhile theory if it defines the range of justice more in accordance with our considered judgments than do existing theories, and if it singles out with greater sharpness the graver wrongs a society should avoid. [137]

The President's Commission shares this view: "For the purpose of health policy formulation, general theories as well as ordinary views of equity do not determine a unique solution to defining adequate care but rather set some broad limits within which that definition should fall. It is reasonable for a society to turn to fair, democratic political procedures to make a choice among just alternatives." [138]

While the appeal to democratic political procedures appears attractive, the examination of the hypothetical choice procedure emphasizes the need to elucidate vague proposals before they can be endorsed. What is the conception of democratic political procedures being advocated? Are the proposed procedures consistent with our ethical judgments?

The Liberal Conception of Democratic Political Procedures

The appeal to democratic procedures by liberal philosophers tends to follow an unfortunate pattern. Toward the end of an argument, democratic political procedures seem to be invoked to resolve all remaining problems. Characteristically these invocations are short, ending without any elaboration, examination, or justification of these democratic political procedures. It seems that such procedures are assumed to be self-defining and self-justifying. [139] To continue this inquiry, therefore, it is necessary to elaborate the implicit conception of democratic political procedure being advocated.

One might distinguish two conceptions of democratic political procedures: electoral democracy and deliberative democracy. In electoral democracy the ideal is majority rule. Here the democratic political procedures consist of voting at the ballot box for representatives who then draft legislation and formulate policies. What counts in electoral democracy is the "relative power of some (even all) citizens" in shaping laws and policies.[140] The appeal of electoral democracy is twofold. First is the appeal based on size: in large nation-states voting seems to be the only efficient mechanism for popular participation in politics. The second appeal is that of closure. Voting is the ultimate "Fix-It Up Machine"; with voting there can be a final, definitive way of selecting laws or policies.

By contrast, in deliberative democracy the ideal is public participation in debate and persuasion. Here the essential political procedure is not voting but some form of collective practical reasoning, the comparison of competing visions. What counts in deliberative democracy is not majority rule because it is the majority, but argument and persuasion. The appeal of deliberative democracy is more philosophical than practical; it rests on a view of free and equal persons collectively participating in self-rule and, through it, self-development.

Which of these conceptions of democratic political procedures do liberals advocate? Initially the deliberative conception seems to be favored. Rawls, for instance, argues that while the principles of justice do not single out a precise policy for basic health care services, they are to serve as "guidelines for deliberation."[141] Similarly, in *A Theory of Justice* his aim seems to be "to formulate an ideal constitution of public *deliberation* in matters of justice, a set of rules well-designed to bring to bear the greater knowledge and reasoning powers of the group" in the enactment of laws and policies.[142]

But this initial impression is misleading. While liberal political philosophers may aspire to deliberative democracy as the ideal, it is not consistent with the tenets of liberalism. What are the form and content of such discussions and debates in a liberal polity?

One of the advantages of electoral democracy is that its form, periodic elections, is well understood, easily instituted, and already extant. Advocates of electoral democracy need offer no detailed elaboration of the institutional structure of their political procedures. But the institutional structures necessary for deliberative democracy are neither obvious nor extant; they must be imagined and specified. Yet the advocates of liberalism are virtually silent on the institutional structures necessary to create and foster forums for such deliberations. Traditionally, liberal philosophers have been more preoccupied about securing individual rights than about devising the institutions which might foster democratic deliberations.

In the liberal view, schemes of health care services that fulfill the principles of justice by promoting fair equality of opportunity are deemed "equally just." These are the schemes to be submitted to democratic political procedures. On what basis will citizens in a liberal polity discuss these "equally just" schemes of basic medical care services?

To deliberate on laws and policies requires some basis for discussing, arguing, and persuading. When the laws and policies concern different schemes of basic medical services, the basis for discussion seems to be of three types: the justice of the schemes, the good of the schemes, and the interests of participants in the schemes. Clearly, in a liberal polity, the citizens cannot compare the justice of the schemes. The schemes have been designated "equally just" because they all promote fair equality of opportunity. There is no additional way of comparing and ranking them on the basis of justice; there is no category "more just." Indeed, in a liberal polity, the reason for turning to democratic procedures was that the principles of justice were indeterminate among these different schemes.

Citizens can discuss and debate different health care schemes by comparing the importance of the opportunities secured by each scheme and the conception of the good life that informs each view. In advocating and justifying their view, the citizens would have to appeal to some conception of how these opportunities fit into a human life, why they are urgent, and why the collection of services expresses the polity's conception of justice. Indeed, in outlining the four conceptions of the good life that justify the four different health care schemes, I showed how citizens might begin to articulate arguments for one set of services rather than another. But because such discussions rely on invoking particular conceptions of the good life to justify policies, they cannot be tolerated in a liberal polity.

If citizens are unable to debate either the justice or the goodness of these various health care schemes, what is the substance of their discussions? Only interests seem to remain. Indeed, Ronald Dworkin explicitly argues that in a liberal society individuals should assess different policies by how they affect their personal interests and not whether they are worthy or how they distribute goods to others. For individuals to assess policies by their goodness or how they distribute opportunities and resources to others would be, in his view, to violate basic liberal tenets and fail to respect individual rights.[143] According to Dworkin, then, policy debates in a liberal polity should focus on individual interests, not on the justice or the goodness of the policies. And obviously this is easily accomplished; citizens can compare different health care schemes by determining how they affect their personal access to particular health care services. A patient with renal failure, for instance, can evaluate the schemes by whether they guarantee dialysis. Similarly, people in need of nursing home care—or with relatives in need of such care—can evaluate the schemes by determining whether and how well they provide such care. The political deliberations that liberal philosophers envision thus seem to consist of bargaining over interests and preferences. But there is no reason to elevate such bargaining as an ideal or to call it deliberation. Nor is there any reason to suspect that such bargaining will produce the best scheme of basic medical services or rich deliberations.

Respecting the liberal ideal of neutrality eviscerates democratic political procedures of moral deliberation. Without the possibility of appealing to particular conceptions of the good life as reasons for implementing a law or policy, the substance of citizens' discussions can never rise above selfish interests. Thus no matter how much liberal philosophers may wish for political deliberation on laws and policies, their political philosophy negates such a possibility. Liberalism makes democratic political procedures an elaborate euphemism for voting. And Rawls may be implicitly admitting this when he suggests that the selection of just policies ultimately depends upon the legislature's vote: "On many questions of social and economic policy we must fall back upon a notion of quasi-pure procedural justice: laws and policies are just provided that they lie within the allowed range, and the legislature, in ways authorized by a just constitution, has in fact enacted them."[144]

Electoral Democracy and Our Ethical Judgments

Does this vision of electoral democracy for determining basic medical services match our actual judgments and practices? Advocates of different schemes of "truly" basic health care services do not simply articulate their scheme and then urge voting. Nor do they simply encourage people to support their scheme because it will promote their interests. Instead people argue about which scheme is more just and worthy. For example, the legislatures of both Oregon and Arizona have decided not to fund organ transplants with Medicaid funds and to increase spending for prenatal care.[145] These policies are justified by arguing that organ transplants help only a few people, while many others are denied basic medical care. In addition, while organ transplants may extend life for an average of five years or so, prenatal care can avoid lifelong suffering by preventing the creation of infirmities and handicaps at birth. The resulting public debates have not simply appealed to interests or called for a referendum, but have instead focused on justice and the worthiness of different opportunities. Similarly, the advocates of what I called scheme 2 have explicitly argued for their scheme by articulating a conception of the good life and suggesting it is more worthy because it recognizes aging and death as inherent, natural facts and tries to give them social meaning and honor. In addition, the advocates of scheme 2 maintain that it better secures intergenerational justice, by spending more for the young than the old.[146] Indeed, Daniel Callahan is explicit about the need to debate competing conceptions of the good life in designing a just health system: "The most important task [in the constructive work of developing an alternative health care system] is to present a societal perspective on health, one that can provide a solid foundation for a way of life that will give a sensible and proper place to health in our common existence. To achieve this, we must try to determine appropriate goals and ends for biomedical enterprise in the context of an examination of what constitutes the human good."[147]

Current debates about "truly" basic medical care services attest to the belief—in practice—that there are ethical grounds for comparing the justice and worthiness of different schemes. These grounds are assessments of the different conceptions of the good life that inform each scheme. In such examples, electoral democracy does not seem to match our practices.

Despite the fact that liberals wish for something different, something more, their appeal to democratic political procedures is actually an endorsement of voting and the relative power of the majority. But this liberal vision of democratic political procedures seems neither philosophically necessary nor practically accurate. There are principled ways to debate the justice of different health care schemes that promote fair equality of opportunity. And we do argue in our public life.

What is this alternative, deliberative democracy? What institutional arrangements are necessary to foster such public deliberations on laws and policies? These are questions which liberals have avoided, but which we must confront. For only by answering them can we hope to address the most pressing medical ethical dilemmas confronting us.

The Cost of Not Specifying Basic Medical Services

Everyone from congressmen to citizens rightly sees the need to change the current distribution of health care resources. The agglomeration that is the American health care system is capable of delivering the most sophisticated medical care available anywhere. But not to all. And what is equally important, its costs are escalating with no apparent end in sight. We need an alternative that is both practical and just. It is for guidance in constructing such an alternative that we have turned to theories of justice.

The costs of the health care system must stay within the resource limits established at the political level while satisfying the principle of equal access at the patient-centered level. These requirements, however, pull in opposite directions, generating the need for a third requirement, distributive decisions at what I have called the *medical* level. Such a distribution must identify the range of basic medical services that society will guarantee citizens as a matter of justice.

My investigation has revealed that liberal theories of justice cannot provide a suitable framework for distribution at the medical level, for defining basic medical services. It is possible to specify a scheme of basic medical services that society should guarantee citizens as a matter of justice, but only by invoking a particular conception of the good life and contravening the tenets of liberalism. This failure has both practical and philosophical consequences. The practical consequences are clear: the expensive, inequitable health care agglomeration that we currently have, without prospects for agreement on substantive aspects of its reform or replacement. In addition to the practical consequences, however, there are important philosophical consequences of this failure.

The objective of liberal political philosophy is to provide a framework for addressing practical ethical problems, especially matters of justice. In health care, a theory of justice should help to guide us in weighing and balancing the various health care services, to specify those services that are most urgent and that should be funded within the political resource limit. But, as I have argued, liberalism appears to preclude the weighing and balancing of opportunities secured by various health care services to determine which scheme is most just. Daniels seems to acknowledge this point in a footnote:

> [Rawls's] principles of justice do impose some substantive constraints on the fleshed-out principles of justice, even if the details of [weighing] the index [of primary goods] are not known: the worst off, however determined by an appropriate index, must be maximally well off. But this advances little toward a substantive theory for health care. All we know is that our fair share of social goods will be weighted according to some appropriate consideration of our health care needs, given social conditions, etc. If this is *all* that emerges from the contract theory then we have not moved very far toward knowing what our entitlements to health care are likely to be, which was the point of turning to the theory in the first place. (emphasis in the original)[148]

This point has implications beyond justice in health care; it signals a more central failure of liberal political philosophy. The need to weigh or balance diverse demands is fundamental to many other matters of justice; balancing competing demands is, after all, most of what concerns legislators. For instance, weighing various primary goods—the good of income and social bases of self-respect—is necessary to resolve the question of whether justice requires a capitalistic system of private property or democratic socialism.[149] More important, such a weighing is at the heart of determining the just distribution of resources at the political level. For only by knowing how to weigh the various demands on social resources, from defense and foreign aid to income support and disability programs, to support for the arts and education, to housing and infrastructure, can we know what constitutes the just distribution of social resources.[150] Rawls himself acknowledges the importance for political philosophy of providing a framework for weighing when he criticizes utilitarianism:

> Different political views, however, balance these ends [—greater average well-being and a more equal distribution of resources—] dif-

ferently, and we need criteria for determining their relative weights. The fact is that we do not in general agree to very much when we acknowledge ends of this kind. It must be recognized that a fairly detailed *weighting* of aims is implicit in a reasonably complete conception of justice. In everyday life we often content ourselves with enumerating common sense precepts and objectives of policy, adding that on particular questions we have to balance them in light of the general facts of the situation. While this is sound practical advice, it does not express an articulated conception of justice. One is being told in effect to exercise one's judgment as best one can within the framework of these ends as guidelines. (emphasis added)[151]

Despite its importance, liberal philosophers have assiduously avoided indicating how such a "fairly detailed" weighing should occur within a liberal political philosophy. Often the problem is abstracted away. For instance, Rawls almost always simplifies his considerations of how the primary goods are to be weighed.[152] At other times the problem is relegated to politicians for resolution.[153]

The method of avoidance cannot be applied to this problem. As my analysis of the details of the liberal legislator's deliberations suggests, there is an irreducible contradiction between weighing various goods and liberal political philosophy. A framework for weighing can be elaborated only within a political philosophy that does not affirm the ideal of neutrality. Consequently, to resolve many important matters of justice, including what health care services society should guarantee citizens as a matter of justice, we need to outline a political philosophy that permits invoking a conception of the good life in the justification of laws and policies.

5

The Liberal Communitarian Vision

The acute and interminable irresolution surrounding medical ethical questions in the United States arises not from advances in biomedical technology but from the tenets of liberal political philosophy. As the investigation of the problems of terminating medical treatments and the allocation of medical resources revealed, without invoking a conception of the good life, there can be no framework for principled public resolution of such issues. Resolving these issues will require more than technical solutions, more than another interpretation of the patient's best interests, more than a refined version of cost-effectiveness analysis, more than the elimination of unnecessary care; it will require rejecting the liberal ideal of neutrality.

But such criticisms are insufficient. Like utilitarianism before it, liberal political philosophy may persist despite inherent ethical difficulties unless there is an alternative vision. The necessary complement to these criticisms, therefore, is a constructive alternative political philosophy that recognizes the role of conceptions of the good life in justifying laws and policies. Only such a political philosophy can provide a framework in which medical ethical issues can be addressed. In this and the following chapter I begin the constructive endeavor by outlining the theoretical claims of this alternative and how it might structure a new medical care system. This attempt constitutes the beginnings of an alternative vision.

Background Tenets for Political Philosophy

In Chapter 2 I suggested that there appear to be three basic tenets that define the practical and philosophical background for *any* political philosophy: pluralism, the justification by reflective equilibrium, and the aim of addressing practical public controversies. The distinctive

155

characteristic of liberal political philosophy is its understanding and approach to pluralism. But for the purposes of medical ethics, an adequate political philosophy will have to accept these background tenets but reject the liberal approach to them. To be specific, it will have to affirm pluralism but simultaneously affirm the need to appeal to conceptions of the good life in justifying laws and policies. How can this be done?

To many, especially medical ethicists, there seems to be a natural answer to this question: utilitarianism. Rejecting liberalism, a form of deontology and one of the two dominant ethical theories, naturally implies turning to utilitarianism, the paradigmatic form of the other type of theory, consequentialism.[1] More important, utilitarianism seems to accept both pluralism and the fact that public laws and policies must be informed by a conception of the good life. By accepting a subjective conception of well-being, that individuals have different preferences and views of happiness, utilitarianism seems to accept pluralism. In addition, the fundamental principle of utilitarianism is that the best action, for our purposes the best laws and policies, should be chosen based on the aggregation and maximization of the good, however this is conceived.

It is beyond the purpose and scope of this work to criticize the suitability of the utilitarian vision. In any case, others have done this more thoroughly than I could.[2] Instead the aim is to offer an alternative vision. This alternative is not primarily a distinct conception of the good life, but a political philosophy to ground our political institutions. At the moment what is needed is not a philosophy of the good life, but a philosophy for creating a political framework within which people pursue a plurality of conceptions of the good life and yet which recognizes that policies will have to be justified by appeal to a particular conception of the good life. What is now needed is a view that incorporates the partial truths of both liberalism and utilitarianism in a systematic manner while avoiding the fundamental defects of each.

The Ideal of Liberal Communitarianism

I call this alternative view the liberal communitarian vision. The ideal of this vision is a political community characterized by public deliberation about a conception of the good life, which, in turn, serves as a guiding ideal for the formulation of laws and policies to regulate communal life. The political ideal is one of a deliberative democracy in which citizens interpret and create the community's values and specify how these are to shape specific policies.

Informing this ideal is a vision of a person who is (1) autonomous, (2) with fully developed capacities, including those capacities that can only be fully developed through participation in democratic deliberations, and (3) who has transcended his contingent existence through participation in the shaping and sustaining of his community.

We can imagine a community of individuals who recognize one another as citizens and come together to shape the common institutions and policies that create the conditions in which they live. Each citizen is committed to sustaining the community not just for himself, but for his fellow citizens and for the future generations. His primary intent is not to further his own particular interests, but to do what is best for the community taken together, to sustain the common institutions, and, thereby, to secure his own interests. In the deliberations with his fellow citizens he aims to explicate their shared vision for the community and specify what policies should be enacted to realize this vision. Engaging in communal deliberation is seen by the citizen as valuable because it grants him direct control over the institutions in which he lives but also because it elicits certain capacities that are otherwise underdeveloped or not developed; a citizen views the deliberations as self-enriching. Finally, a citizen finds participating in such deliberations elevating because in the process of exchanging views and forming policies with his fellow citizens, he becomes bound together with them in an ongoing community which seems to enlarge each of their beings, ensuring that some of their being will persist after their lives.

To elaborate this image: An individual is born into a social world and inherits a tradition and a past that he has neither chosen nor created. This is trivially true as a matter of sociology; there is no other way for one to develop as a person. But it is also profoundly true as a matter of philosophy, for it means that a person's identity is inseparable from these inherited factors. A person cannot understand himself apart from his cultural inheritances.[3] But a citizen has not chosen these inheritances; they are given to him. In this sense a person begins unfree, subject to social conditions and political laws that he did not create. Part of the inspiration for the liberal communitarian vision is that it creates the possibility of overcoming—although not escaping—this condition of being unfree—radically situated—subjects in two ways. The first is that the liberal communitarian vision permits the possibility of reflection on and thus distance from these inheritances. Of course, personal reflection, alone or with friends, is possible under a variety of political systems. It does not require participation in democratic deliberations. Through personal reflection an individual can explore his life, its history, meaning, and purpose, as well as what he understands the communal life to be. The liberal communitarian vision adds communal reflection, which is necessary to explore and establish the history and meaning of communal life, to reveal what the community conceives itself to be. Ultimately it is only by knowing what the community is, what the community takes itself to be, that an individual can know himself. For it is precisely by knowing this that an individual knows his inheritance. This reflection is one way the individual can distance, although not separate, himself from what he has been given.[4] And this never-separate, attached, reflective distance is necessary for freedom, for knowing what has shaped our identity and determining how we stand in relation to it.

But, more important, participation in communal deliberation permits the possibility of controlling and shaping the social world in which we live. Social conditions and political institutions are given to a citizen and shape the world in which he leads his life. Part of freedom is being able not just to choose and pursue one's individual conception of the good life, but to shape the social and political structures in which these choices and pursuits occur. Political participation in democratic deliberations permits the individual to create his social world. Of course, this control over his world is not absolute; he inherits existing institutions and practices. But through participation in democratic deliberations an individual can alter or refine these institutions and practices and create new ones. In this way, the individual does not just make his own life within structures made for and given to him, he lives under laws and, thus, social conditions that he legislates with others. Thus in liberal communitarianism, the citizen is capable of realizing a higher level of freedom. He is personally free in being able to pursue his own conception of the good life. But he is free in an additional, political sense because he can create and pursue the conditions within which this good life is formulated and pursued. The liberal communitarian vision makes this political autonomy possible. And through this a person can cease being subject to an inherited world. Thus participation in communal deliberations permits personal autonomy—knowing our identity and its sources and thereby being free by a kind of attached, reflective distance—and political autonomy—shaping our social world and therefore being free through control of the conditions in which we form and pursue our life plans.

To this political autonomy made possible by participation in democratic deliberation is added a more developed person. Such participation engenders distinctive human capacities. To be able to live in a social world that is given, to understand it and one's relation to it, to shape its institutions and practices, develops an individual's capacities and virtues. In part, this participation extends capacities nurtured within family and friendships and, thereby, transforms them by bringing them into common life. Among these developed capacities are a sense of empathy and commitment and a sense of responsibility for creating the future. As an individual lives his life in the community of others, he develops the capacity to understand the views of others and to make his decisions not against them, but with them. In this sense, participation develops the capacity to specify interests so they cohere with those of others, to see one's good in realizing the good with others. The individual does not compromise his interests, merely sacrificing them to the good of others, but he sees them differently; he changes his interests because of his communal relations. Participation in democratic deliberation thus transforms what is expressed in the family as love into communal empathy and commitment. Similarly, as the individual lives and participates in the formulation of laws and policies, he shapes the social and political conditions that will be given to future generations. In this sense participation develops the capacity of being responsible not just for oneself but for others. Participation in democratic deliberation thus transforms what is expressed in the family as caring for children into communal responsibility for future generations.

Beyond developing the capacities that originated in the family, participation in democratic deliberation develops at least one unique capacity: moral reflection. In many other aspects of life there rarely is a need to provide a justification of one's views and actions. The need for public persuasion in deliberation requires justification and thus moral reflection. This requirement combines the other capacities; persuasion and justification require the individual to interpret his communal past, empathize with his fellow citizens, and specify what should be jointly created in their mutual interest. In addition, engaging in moral deliberation on public matters that will affect a large community means that the range and nature of the subjects are radically altered and expanded. For instance, in her personal life a woman might reflect on whether to participate personally in, say, surrogate motherhood, whether as a surrogate or a purchaser of the surrogate services. But in public reflection the range of issues related to this subject is greatly expanded, for what is at stake is not merely a personal choice but the communal meanings of institutions such as the family. Deliberations within a political community thus make the most wide-ranging moral reflection possible and indeed inescapable. In developing the capacity for deliberation, participation in democratic deliberations forces individuals to lead deliberate lives.

Finally, participation in democratic deliberation permits the individual to transcend his contingent, individual existence by becoming part of an enduring community, a people with a past and a posterity. An individual possesses limited capacities; his temporal finitude means he cannot even fully develop the capacities he actually possesses. Existence, and whatever is done in it, is ephemeral. The only way to overcome these limitations of capacities and time is through union with other people in a community that develops the full range of human capacities and that continues the traditions and ideals after each individual has died. Through participation the individual contributes to the goods realized by the community, which far exceed his own contribution. In union with others the range of human capacities is realized.[5] Moreover, by uniting with others in a community, a person is able to transcend his mortality. The possibility of an individual's creating and contributing to something which endures beyond his life, and even his children's lives, to a people, can be realized only through political institutions and communities. By participating in creating and sustaining his community, he has the possibility of making the world different, better, for having lived. He thereby secures the community and its traditions for posterity. In doing so he recognizes himself as part of an enduring people. And in this way, he can be said to live beyond his own life.

Thus it is only through such deliberations that we can achieve political autonomy, develop distinctive human capacities, and contribute to an enduring world, a people and its posterity, which lives beyond our death. It is the possibility of creating conditions in which these three ideals can be realized that inspires the liberal communitarian vision.

How does this liberal communitarian vision fulfill the background tenets of political philosophy? In this view citizens collectively articulate their shared conception of the good life and the policies that are informed by this conception and govern their lives. More important, the pluralism affirmed in the liberal communitarian vision is richer than the pluralism of liberalism.

The liberal view adopts a pluralism of avoidance: pluralism is a historical fact, and it is affirmed to avoid the autocratic use of state power.[6] By contrast, the liberal communitarian vision adopts another formulation: pluralism of affirmation. On this view, pluralism is accepted as a philosophical tenet about the diversity of goods and worthy lives, and it is affirmed to realize the various possibilities of human existence, the full range of human goods. The pluralism of affirmation does not require accepting that all the conceptions of the good life that people pursue are worthy. Indeed, many of these conceptions—professional wrestling, grass counting, purveying pornography, to give a few examples—can be not only foolish but despicable and contemptible. Rejecting certain life plans as degrading, however, still permits us to recognize that there is more than one way to lead a worthy, meaningful life. Human life is composed of incommensurable goods; people can lead worthy lives in which these goods are ordered differently and even in a conflicting manner. Two lives can be incommensurable and yet both can be worthy.

To realize the pluralism of affirmation requires recognizing a plurality of communities of deliberation. The pluralism of liberal communitarianism is realized not by simply permitting pluralism in private affairs but by permitting a diversity of political communities pursuing different conceptions of the good life. Political philosophy can, therefore, affirm pluralism not for negative reasons, to avoid the autocratic use of state power, but as a positive, affirmative ideal, as the way of realizing the multiplicity of human goods.

I claim no originality for the liberal communitarian ideal or its inspiring vision. They have a long philosophical tradition, and they have formed part of American political culture and practices.[7] The articulation offered in this and the next chapter is derived from this tradition; it is meant to answer the objection that this ideal is vague, undeveloped, undefended, and worst of all, impractical. To meet the objections I will try to specify explicitly the underlying ethical conceptions, especially those of deliberation and of a person, and to see how such a vision might be plausibly and practicably constructed.

The Conception of Deliberation

The conception of deliberation in the liberal communitarian vision has four distinctive features. First, in part these deliberations aim at creating or articulating a conception of the good life. The conception of the good life must not be viewed as something that can be captured by listing a few principles valid for all times. Rather, the conception of the good life is a complex picture of ends, attachments, virtues, and desires that are deemed worthy and worth aspiring toward. It contains many elements, some of which involve the public realm and some of which are purely private. The degree of detail in a conception of the good life will vary among different conceptions; thus the good life for an Orthodox Jew is much more detailed than the good life for, say, a democratic individualist influenced by the American transcendentalists.[8] This is not just an accident of history, resulting from the fact that one conception has had more time to be developed and refined; it also derives from the internal ideals of the two conceptions.

A public conception of the good life is neither definitively codified nor created *ex nihilo*. It is a construct, given form and content by a cluster of four elements of a shared social life: accepted moral ideals, traditions and customs, accepted practices, and paradigmatic precedents of history, that is, stories. Some of these elements will be shared between different communities within a society, but others will be distinctive to a particular community. Communal deliberations reconstruct these shared elements into a publicly accepted picture of the good life. The nature of this reconstruction will differ among communities depending upon their conception of the good life. In some communities with more detailed conceptions of the good life, such as Orthodox Jewish ones, the emphasis will be on interpretation of these elements; in other communities with less detailed conceptions of the good life, such as democratic individualist ones, the emphasis will be on creating collective values.

The publicly accepted picture of the good life is in outline, never fully specified, never "settled" or "established."[9] Even a detailed conception of the good life can never be summarized in a list of principles, and it is never exhaustively established to be followed like a recipe.

Public deliberations are necessary to illustrate and to provide detail in the picture of the good life because this picture can never be complete or its meaning beyond dispute. Indeed, there will always be the need at least for specification and articulation of certain ideals, traditions, and practices; for extension of the conception into new realms not considered before; for evaluating real and apparent contradictions between different ideals, traditions, and practices; and for responding to challenges from alternative conceptions found in neighboring communities. As many traditions reveal, even a detailed conception of the good life requires ongoing deliberations. To note a specific example relevant to medical ethics: within the Orthodox Jewish community there is a debate about brain death and harvesting organs for transplantation.[10] In debating, both sides draw on their shared traditions and ideals to elaborate their points; the tradition is not "settled" but constantly being reconsidered: "When a tradition is in good order it is always partially constituted by an argument about the goods the pursuit of which gives to that tradition its particular point and purpose . . . Traditions, when vital, embody continuities of conflict."[11]

Thus a conception of the good life is not specified in advance, ready to be applied to situations in some mechanical manner. We are often uncertain about our own conception, and deliberations serve to clarify it. In this sense our desires, preferences, and ideals are not given or fixed but often discovered or only partially articulated, in need of finer formulation, specification, and elaboration. The centrality of deliberations in politics emphasizes that conceptions of the good life are not settled or fixed or given, that they are in some deep way constructed from the materials of a shared life.[12] Because of the necessity for deliberations on the good life, affirming the worthiness of public deliberations is integral to any vital conception of the good life.

Second, since deliberations will be about conceptions of the good life they will be about fundamental ideals. Of course, they may focus on many things, whether policies are more efficient or induce less evasion and the like. But recognizing that public deliberations can include fundamental ideals affirms the possibility of reasoned discussion and judgment about such ideals and rejects skepticism about deliberations on them. To affirm reasoned discussion on fundamental ideals is not to suggest that there is only one true set of ideals or only one true interpretation, only that it is possible to discuss ethical values rationally.

As I have said, these ideals and their interpretation are neither given nor matters of naked choice; deliberations on them are neither vacuous nor meaningless. Deliberations on fundamental ideals aim to find the best fit of ideals, judgments about particular cases, and considered intuitions. However, new situations will arise, views may change, conflicting principles may be resolved. These changes might necessitate the creation or articulation of new ideals. Hence in aiming to fit ideals and judgments, there may be the need to elaborate new ideals. The justification for a particular collection of fundamental ideals and their interpretation is "reflective equilibrium," or something analogous, in which ideals, judgments, practices, and intuitions cohere in a consistent whole, or in Dworkin's phrase, a "seamless web."[13] This suggests that there are better and worse interpretations of coherence among ideals. Public deliberations aim to achieve reflective equilibrium, to define the best fit. The results of public deliberations serve as the collective standard.

The justification of public values offered in liberal communitarianism is identical to the justification found in liberal political philosophy. The main difference is that liberalism constructs and justifies the principles of justice, while liberal communitarianism does not limit public values to justice. One of the distinctive features of liberal communitarianism is the recognition that both questions of the good life and "questions of justice are endlessly contested and debated" in our society.[14] This means that public construction extends beyond justice to include shared elements of the good life. Liberal communitarianism takes as relevant factors that must be considered and fit into a seamless web a wider range of publicly shared ideas, traditions, and practices.

Further, liberalism recognizes two bases of criticism of institutions. They might be evaluated by whether they are justified, that is, correspond with our ideals, convictions, and traditions, and by whether they realize their objective, that is, can provide a framework to solve practical problems. The same is true in the liberal communitarian view; the bases of criticism are the ideals, traditions, and practices of the political community itself. For these important reasons, the matter of justification for the public deliberations does not distinguish liberalism from the view outlined here.

Third, it is possible to distinguish conceptually two levels of deliberations: there are deliberations about conceptions of the good life, and there are deliberations about specific laws and policies. This distinction is somewhat idealized, since often actual deliberations are not distinctly demarcated but interweave these two levels. Furthermore, deliberations are, in a manner of speaking, bidirectional—that is, dialectical. We do not settle questions about conceptions of the good life or justice and then somehow mechanically apply such a view in formulating laws. Deliberations about conceptions of the good life often suggest specific laws that need enactment or repeal. It is equally true, however, that deliberations about specific laws and policies suggest reinterpretation, additions, revisions, or qualifications of the conception of the good life. Such reciprocal revisions form part of the process of achieving reflective equilibrium. They are also one of the reasons for public deliberations.

Fourth, it is necessary to emphasize that the deliberations on the good life and policies are not merely instrumental. The noninstrumental objectives of public deliberations derive from the vision that informs liberal communitarianism.[15] Public deliberations aim at what I have called political autonomy, that is, having citizens decide what laws, policies, and social conditions will govern their lives. Thus, deliberations are initiated by a problem, the need to address a specific theoretical or practical issue. In the deliberations, the citizens reason through how the ideals, traditions, and practices suggest approaching the problem. While the problem usually is pressing, and there is need for closure, some policy or law to settle the problem, this resolution need not be definitive; considerations can be reopened and the policy subjected to further deliberations. Indeed, difficulties discovered while implementing the policies may suggest specific matters in need of further elaboration. In some sense this aim is instrumental, to set a policy for regulating some good. Yet it also goes beyond this because the aim is not just to have a policy, but, what is equally or more important, to have citizens themselves actually participate in its formulation. The writing of the law is as important as having the law itself. This makes political autonomy possible.

Another noninstrumental aim of deliberations is what might be called self-development of the citizens. Participation can elevate a citizen's perspective beyond his own self-interest, requiring that he consider the good of the entire community. Similarly, participating in democratic deliberations forces individuals to engage in moral reflection, justifying their views on an extended range of issues and ideals. Democracy is valued then for its effects on ordinary human beings, raising them from passivity and dependence to autonomous, deliberate citizens.[16]

Deliberations also aim at what might be called the establishment of a common life, the formation of a people with a posterity. This balances individual self-development. Deliberations aim to create a public realm, to identify shared ideals and traditions, to craft a joint vision. They do this by having people articulate, specify, and reformulate their ideas to determine what the community collectively values and how it values these things. To put it another way, deliberations reestablish a communal reflective equilibrium. Further, they define a common life in the actual process of coming together for public deliberation. As citizens deliberating with others about our communal life, we are not just interested in our own lives. We express our views to others; this both assumes and expresses a common life. The communal act of reasoning, the collective examination of ideals and traditions, is a distinctive characteristic of democratic deliberations. In the coming together, the attachment of the individual to the community, the joint enterprise is expressed.

Two final points: This liberal communitarian vision does not define democratic participation in public deliberation as *the* good life, as *the* way of life. Politics and political deliberations do not constitute all aspects of human life; they are not a comprehensive moral ideal. A conception of the good life contains many different elements. Some of these will be defined by the political community, others will be private. Where the line between these two falls is a central matter of public discussion. Regardless, certain fundamental aspects of a person's conception of the good life will remain for the individual to articulate and affirm. At a minimum, it seems that these personal elements will include things such as vocation, avocational pursuits, family decisions, and the like. In addition, since the individual can refrain from participation in political life, a major aspect of the conception of the good life is left to individuals. The public aspects of the conception of the good life distinguish different communities and give distinctive character to the lives of individuals in different communities, but they can never constitute an exhaustive conception of the good life. Men and women should not lead one-dimensional lives, and their lives would be no less one-dimensional if political affairs rather than personal affairs were the only dimension. Consequently, this ideal takes democratic deliberation as necessary in articulating a conception of the good life for political purposes, but it does not make politics *the* way of life, or a comprehensive ideal. For it neither expresses a "conception of what is of value in human life . . . that [is] to inform much of our *non*-political conduct" nor covers all elements of human life. [17]

Finally, embedded in this vision of deliberation is a conception of political community. A political community is a group of citizens mutually committed to one another in the ongoing process of deliberation in elaborating their shared conception of the good life and specifying laws and policies. On this view the relevant community is characterized not by a moral principle or by being in some particular location or by an arbitrary historical boundary. Formally, a community is defined by the people who are eligible to participate in the deliberations, where the primary, although not sufficient, requirement of eligibility is some commitment to recognizing, elaborating, affirming, and abiding by the community's particular conception of the good life. There will be other requirements for eligibility, often specified by a community's particular conception of the good life, but this commitment is fundamental. Practically, shared traditions, customs, religions, occupations, and the like define many communities because these are the sources for articulating conceptions of the good life. But communities are often formed on the basis of a newly acknowledged common commitment to some vision of human life.

In important ways, this conception of political community is distinct both from the utilitarian view, which expands the relevant community to encompass all sentient beings, including animals, and from the liberal view, which, if it is not universalist, defines the relevant political community in vague terms, as a community having a democratic public culture.[18]

The Conception of a Person

A citizen is a potential participant in democratic deliberations. For a citizen's participation in public deliberations to be meaningful, he must be capable of (1) conceiving, articulating, and justifying a conception of the good life, (2) evaluating and judging the contributions of others in reasoned argument, and (3) affirming and abiding by political decisions, laws, and policies as his own. Having these capacities and having society ensure the opportunity to exercise these capacities in the public deliberations is one element of freedom.

A second element is to live under social conditions that one has helped to create by participating in democratic deliberations. I have described this aspect of freedom as political autonomy. It is significant that citizens cannot be required to participate in communal deliberations: part of being a free citizen means that "citizens always have the right to choose between participation and passivity."[19] Non-participation may be a form of protest against the actions of the polity; it may also express a person's valuing other admirable goods which cannot be realized in politics, such as solitude or love.[20]

Persons as citizens are equal in having an equal opportunity to exercise their capacities, in particular to formulate and to express in public deliberations their conceptions and judgments, and equal opportunity to shape their community. This equality of opportunity, of course, does not mean that each citizen will exercise his capacity in strict equality with other citizens. In deliberative democracy, equality "is not power that is shared, but the opportunities and occasions of power. Every citizen is a potential participant."[21] Some citizens will naturally be more articulate, more energetic, finer judges, and therefore might well participate more. Equality among citizens ensures that none is arbitrarily excluded or is excluded because of his views.[22] Clearly, equality must include some resources to ensure that citizens can exercise their capacities for participation in deliberations; otherwise the ideal is formal and hollow.

A further element of the conception of persons as citizens is that they must have a basic commitment to their political community. Part of this commitment is captured in the option to participate, another part in the affirmation and acceptance of political decisions. Citizens are committed to the community for, among other things, its shared life. The public deliberations reveal and express the citizen's understanding of what is worthy in the community's common life. But a deliberative democracy is not necessarily a homogeneous group, although it may be that. Suggesting that there will be commitment and identity between community and individuals raises the specter of suffocating, ritualistic small groups—a prospect rightly deplored.[23] A conception of deliberative democracy cannot require or impose consensus and rule out conflict. As I have noted, conflicts and varying interpretations are inevitable, even healthy. But two types of conflicts need to be distinguished: the resolvable and the fundamental. Resolvable conflicts can occur between people who share a basic commitment. They can disagree, each thinking that the other's view or interpretation is wrong or mistaken. However, the disagreement is over an issue which does not call into question the commitment. It is a resolvable conflict not in the sense that there may be an answer which both will agree to, but that adopting either's view does not endanger the common commitment and otherwise shared viewpoint. Conversely, fundamental conflicts suggest that there is no common commitment; the issue over which there is disagreement is fundamental, and the persistence of disagreement undermines a shared viewpoint and the possibility of community. To return to the example of the Orthodox Jews disagreeing over brain death and harvesting organs for transplantation: As long as those debating appeal to recognized authorities, traditions, and texts, Halakah, but disagree over their interpretation and specification, there is a resolvable conflict. If the conflict arises because one participant questions the authority of Halakah, then there is a fundamental conflict. In this way, resolvable conflicts are inherent and integral to deliberative democracy, the basis of deliberations. But no political community can withstand persistent fundamental disagreements. For these reasons, commitment cannot be coerced. Hence, when a citizen detects a pattern of public decisions which he feels are grossly mistaken and attempts at reform have failed, when a citizen perceives fundamental conflict with the political community, freedom requires the option to leave the community.[24]

Political Rights and Goods

The liberal communitarian vision requires the guarantee of rights and opportunities to citizens; otherwise the possibility of deliberation would not be real. Two types of rights need to be distinguished: general and communal rights. General rights are political rights necessary to secure political participation; therefore they are common to all deliberative communities. They include the rights to (1) speech and expression; (2) association, both public and private; (3) free movement and, in the extreme, exit; (4) voting; (5) bodily and personal integrity; and (6) safeguards for criminal proceedings. This is not an exhaustive list but is intended to specify key political rights that must be guaranteed to all citizens.

In addition, there are specific communal rights, rights that a particular political community will recognize depending upon its particular conception of the good life. Thus, we can imagine a community guaranteeing the right to animal sacrifice while another might prohibit any use of animals, even for scientific research. Similarly, one community might grant a right to euthanasia and another might prohibit termination of care for incompetent patients.

The list of general rights will appear almost identical to a list of rights secured by the principles of justice for a liberal polity. The important point about rights is not their enumeration but the grounds of their interpretation. In a liberal polity, rights are meant to grant individuals the opportunity to develop and "exercise [their] capacity to decide upon and revise, and rationally to pursue, a conception of the good . . . [and to develop] and exercise [a] sense of right and justice."[25] This purpose is critical to their interpretation and adjudication in particular cases. Conversely, in the liberal communitarian vision the aim of general rights is to promote and protect participation in political deliberation. Communal rights will be for the purpose of realizing certain elements of a particular conception of the good life. One example to illustrate how this difference in objective affects the interpretation of rights might be the area of pornography. We can imagine that a community might prohibit the distribution and sale of pornographic books, magazines, telephone calls, and videos, while permitting political speech in public deliberations for legalizing these pornographic materials. Such prohibitions might accord with the interpretation of rights for political participation but not with rights for formulating and pursuing a conception of the good life.

In addition to rights, it is worth stating that the political ideal of deliberative democracy suggests an interpretation of needs that society should provide. Here again particular conceptions of the good life espoused by particular communities will be necessary to specify fully what will qualify as needs to be guaranteed by the polity. But the objective of participation in public deliberations provides part of the grounds for this specification of needs. For example, in the liberal communitarian vision there will have to be some provision for mandating time off from work for participation in critical political forums.

A Federated System

The liberal communitarian vision roughly outlined here raises many questions. By specifying some details of how such a vision might operate in the area of medical care, I hope to answer some of these questions. There is one fundamental question—and criticism—that cannot be deferred: How can such a scheme work in the modern world, made up of large nation-states facing complex problems which impinge on the lives of many people living in disparate areas? As Donald

Keim asks, "Can one realistically expect widespread participation in a country of 200 million people?" [26] Is this not just a "beguiling utopia" made more appealing by its impossibility? [27]

Such questions point to three fundamental issues: size, complexity, and membership. First, if democratic deliberation is to be a realistic possibility, if political participation is to permit political autonomy, to foster individual self-development, to express and create a sense of common identity around a shared conception of the good life, and not devolve into voting, then the political communities of liberal communitarianism will have to be small. How small? And if they are small enough for deliberations, are they viable?

Different forms of deliberation are possible, and different communities may adopt different ones, in part depending upon size, issues to be addressed, and particular views of participation within a community. Several possibilities seem reasonable. One is the New England town meeting format, in which once a month, say, the entire community is collected to discuss communal issues. Options are presented by town governing officials, and a discussion and general vote at the meeting settle issues and policies. A second possibility might be for the community to elect or appoint committees that explore different issue areas, holding open deliberations for citizens who wish to participate. The committees then might recommend to a general communal gathering several options to be discussed and voted on or to be submitted to referenda. A third possibility might be for a community to be subdivided into smaller groups that discuss their views. A single spokesman might then present their collective ideas at an open meeting of all citizens. Such an open meeting might deliberate and resolve issues by a vote of the citizens.

How small do political communities need to be for such deliberations? No precise number can be given, but a good working estimate can be gleaned from New England town meetings, which occur in towns with populations of up to 25,000 or so. For example, "Wakefield, Massachusetts maintains a town meeting of nearly twenty-six thousand" people. [28] This number approaches the upper limit for the size of communities with meaningful democratic deliberations, although in some large, densely populated cities political communities may be made up of slightly more people. Such a size would seem to permit meaningful communal discussions if we remember that communities will include many children and many citizens will choose passivity, although if deliberation can actually be made meaningful, more people may find participation worthwhile. Indeed, in New England town meetings attendance ranges from 25 to "66 percent in moments of crisis." Interestingly, these attendance figures do not seem to deviate significantly from attendance in eighteenth- and nineteenth-century town meetings in Massachusetts.[29] But most important, deliberations require the opportunity to participate; each individual need not personally voice his own position. These factors imply that political communities of this size could permit real deliberations within tolerable time limits. As one participant—and critic—of town meetings writes: "I recall one town meeting with nearly a thousand citizens, and once I found myself presiding over an assembly of some 2,500 faculty and students. In both cases, after about four hours of debate, practically everyone who was present felt, I believe, that his viewpoint had been fairly represented."[30]

Having political communities of this size in the United States seems conceivable within these numerical limits: there would need to be roughly 10,000 communities of 20,000 citizens each. And there already exist many political units of such size. There are more than 19,000 municipalities (only 2,200 have a population of 10,000 or more), more than 3,000 counties, more than 14,000 school districts, more than 3,330 colleges and universities, and more than 5,500 hospitals in the United States.[31] With so many political and other collective entities already extant in this country, the number of communal polities necessary for democratic deliberations is not unreasonable. It seems that an acceptable size for democratic deliberations does not require an enormous number of communities, at least by the standards of existing American political institutions.

There is a negative corollary to the conclusion that it is possible to have enough small communities for democratic deliberations: Can a multitude of political communities address complex issues that seem to transcend small political entities? Or will such issues lead to petty rivalries and philosophical differences without resolution?

The diverse political communities within a nation-state are not to be taken as completely autonomous. They can address a number of political issues that have their primary focus and effects on the locality and that are, to a large degree, already decided at the local level, or could be decided at the local level without significant conflict between communities. Such issues include (1) matters of education—regulating the institutional structure of schools, the content of the curriculum, the allocation of resources among academic and extracurricular activities; (2) matters of the environment—regulating garbage collection, disposal, and recycling, water use and conservation measures, the use of energy sources such as wood-burning stoves; (3) matters of zoning and development—regulating commercial activities and products, the scale of buildings and architectural styles, parking and traffic patterns; (4) matters of public services—regulating police and fire protection; (5) matters of art and culture—regulating support for artists, public displays of art; (6) matters of public assistance—regulating the provision of public aid and public work, the provision of health care.

Clearly many issues from defense and foreign affairs to tariffs and air safety will inevitably transcend the small political community. Some of these issues need not require national intervention but can be addressed by a voluntary federation of multiple small communities with shared concerns and approaches. For instance, many small political communities may share a common interest in protecting certain bodies of water, managing public transit systems, or promoting certain types of development, and these communities could form a federation for such endeavors. But other issues will transcend even such federations, requiring regional or national policies. Therefore a multitude of small political communities must "complement and be compatible with the primary representative institutions of large-scale modern societies." [32] These communities will have to be federated into the larger polities—individual states and the nation-state. And inevitably these will be run as representative democracies. The liberal communitarian vision recognizes the necessity of national politics and the necessity for representative democracy at the national level. There will of course be many matters on which the division of authority between the local political communities and the state or national governments will be unclear and a matter of conflict. Conceptually, this is no different from conflicts that currently arise among cities, states, and the federal government. A system based on the liberal communitarian ideal of democratic deliberation would incline us to favor leaving to local communities what can be done by them. The avoidance of national policies where they can be avoided will permit more communal deliberations as well as a diversity of approaches.

The result is a vision of a federated communal system, or a political union of communal polities. The different communal polities will pursue different conceptions of the good life and thereby realize a wide range of human goods. Further, participation in the overarching political community is necessary to engage in certain political decisions, such as those relating to foreign affairs. Thus, in the political union of communal polities each person can appreciate the realization of many human potentialities. This vision is similar to Rawls's social union of social unions, with the fundamental exception that the liberal communitarian vision recognizes these small entities as political communities with the power to establish laws and policies to govern their common life.[33] Furthermore, because these communities are political, not merely social units, they are given political recognition and public support, both financial and legislative, by the national government.

Finally, there is the issue of membership. One important role for the national government will be in the area of membership and guarantees of participation. Each communal polity will be limited in size, and the members of the community will have to decide who are its members and who are not. At first there will be self-definition. Many people will not want to join communities with certain conceptions of the good life and resultant policies, but will want to participate in other communities with a conception more consonant with their convictions. Inevitably, in some communities more people will want to be citizens than can be accommodated. Determining membership is a substantial political decision and one that is fundamental to any political entity. But its basis is restricted; if citizens are to have the right to free movement and exit, there must be a correlative right to join some communal polity. However, this is not a right to join a particular community. The values of particular communal polities will delimit the commitments necessary for membership. We can imagine that the conception of the good life which unites a community might require certain exclusions. For instance, in the context of medical care, a lesbian community with a shared view of feminism might want to limit its members to fellow lesbians; an Amish community might want to limit its membership to fellow Amish; and an American Indian tribe might well want to make membership in the communal polity coextensive with tribal membership. Thus, communal polities might appear to exclude people on the basis of suspect categories, such as race, religion, age, or sex. But such exclusions will not *ipso facto* be unjust. They will be acceptable when, as I have indicated, they derive from a conception of the good life and affirm shared ideals, tradition, and practices. This, of course, is not to affirm the reverse: that all exclusions on the basis of such categories will be deemed just. If a person is willing to participate in a community, affirm its conception of the good life, and abide by its communal decisions, then there is a presumption that the person is eligible for membership. The valid grounds for exclusion—if for reasons other than size—will have to be integral to a conception of the good life. If they are not, then such exclusion would be unjust.

Further, once a person is a member, the community cannot revoke membership for him if he wants to remain. Ostracism would preclude civil disobedience. Leaving, therefore, is an individual choice; in deliberative democracies ostracism should not be possible.

There are many other important issues relating to size and membership. Some communities can maintain exclusivity by setting a small size limit and by being located in areas where property prices are high, effectively—if not explicitly—excluding people on the basis of economic status and related characteristics. Neighboring communities might adopt policies that could undermine each other. For instance, one community might encourage the development of shopping malls and "warehouse" stores, undermining the small businessmen of a neighboring community. Such problems, of course, are not unique to the liberal communitarian vision outlined here, but are of profound importance nonetheless.

Liberal and Communitarian Facets

From this rough outline, the liberal communitarian vision should be imaginable though impressionistic; many details need to be filled in. At this point it might be worthwhile explaining the reasons why such a political ideal has been called a liberal communitarian vision.

The liberal communitarian vision is a *liberal* ideal for two reasons. First, it recognizes the claim of pluralism. Of course there are important differences between liberalism and liberal communitarianism. Liberalism accepts pluralism as a fact and permits individual diversity, while the liberal communitarian vision affirms pluralism as a positive value enhancing the realization of human potentialities and seeks not only to permit it but to foster it through political diversity. Nevertheless, both political philosophies give a prominent place to pluralism and recognize that any justifiable political vision must accept it.

Second, like liberalism, the liberal communitarian vision recognizes and protects important individual rights. One of the persuasive appeals of liberalism is its emphasis on the rights of justice that protect individuals and members of minority groups from the oppression of social opinions and majority rule. Because these rights seem indispensable, liberal philosophers want to avoid justifying rights, laws, and policies by appeal to conceptions of the good life, calculations of social utility, or some interest of the majority. The list of general rights enumerated in the liberal communitarian vision will be similar if not identical to liberal rights. However, the justification and, therefore, interpretation of the rights will differ from liberalism because in liberal communitarianism rights exist to promote and protect democratic deliberations. Nevertheless, in a liberal communitarian vision the protections afforded by these rights are secure because their justification does not rely on calculations of social utility or the like. Hence the charge that the "liberal politics of rights is morally better than" that of liberal communitarianism seems untenable if the basis of the moral evaluation is the rights and protections of speech, association, personal integrity, and the like.[34] Any political philosophy committed to democratic deliberation as a substantive good will value—and preserve—the individual general rights necessary for participation and will secure these rights, also valued by liberalism, without subjecting them to calculations of utility or other interests.

The liberal communitarian vision is also a *communitarian* ideal for two reasons. First, the liberal communitarian vision recognizes that laws and policies will have to be justified by appeals to particular conceptions of the good life. There is no alternative if there is to be a shared framework for addressing pressing public issues such as ethical issues in health care. Second, because conceptions of the good life must be introduced into politics, democratic deliberations are necessary. And having meaningful democratic deliberations requires the recognition of political communities that can deliberate on matters of the good. At the center of this vision is the ideal of a community committed to political autonomy, the development of certain individual capacities by participation in political deliberations, and the cultivation of a common life. These are fundamental communitarian objectives.

The ideal of politics embedded in the liberal communitarian vision, an ideal of a political community deliberating and articulating a conception of the good life and formulating laws and policies, tries to retain the truths of both liberal and teleological theories. It also tries to overcome their flaws, namely, the tendency to irresolution and to ossified and suffocating collectivities. Whether the liberal communitarian vision can achieve this fusion depends upon its being justified, philosophically plausible, and politically practical. An attempt to offer a full justification of this ideal would require a detailed history and cultural interpretation of our polity that is beyond the aim of this book.

What I offer here is a preliminary outline of liberal communitarianism. Many questions about its substance remain. Rather than addressing these questions in theoretical explorations, I will consider this vision in the medical care context, inquiring whether it might inspire a justifiable and plausible alternative to the existing system that can help address pressing medical ethical issues. By considering a specific example in detail, I hope to anticipate and articulate answers to these questions.

6

A Liberal Communitarian Vision of Health Care

The usual approach to suggesting reforms of the health care system is to devise a scheme "related to existing health financing and delivery patterns and the institutional framework now in place."[1] Such an approach may be politically prudent. Indeed it may be inevitable, if and when actual policy reforms or demonstration tests are implemented. Too frequently, this approach leads to ignoring or compromising moral ideals in the name of practicality. It also encourages piecemeal reform that can ultimately produce no change at all because of the many old elements left intact.

In contrast, I begin by imaging a reconstructive ideal—a health care system organized to realize the liberal communitarian ideal.[2] Such an ideal is not likely to be implemented when reforms are actually made in the health care system. But this ideal should serve as a shared, tangible, coherent, and morally justifiable model of a just alternative to the current system. As such, even if it is not implemented, it can serve as an important ethical guide for policy. In addition, this model should help us in imagining a liberal communitarian polity, thereby answering, at least in a preliminary way, the objection that advocates of such a view have never offered a specific image of their alternative to a liberal polity.

The Basic Structure of Community Health Programs

To begin, let us imagine the United States as a liberal communitarian polity, at least in the area of health. It is divided into thousands of community health programs (CHPs), each made up of a few thousand to a few tens of thousands of citizen-members.[3] These CHPs might be formed around preexisting community hospitals, health maintenance organizations (HMOs), neighborhood health centers, or business or union health programs, or they might be newly constituted. Each CHP would be responsible for guaranteeing and arranging care for the members, although in some cases the actual provision of care would occur elsewhere. To elaborate this vision, it is necessary to specify six aspects of a prototypical CHP: the administrative and deliberative structure; the decisions about membership and enrollment; the arrangements for financing, determining benefits, and regulating costs; the relationship with other CHPs, hospitals, medical schools, and other social institutions; the role of physicians; and the regulation by higher governmental bodies.

Administrative and Deliberative Framework

In an existing CHP, the daily administration for the provision of care would fall on citizen-members whose occupation is health care management. Decisions about capital purchases, hiring, and the like would be made by the administrators. In this sense, the administrators of a CHP would be similar to the existing administrators of hospitals and HMOs, with the same responsibilities and daily headaches. The main difference between the administration of CHPs and that of existing health care institutions would be in the formulation of policy guidelines and objectives. Currently, the policy and major objectives of health care institutions are determined by a hospital's administrators, medical board, board of directors, or the equivalent. The liberal communitarian ideal opposes such a hierarchical approach; it would democratize these decisions through communal deliberations.[4]

Each CHP would proceed in its own way; part of the recognition of pluralism is that different communities would institute deliberations according to their own models. But we can imagine an idealized set of deliberations occurring in a three-step procedure. First, there would be some need for the CHP members to articulate the broad outlines of their shared conception of the good life. In some communities the outlines of this shared vision would be obvious. All members would recognize the same articulation of the vision, and indeed this commonality would be what has brought them together. This would be most characteristic of a religious community, such as a Mormon or a fundamentalist Protestant community, that has a shared tradition, canonical texts, recognized authority figures, fairly detailed views of acceptable medical practices, and, possibly, already existing hospitals that operate according to its views. But it might also be true of communities that share a well-developed secular philosophy. Many communities, however, will have been formed without a well-articulated conception of the good life. In these communities, articulation of a conception of the good life in the abstract will be difficult. Thus they might begin by considering commonly known medical ethical cases or issues; for example, they might deliberate on the *Cruzan* case, *in vitro* fertilization, abortion, Baby Doe cases, artificial hearts, DNR orders, living wills, euthanasia, AIDS testing, genetic engineering, brain tissue transplants, and the like. And, as in good philosophical discussions, changes in details or facts would be used to surround the issues and highlight the points of agreement, uncertainty, and disagreement. The aim of the deliberations at this stage would not be to establish policies, but for the CHP members to voice their views, justify them, and think through the differences. By covering such issues, and related ones, the CHP members would have deliberated not only on the most pressing medical ethical issues, but through them on fundamental ethical matters. For instance, by examining and justifying positions on *Cruzan* and related cases, euthanasia, Baby Doe, and so forth, the CHP members would have gone a large way toward articulating their conception of the person. In particular, by determining when it is justified to terminate medical care to incompetent patients, the members would have to determine when a patient could no longer realize fundamental human goods. And this would entail specifying such goods and how they relate to fundamental characteristics of persons, whether feeling emotions was essential or self-consciousness or the possibility of autonomous living. By extending this view to other situations, such as Baby Doe cases, and revising it in light of particular judgments of those situations, the members would begin to articulate their conception of a person and the fundamental elements of a human life.

Having deliberated on a conception of the good life by considering particular medical ethical issues, the CHP members could proceed to the second step, the formulation of specific policies. The CHP might establish four different committees made up of about twenty people each. The committees would be composed of administrators, physicians, other health care workers, and members of the CHP. Any medical or financial expertise needed in the deliberations of a specific issue should be provided by appropriate committee members. Thus a committee discussing policies on termination of treatments to incompetent patients might have a neurologist and a critical care physician as members to provide important facts when needed. A different committee would focus on each the four main areas of medical ethics: the physician-patient relationship, the selection of medical interventions, the allocation of resources, and personally transforming technologies. The committees would hold deliberations, open to the entire CHP membership, which would occur over many months. The role of the committees would not be to hold hearings or to dominate the deliberations, but to provide information relevant to the policy questions, to focus the deliberations on specific policy issues, to ensure that all important policy matters were examined, and to distill the deliberations into specific policy recommendations for deliberation by the larger community. In addition, the committee devoted to allocation of resources would submit one—or several—proposed budgets for the CHP.

Thus the committee on the physician-patient relationship might consider the types of informed consent forms to be used and design forms for common treatments; they might also consider the storage of patient information, who should have access to it and under what circumstances. The committee on selecting medical interventions might consider criteria for treating incompetent patients, whether or not to use some experimental therapies or drugs, criteria for provision of commonly used and expensive services, whether to permit abortions, whether the CHP members should be tested for HIV. The committee on allocation of resources might consider what proportion of the CHP's resources should be devoted to nursing home care, drugs, bone marrow transplants, dialysis for patients over age 65, or clinical research. The committee on personally transforming technologies might consider policies relating to brain tissue transplants.

Consider a specific issue: living wills. The committee might begin with the suggestion that the CHP use an existing living will, like the one from Concern for Dying, or draft its own type of living will. The committee might then propose three different uses of the living will. First, each member might be sent a living will, but not be required to use it. Second, each member might be required to fill out a living will form at a scheduled visit to his or her physician; this form would then become a permanent part of the patient's record, to guide physicians and a designated proxy if the patient ever became incompetent. Or third, each member might be required to fill out a living will form during each hospital admission, with the old form being updated after the first admission. Different members of the community might address each option, defining the types of items to be included in the living will, the different scenarios that might be addressed, and how the living will might affect DNR orders, or extending discussions into areas of euthanasia. In the end the committee might draft several different living wills and propose several different ways in which they could be implemented.

After each committee had covered the range of medical ethical issues under its auspices, the recommendations would be brought before meetings of the entire CHP. The recommendations could be described and the rationale for each given. There might be conflicting recommendations from the different committees in need of resolution. For instance, the committee on allocation of resources might not include funds for home health care in its proposed budget, but the committee on selecting medical interventions might recommend the extensive use of home health nurses and aides for the treatment of many illnesses, ranging from uncomplicated myocardial infarctions to infections requiring intravenous antibiotics to the monitoring of hypertension. Over several months the recommended policies and proposed budget would be discussed and approved by consensus or a vote of the CHP members at general meetings. The approved policies would guide the CHP administrators, physicians, health care workers, and members in providing and seeking health care. No doubt individuals would disagree with various specific policies. But most disagreements should be resolvable, although some members might find their disagreements fundamental and leave the CHP for another one.

The third step is a continuous review of these various policies. Implementation of the policies would reveal inadequacies in need of clarification or revision and simple gaps in need of filling. Physicians might find certain policies too cumbersome to implement; members might find some policies offensive or intrusive; new therapies or interventions might require new policies; and budget problems— overspending, underspending, or maldistribution—might require revision of the budget. To address these various problems, the committees might hold periodic discussions and make policy recommendations to the larger CHP.

This is an idealized procedure. Yet, as described, the deliberations on and formulations of CHP medical policies would not be very different from the types of deliberations that currently occur at many HMOs and hospitals that require their own policies in each of these areas. The substantive difference between existing deliberations and those imagined here is in the parties to the deliberations. In existing institutions these deliberations occur in designated committees, often without community representation. The vision suggested here democratizes such deliberations to provide an opportunity for all CHP members to participate in formulating the policies to govern their own medical care. Of course, it must be admitted that even as described in an idealized model, the process of deliberations and policy formulation will be longer and more clumsy than it is currently. Indeed, many of the CHP members may lack information or have faulty information on relevant issues; they may be relatively inarticulate; they may be impassioned about minor issues; they may lack the knowledge or skills to develop coherent policies. Consequently, a significant proportion of the initial deliberations may be spent educating the participants. But the criteria of efficiency are not the only or the highest standards. Whether the inefficiencies are justified in attempting to realize the ideals of the liberal communitarian vision is a moral issue not settled by appeal to efficiency itself.

This view of deliberations in CHPs to devise health care policies suggests that CHP members are not what we ordinarily conceive of as patients or members of a health care group such as an HMO. In fact, it is appropriate to describe CHP members as citizen-members. Use of this phrase is a direct consequence of the endorsement of democratic decision-making. Members of CHPs are not simply provided health care services for an annual fee. Instead, they are responsible for deciding various aspects of the CHP's policies, ranging from what services will be provided to what informed consent procedures will exist. Mandating that such decision-making be democratic, that CHP members have responsibility and authority for fundamental policy choices, transforms CHPs from mere medical service institutions to political institutions. And this in turn makes members not just recipients of services conceived and administered by others, but participating citizens determining the health care policies they will receive. Hence the notion of citizen-members, which suggests the creation of a new type of medical care institution with a new framework for decision-making which is modeled on democratic procedures.

Membership and Enrollment

Each CHP would determine the size it wants to be and devise policies on membership and enrollment. Obviously, if deliberations are to occur there must be some limit on total membership; I have suggested an upper limit of 20,000 to 25,000. Some CHPs might prefer to remain smaller to permit more participation in deliberations. Others may wish to be large to ensure sufficient funds for the provision of a more extensive range of services. Every five years, to coincide with the financing arrangements, each CHP could revise its target size, but it could not exclude existing members. Any unfilled spaces below the target size would have to be open to new enrollees. Candidates for membership could apply as single individuals, families, or groups that have come together because they share the same vision, place of work, or some other characteristic. If the applicants are willing to abide by the CHP's policies and participate in its deliberations, then they are suitable candidates for membership. In considering enrollees a CHP may only use criteria which are informed by its conception of the good life. Criteria such as race, sex, age, occupation, economic status, and the like are not automatically prohibited as being suspect categories. Such criteria can be the basis of admission when related to a CHP's conception of the good life, as in the case of a religious community or a community affiliated by a view of aging or a community affiliated by employment and employment-related health concerns. The use of preexisting physical handicaps, medical illness, or screening health tests as criteria to deny admission should be prohibited. Further, the use of geographic location as an admission criterion should be limited since it can easily be a marker for other characteristics, especially income. Nevertheless, a CHP should be able to limit its geographic size for various reasons related to providing health care services, such as home health care, various public health measures, and educational programs. Discriminations on the basis of some criteria are ruled out, especially, in this context, the health-related criteria, since they would permit certain CHPs to segment the market and to exclude high-cost patients from their membership. This would undermine the ideal of equality. The grounds of discrimination currently employed in the provision of health care would probably not operate—or would be attenuated—with CHPs, because the financing provisions would eliminate the large financial benefit derived from excluding high-cost patients from membership.

There can be formation of new CHPs at any time. This grants people who are dissatisfied, but who do not find other CHPs congenial to their philosophy, the possibility of forming their own CHP. Of course, there would be many practical difficulties in forming new CHPs, but they hardly seem insurmountable given the rate of formation of new HMOs. In 1986, for example, 146 new HMOs were formed, a 30 percent growth in the total number of plans over just one year.[5] Further, it is doubtful that many CHPs will have closed memberships. With about 25 percent of the American population changing residences each year, there should be sufficient movement to ensure open places in many CHPs. Finally, with the size of CHPs being relatively small, citizens in urban, suburban, and even many rural areas should have many different CHPs to choose among for their affiliation. Only in fairly sparsely populated areas would citizens have a very limited choice among alternative CHPs.

Health Care Financing, Benefits, and Cost Control

Each person or family in a CHP would receive a voucher from a federal board. The voucher would represent five years of payments. A person or family would give this voucher to their CHP, which in turn would receive annual payments for five years from the federal board based on the voucher. No additional money would be available from the government, although CHPs might decide that members should contribute more money to provide additional medical services. The five-year time period for vouchers should permit longer-range planning, especially in the areas of capital equipment and training of employees. A CHP would be responsible for determining what benefits to provide its members, what care is most important, and which services will not be provided by the CHP. In deciding how to structure the provision of its health care services, the individual CHP will also have full responsibility for determining cost control programs. To elaborate the financing and benefit arrangements of CHPs, five questions need to be addressed.

First, where would the funds for the vouchers come from? Currently the United States spends in excess of $600 billion per year on health care. The identical pool of resources could be available for any new health care system without any redistribution of resources from other social programs or additional burden to individuals and private corporations. To establish this voucher scheme, there would have to be a shift of funds. In the current system, the government pays about 41 percent of the health care budget through Medicare, Medicaid, and other programs, such as Veterans hospitals. About 31 percent of the funds come from premiums to private health insurance programs, and another 25 percent come from direct patient payments for health care services.[6] Under a voucher system, all resources would need to be pooled into some sort of health care trust fund. There are many good practical arguments against making such a trust fund a governmental responsibility, especially the reluctance of congressmen and senators to be responsible for a growing federal budget and for setting the premiums.[7] Nevertheless, to dissociate access to health insurance from jobs and the ability to pay, to ensure equitable payments to all, will necessitate redistribution of resources. This makes a significant federal role in a health care trust fund inevitable. Thus a federal health oversight board would seem a desirable part of the financing structure of this view. The federal board's responsibilities would include establishing a health care trust fund, collecting funds, and disbursing vouchers. Precisely how these funds would be collected, whether through a progressive payroll tax or some combination of business tax and other taxes, is not of particular concern here. However, the fund-raising mechanism should be progressive, and, at least initially, the fund should not consume additional resources from other sectors of the economy.

In addition, the federal health oversight board would allocate monies to health care research. Leaving each CHP with the complete responsibility for determining what proportion of funds will go to research might well create a "free rider" problem: some CHPs might contribute little and use the medical discoveries financed by others.[8] Hence, it might be best for the federal board to simply reserve, say, 5 percent of all health care funds for research. These funds then might be distributed to specific researchers through a single granting body. This would not be dissimilar to the National Institutes of Health granting program. In addition, individual CHPs still would have the option to contribute their own funds to research, even to specific research programs. This two-tracked system would permit individual CHPs to express their priorities on research programs through their contributions to research, without compromising research through the "free rider" problem.

Second, what would the value of the voucher be? Currently the

United States spends about $2,000 per person on health care. In 1986, Medicare covered 31 million elderly and disabled people with greater medical needs at a cost of $78 billion, or about $2,500 per beneficiary.[9] There is nothing special or morally mandated in such figures. Indeed a lower figure, about $1,600, could be justified by considering the well-known linear relationship between per capita gross national product and per capita health.[10] The current spending provides a suitable standard for the value of vouchers without adding any additional burden to the economy. Further, we might establish a sliding scale for the vouchers, providing more funds for the elderly than for adolescents because of the increased illness and use of resources. The aim of such a sliding scale would be to ensure that a CHP does not have an incentive to exclude elderly members because they might use more services. Such a sliding scale should ensure the principle of equal access. For instance, we might establish the value of a voucher for those over age 65 at $3,000 per year, for those between 45 and 65 at $2,000 per year, for those between 18 and 45 at $1,500 per year, and for infants to age 18 at $2,000 per year. These prices are based on 1986 costs; the total cost should approximate what the country currently spends for health care. Finer gradations or slight increases in the value of the voucher for the elderly might be necessary adjustments which the federal health oversight board could implement.

This allocation of resources is generous, devoting in excess of 11 percent of the nation's GNP to medical care. Overall cost limits would be established not by reducing this amount, but by limiting future increases. Clearly the voucher value should increase with inflation. But if there is to be an effective ceiling on total health care cost to the nation, the increase should reflect the consumer price index, not the more inflationary medical care "market basket." If individuals want to spend more because their conception of the good life puts a higher priority on physical health than on other goods, they should be able to do so. But the nation should not be forced to supplement this additional expenditure.

Third, how would the vouchers be used? Each person or family would be granted a voucher. Vouchers are usually the mechanism favored by conservatives because they permit individuals to choose among services in the free market, negating the power of governmental bureaucracies. Some liberals have endorsed the idea of vouchers in education, for instance, as a way of overcoming "state bureaucracies and . . . mobili[zing] parent/student constituencies in a fashion that also serves to mobilize citizenship."[11] But most liberals are rightly suspicious of them, especially since they seem to encourage private, market choices rather than communal deliberation and action. I shall not defend the use of vouchers in general. But it is worth noting two points. First, the scheme being outlined is not a voucher plan alone; it involves an entire institutional framework within which vouchers are to have a role. Thus the proposed system is not a free-market one, with vouchers functioning as money. The institutions provide certain constraints on the use of vouchers. Second, in the area of medical care the use of vouchers may not be as threatening as in other public services. Unlike the area of education, medicine has not been thought of as a public good; the government has never assumed responsibility for providing medical services for all regardless of income. And unlike education, medicine has not previously been associated with geographic neighborhoods and local control over schools. Medicine has always involved travel to hospitals and physicians' offices. Most important, it seems that vouchers are the only way to ensure simultaneously the redistribution of health care resources for equal access and communal decisions about allocation of resources in medical care. Indeed, without some kind of voucher plan, it seems impossible to have a health care system which fosters communal deliberations on health care matters. Conversely, the worst aspects of a voucher system—its undermining of communal association and decision-making—will be limited in this liberal communitarian ideal because the vouchers will be valid for five years, engendering a commitment to a single CHP, and because individuals and families will not just be purchasing a good, but will be participating in deciding policies under which they will receive their medical care. While the choice to join a particular CHP will be private, the way a CHP makes decisions regarding the provision of health care services will require citizen-members to participate in communal deliberations.

The government's contribution for the voucher would represent the total amount the government would contribute for health care. A CHP of 20,000 members would have about $40 million per year in voucher funds to provide for health care. (This is an approximation, since the amount depends upon the particular age mix of a CHP.) Each CHP will decide how it wants to allocate its resources, that is, what services are basic medical services that should be provided to its members. Consequently, the number of basic distributive decisions confronting each CHP will be quite large. To take just a few examples, a CHP would have to decide whether to provide nursing home care, or leave it to individuals or families; whether to pay for pharmaceuticals, eyeglasses, and other medical appliances; what proportion of the CHP's resources should be spent on preventive, acute, and chronic care; whether to cover expensive items such as organ transplants; whether to provide services in hospitals or through home health care services; and so on. Further, each CHP will need to devise a scheme to limit unnecessary use of services and to ensure that costs do not escalate beyond the budget limits. Again, many options are available, from patient co-payments at the time of use of services, to education of physicians and health care staff, to simply cutting services. Different CHPs will make very different choices; the final health care schemes will reflect differences in the conceptions of the good life as embodied in medical care policies.

In addition to determining what health care services the CHP should provide and what cost containment policies should be implemented, a CHP will need to decide the amount of resources it will contribute to research and what research efforts should receive high priority. Again, such decisions will reflect the particular values a CHP espouses. Some CHPs may contribute a high amount of their funds to research, say 10 percent of total health care resources; other CHPs may not want to contribute to research at all. Similarly, certain CHPs may collect monies for basic scientific research into genetics; others may refuse to fund development and testing of life-saving interventions but will fund treatments for chronic diseases of the elderly; other CHPs may find a particular disease, such as AIDS, of particular importance and in need of all their research resources; others may find having children a critical good and generously support research into reproduction. Ultimately, because CHPs embody self-rule, it will be the members of each CHP who decide what benefits they receive and what mechanisms will be implemented to limit costs.

Fourth, how will CHPs be able to spend more or less than the voucher amount? Presumably, most CHPs will work within the generous financial limits generated by voucher income, ordering programs from high priority to low and allocating the existing monies accordingly. Some CHPs, however, may feel that additional health care is more valuable than alternative uses of their resources and might increase their total health care expenditures over the voucher amount by imposing additional health care taxes on CHP members. Other CHPs might view alternative uses of their voucher money as more valuable than health care and would decrease their health care expenditures to a level below the voucher amount, rebating the conserved resources to members. In the extreme, free-market CHPs might give each individual member the full value of his voucher in cash, leaving him to find medical care in the market on a fee-for-service basis. The options of raising additional money by taxing and of disbursing unallocated funds are necessary if we are to realize the liberal communitarian ideal of having communities decide their conception of the good life and the policies that flow from it. This option permits individual CHPs to determine for themselves how important health care is compared to other uses of their resources, and how urgent the various health services are.

To ensure that the additional taxing mechanism is not abused to exclude the poor, the disabled, and those with few resources, some restrictions will be necessary. For instance, any CHP that imposes a tax on itself might be required to set aside at least 20 percent of the taxed income in a reserve for grants to those unable to afford the tax. Standards for determining what is affordable could be set by the regulatory boards. One possibility might be that any family which earns less than 250 percent of the poverty level would receive a grant, and the grants would be distributed on progressive sliding scale. Further, no new applicants could be excluded for membership in a CHP because they could not afford any additional taxes. The tax would have to be high enough to ensure that those who could not afford it would receive grants. Any unused portion of this reserve for grants—which, in wealthier CHPs, might be the entire 20 percent—should be given to a national or state fund for medical research. This is to ensure that CHPs with only rich members do not tax themselves and then retain the 20 percent set aside for grants, since they have no poor members.

Fifth, how will the citizen's right to leave be accommodated? While the vouchers would be for five-year periods, the money would be disbursed on an annual basis. The aim of using a long-term voucher is to engender a commitment to a particular CHP. However, citizens may need to leave a particular CHP because of fundamental conflicts with the CHP philosophy, changes in employment location, or other obligations. Consequently, there must be a mechanism for these people to obtain a refund from their current CHP and a voucher for submission to their new CHP. This function might be assigned to a state health oversight board. The process should not be too onerous, since all citizens have a right to leave. However, this option should not encourage frequent changes based on whim or, worse, attempts to find a new CHP which provides a service the patient currently needs but which has not been included as a basic service by his CHP. (I address this issue later in this chapter, in the section on excessive pluralism.) Thus part of the state health oversight board's responsibilities would be to review the grounds for switching CHPs.

Before concluding this section it is worth highlighting some of the important advantages of this type of financing and benefit scheme. To put it simply: Through democratic deliberations on health care services, this scheme combines the advantages of a central financing mechanism, a large enough pool of patients to spread risks and costs, and the acceptance by citizens of limits on health care services. In particular this scheme should foster a strong incentive to limit waste and to encourage physicians to eschew expensive but marginally beneficial interventions. In the current system savings from health care are not retained for other health care programs but lost to insurance company profits or in the larger government budgets to non-health-related programs, which often do not directly benefit those saving the health care funds. With CHPs any financial savings in one area will be transferred to provide another urgently needed service to the CHP members. This scheme therefore has the advantages of a single payment mechanism which can limit costs and ensure priority in funding more urgent services.[12] Further, citizens themselves will have a strong incentive to limit their own claims for resources, knowing that spending on a relatively minor or marginal service will deplete the overall pool of resources, and thus reduce services available to them through the CHP. Thus the size of the CHPs and the single fund of health care resources for all CHP services should provide a practical way of harmonizing the abstract social interest in efficient use of resources with the physician's and patient's concrete self-interest in providing an extensive range of good medical care. It does this without using the fee-for-service market incentives that discriminate against the poor and can prevent people from seeking necessary medical care.

In a related way, there should be widespread acceptance of the scheme of services provided and the attendant limitations on particular services. The current system encourages citizens to view limits on health care services as externally imposed and to petition politicians for increases regardless of the effect on other governmental and social services. Self-rule by the citizen-members of the CHP makes any limits on health care services self-imposed. If the members do not find the distribution of resources and limits on services acceptable, they can alter the services provided and tax themselves for additional resources. The grounds for complaining to others will be very limited.

Finally, the size of CHPs should grant them some important bargaining power with providers of specific health care services with whom they may contract for services. Like HMOs in the current system, these CHPs should be able to obtain lower costs from hospitals and others in exchange for their fairly predictable demand for services.

Relationship to Other Health Care and Social Institutions

Clearly a CHP composed of 20,000 people and roughly fifty physicians, with a budget of $40 million, will not be able to support all the subspecialists and sophisticated technologies of modern medical care that the CHP members may find important. This implies that CHPs will have to coordinate and associate with other health care institutions. As with all CHP policies, the precise form of the relationships will depend upon the particular CHP's views and interest in associating with other institutions. But we can imagine some of the relationships that typical CHPs might seek.

First, recognizing that its relatively small group of physicians cannot provide all possible medical and surgical services, the CHP would probably seek relationships with nearby hospitals. At one level, a CHP would probably affiliate itself with a community hospital to provide routine in-hospital treatments such as appendectomies. At another level, a CHP might affiliate itself with a tertiary care center to provide more complex diagnostic tests and treatments, ranging from magnetic resonance scans and cardiac catheterization to open heart surgery and experimental cancer therapies. The CHP would negotiate the types of services it wanted access to and the desired payment arrangement.

Further, the CHP might want to associate with other CHPs to provide a range of outpatient, nursing home, and home health care services that each could not afford separately. For instance, several CHPs might establish and jointly administer a facility to perform the growing number of outpatient surgical operations, such as hernia repairs or cataract operations. Similarly, several CHPs might agree to purchase a CT scanner among them, housing it at one CHP facility for their common use. Other CHPs might agree to establish jointly an outpatient cancer treatment center. Such joint projects could extend to the establishment, financing, and operation of a shared nursing home, rehabilitation and occupational therapy center, or home health care service. The individual CHPs would participate in such joint arrangements, while maintaining their distinctive visions by offering different services and care programs in the areas outside the joint projects.

In addition to affiliations with hospitals and other CHPs for the provision of care, some CHPs may want to be affiliated with medical schools. Such an affiliation might be desirable because it would permit CHPs to participate in developing particular therapies that they think are needed, to bring additional physicians to their patients by training medical residents, and to establish a continuing education program in conjunction with the medical school for their own physicians.

Such coordination and association are not novel. Currently many HMOs and neighborhood health centers have affiliations with particular hospitals for inpatient treatment of their members. HMOs and neighborhood health centers also maintain affiliations with medical schools. Indeed, in some instances medical schools actually have established HMOs and neighborhood health centers. Similarly, community hospitals have relationships with tertiary care institutions to provide certain sophisticated treatments that can be administered only at large medical centers. The types of associations formed by CHPs would build on these preexisting ones.

Finally, it is important to acknowledge that health status is affected by many factors besides medical care services. Conversely, many social problems, such as homelessness, are related to the availability of medical care services. To be effective, therefore, medical care institutions cannot be autonomous, but must be coordinated with schools, housing, work sites, sanitation facilities, and other social institutions. Ideally, CHPs would be coextensive with local governments responsible for these other social institutions. In such circumstances, the comprehensive coordination of policies throughout all social institutions born of a common conception of the good life would be easy.

But this is unlikely, and the scheme developed here does not assume such ideal circumstances.

This liberal communitarian scheme does allow for the fact that CHPs may develop relationships with these other social institutions. Indeed, they may find these relationships indispensable to securing health. For instance, a CHP might want to encourage its members to engage in regular exercise and other health promotion activities. To this end it may want to establish work-site recreational and health promotion facilities.[13] Given the diversity of workplaces for CHP members, this may be difficult, but if many CHP members work at, or near, a particular factory or office building it may be possible to establish such a recreation and health promotion site in conjunction with the factory or office. Similarly, some CHPs may find teenage sex, contraception, and pregnancy counseling important and may try to establish a school-based clinic in conjunction with the local high school. Still other CHPs may find that certain housing conditions, lead water pipes and lead paint, for example, threaten their children members and might try to work with the public housing authority or local landlords to eliminate such health risks.

On another level, CHPs that have retarded members might find it important to have comprehensive social programs, such as protected housing and jobs, for such people. They might try to develop such programs, or where they exist promote them. CHPs with physically handicapped members may find that the health and overall well-being of their handicapped members require greater social activity, both in job opportunities and recreational options. The same would be true of CHPs that had a significant number of elderly members whose health would benefit from participation in volunteer jobs and other social activities. Thus the CHPs may try to work with local businesses and government agencies to create such jobs and recreational opportunities.

One of the effects of such efforts at coordination might be for CHP members to build more systematic and comprehensive political structures to coordinate these social institutions in order to realize the various facets of a conception of the good life. CHPs may work with centrifugal force, expanding liberal communitarianism from health care outward to other social institutions. If the hope of systematically instituting participatory democratic institutions in one step is unrealistic, CHPs—to change the metaphor—may provide the nidus for the crystallization of participatory democratic institutions in other areas.[14]

The Role of Physicians

With the existence of CHPs, there would be three different forums for physicians to practice in. Most commonly, physicians would be affiliated with CHPs. They would participate in formulating, implementing, and refining the CHP policies. But clearly their primary function would be to care for CHP patients within the policies they help establish. This role would be similar to the current role of physicians within hospitals, HMOs, and neighborhood health centers. CHPs, however, would be more democratic, and physicians would participate as members with important expertise and insights into making policies for health care. The salary for these physicians would be determined and paid for by the CHP.

In addition some physicians, notably subspecialists and physicians in hospital-based specialties, would be based in hospitals. They would provide services to members of CHPs who came to the hospital for specialized care under some formalized relationship between the CHP and the hospital. For example, cardiac surgeons would operate on patients from CHPs that contracted with the hospital to provide certain cardiac operations; oncologists might work at a hospital treating CHP members with experimental therapies; cardiologists might work at a hospital providing angioplasties. The salary for these physicians would be determined and paid for by their employing hospitals.

Finally, there would be independent physicians operating their own medical practices. They would contract with individual CHPs for their services. Thus a physician with a particular expertise, such as the care of one disease entity or one diagnostic technique, might have an independent practice which serviced many different CHPs. These independent physicians might also treat patients who paid for care out of their own pockets. Such patients might come to receive care not provided by their CHP, such as cosmetic surgery, or they might come seeking a second opinion outside their CHP. In either case the individual patients would personally pay for the physician's services. These physicians would be paid both on a fee-for-service basis and through their CHP contracts.

Oversight and Regulatory Boards

There would need to be several different regulatory functions to ensure that the liberal communitarian ideal is actually realized by the

CHPs. One important oversight function would be to ensure that every citizen is a member of a CHP. Depending on the number of CHPs and their size, this may require the regulatory boards to encourage CHPs to admit more members or to encourage individuals or groups to establish additional CHPs. Another related oversight function would be to ensure that applicants for membership in a CHP are not discriminated against on the basis of race, age, sex, financial status, handicaps, screening health tests, and the like. Third, a regulatory board would have to ensure that the rights to participate in CHP decision-making are respected. This would require scrutinizing CHP plans for policy formulation and review. And finally, a regulatory board would have to oversee CHPs that impose additional taxes on themselves to provide for extra services. The board would have to ensure that these CHPs place money in a reserve fund for grants to those members unable to afford the tax and donate unspent reserve funds to the national fund for medical research.

In addition to overseeing issues of CHP membership and participation, a regulatory board might also be necessary for other functions. For example, conflicts might arise between different CHPs and between CHPs and hospitals over the coordination and provision of services. A regulatory board would be in the best position to mediate such conflicts while ensuring that CHP members continue to receive the necessary medical care.

These regulatory functions are probably best done close to local CHPs. To endow one national regulatory board with powers to oversee 10,000 CHPs, each organized distinctively, with different policies and services, seems a sure way to create an unresponsive, resented bureaucracy. It would be much more tolerable and responsive to the desirable diversity of CHPs to have state regulatory boards. As one health economist put it: "Homogeneity has given way to [differences in health care provisions.] The individual patterns found across the land are best understood and best addressed at a locus of control that is closer to those delivery systems and to the people they serve. California is not the same as West Virginia."[15] These state health oversight boards (SHOB) should ensure that the CHPs are actually adhering to the liberal communitarian ideal. However, the history of state discrimination and denial of civil rights suggests that a federal health regulatory board overseeing the individual state boards and setting guidelines on participation and membership discrimination may also be desirable.

Besides ensuring that SHOBs are enforcing appropriate membership and participation practices, there is another, independent reason for a federal health regulatory board that I have already noted: to oversee the voucher financing aspects of the scheme. A federal board would have to (1) collect the money to finance the vouchers, (2) disburse funds in exchange for the vouchers, (3) operate the refund program for people who switch CHPs, and (4) manage the fund for research derived from the unspent reserve fund from CHPs that taxed themselves to provide additional services.

This two-tiered regulatory structure, with the federal board establishing guidelines for membership and participation as well as collecting and disbursing funds, while the state health oversight boards scrutinize the practices of individual CHPs, is similar to that which currently exists in Medicare and other social welfare programs. It seems the most desirable structure to ensure sensitivity to differences among CHPs, while ensuring the uniform protection of the fundamental rights of participation.

In order to demonstrate that the liberal communitarian ideal is a viable theory, I will focus in the following three sections on the justification, the philosophical plausibility, and the political practicality of this ideal. Again, I am not attempting to justify or demonstrate the practicality of this vision generally. Instead, I am limiting the discussion to the medical care area. But this should serve as a paradigmatic example for the larger polity.

Justification of CHPs

Can the liberal communitarian vision be justified in the area of medical care? The form of justification is identical to the reflective equilibrium invoked in liberal political philosophy; it is necessary to show that the liberal communitarian ideal coheres with the explicit or latent ideals, principles, and practices of the medical system.

The existing health care system lacks a coherent set of objectives and policies justified by a single conception. Many institutions and practices have assumed their shape and function through historical accident, power struggles, and accommodation to conflicting values and thus have one set of explicit objectives and yet contradictory policies or financial incentives. Often no one finds these institutions or practices valuable or acceptable; they continue to exist by inertia, not by choice.

The combination of private health care institutions and insurance coverage unrelated to specific institutions undermines the institutional arrangements necessary for communal discussion and control over health policies. Governmental input, in Medicare for instance, has largely been limited to paying for the care of a particular class of patients, not in policymaking. Private hospitals, HMOs, nursing homes, and other institutions formulate their own policies. Although they serve critical public functions, their finances and governing structure are not determined publicly. Alone, this situation does not exclude communal participation in decision-making, but combined with the existing medical finance system it does. Current medical insurance, reimbursement, and regulatory structures tend to discourage a stable pool of members or patients associated with a single medical institution who might participate in policy deliberations. For instance, with private insurance, a family may go to one hospital for obstetrical care and adult health services, to another for pediatric care, and to a third for emergency services. Such institutional arrangements preclude communal involvement in the formulation of policies at hospitals, HMOs, nursing homes, and the like, even when such involvement is valued.

The point of this survey, then, cannot be to show how liberal communitarianism permeates the existing system, but rather to show that various traditions and practices of this system are consistent with the communitarian vision, even if current institutional structures undermine its realization. Further, the survey can show that this vision, although not fully developed in the current system, plausibly integrates principles and practices of the existing medical care into a coherent and consistent whole and also resolves issues that have been in dispute.

To proceed, I distinguish two facets of the liberal communitarian ideal in medical care: local control over and communal deliberation on medical practices and policies.

Examples of Local Control over Medical Policies

National health care policies are almost completely limited to Medicare, the financing of care for the elderly and the disabled, and research through the National Institutes of Health. By contrast, the tradition of local control over medical policies and practice is enduring. In part this tradition is reflected in and sustained by the American health insurance policy, which leaves individuals free to find their own physicians and hospitals and leaves to hospitals and other medical care institutions the authority to formulate policies with limited governmental guidance.

In the area of selecting appropriate medical interventions, one might note two examples of local decision-making in which different communities have established different policies to express their particular values. Abortion clearly reflects such local decisions. Since 1973 a woman's right to an abortion has been constitutionally protected. But variations among states in the regulation of this right have existed, and the Supreme Court has clearly stated that such variation is permissible. The variation, however, is even more decentralized since medical institutions are not required to perform abortions. Most hospitals offer abortion services, but many individual hospitals prohibit them because they find them unethical. Of course this is most obvious in the case of Catholic hospitals that deem abortion contrary to their religious teachings on family and the role of procreation. Other religiously affiliated hospitals have made similar decisions.

Such choices are, however, not limited to religiously affiliated medical institutions. After *Roe* v. *Wade*,[16] secular prepaid health groups were forced to confront the ethical issues of abortion in the guise of whether they should pay for them. For instance, Group Health Cooperative of Puget Sound, the nation's eighth oldest health maintenance organization, founded in 1947, had to decide whether abortions and contraceptives should be included as part of its standard services to members or whether to leave these services to individual preference and payment. Since the original decision to include abortion services, the question of whether to provide abortions has recurred. The debates have concentrated on two points: the ethics of abortion, and the question of whether a whole community, many of whose members do not find abortions ethical, is obligated to pay for such an intervention.

A second type of intervention in which different ethical views have led to the establishment of different policies in different institutions and localities is the termination of medical care. General policies about terminating care are made at the state level. And there are variations among states. For instance, many states have recognized that the right of patients to refuse life-sustaining treatments includes the right to refuse artificial nutrition and hydration, whether by intravenous infu-

sion or by a tube into the stomach or intestines. But other states have
adopted different policies. Oklahoma, for instance, passed the Nutrition and Hydration for Incompetent Patients Act, which prohibits an
individual from requesting the termination of artificial feedings and
water in a living will.[17] Within states, individual medical care institutions have also established their own policies on terminating artificial
nutrition and hydration. Some hospitals and long-term care facilities,
for example, object to terminating artificial nutrition and hydration
and have refused to honor a patient's request to terminate such treatments. Generally these hospitals and nursing facilities believe that the
termination of artificial nutrition and hydration displays disrespect for
human life, sanctioning suicide or the killing of a human being. If
patients or families have wanted termination of artificial nutrition or
hydration, the patients have been transferred to other medical institutions that do not find terminating such treatments unethical.[18] The
point is neither to catalogue the variations of policies nor to judge
which policies are right, but to note the tradition of state and institutional local control over the selection of medical interventions to reflect different ethical judgments.

Local control is also pervasive in the area of allocating medical resources. One example comes from the United Mine Workers of
America's health fund. In 1949 this fund began a general medical care
program for miners and their families. As initially envisioned, the
program was to be comprehensive, covering all medical care services
from dental care and pharmaceuticals to home and office visits and
hospitalization.[19] The poor health of many miners overwhelmed the
supply of services and resources. Thus the union was forced to revise
its plan, allocating its resources to what it considered the most urgent
medical needs. The union's health care fund stopped covering "home
and office visits, drugs, mental hospitalization, routine dental and eye
care" while maintaining rehabilitative services for ex-miners who had
work-related disabilities, especially respiratory problems.[20] Clearly
this is an instance of local decision-making concerning the allocation
of health care resources, defining those basic medical services and
those aspects of care that the community deemed less urgent to be
paid for by individuals and families. And the conscious decision to
provide rehabilitative services to miners injured or disabled from min-
ing rather than routine health care for working miners and their families constituted a decision about justice: those injured in the course of
work were owed care and services before those still working.

A second historical example comes from the provision of dialysis to patients with chronic renal failure. Before the federal government assumed full funding for dialysis in 1974, individual communities and local hospitals had to decide how much to spend on dialysis and how to select the patients. Dr. Scribner at the University of Washington developed the arterio-venous shunt that made chronic dialysis possible. Consequently, Seattle was the first community to grapple with the issue of resource allocation and patient selection in dialysis. The simple fact that decision-making regarding dialysis initially occurred in Seattle—not in Washington, D.C.—highlights important elements of local control in such policies. The details are also illuminating.

In the 1960s, the entire Seattle community prided itself on its Artificial Kidney Center. Seattle's financial support, through gifts by local corporations and community fund-raising, even during recessions, was vital to the Center's existence, supporting almost 20 percent of its annual operating budget.[21] Because funds and trained personnel were scarce, selection among the potential candidates had to occur. The Seattle Center established an Admissions and Policy Committee composed of local residents and physicians to articulate selection criteria and to select patients. Community members were included in the selection committee to bridge the community and the dialysis center, providing a perspective to both parties from the other side. The intention was to include certain elements of democratic decision-making.[22] Viewing it as an evasion of their duty, the Committee explicitly rejected using a lottery for patient selection among medically eligible candidates.[23] Instead, the Committee established selection criteria that reflected specific ethical judgments. For instance, in recognition of the value of community solidarity—that community members should benefit from community sacrifices—only Washington state residents were considered. Similarly, finding the family an important institution to be sustained, the Committee established marital status and dependents as critical selection criteria.

Prior to 1974, Seattle was not the only case of local control over dialysis. Most dialysis centers were established with substantial local financial support because the community deemed it an important service to provide to some, even if it could not allocate enough resources to provide dialysis to all medically eligible patients. But local control extended beyond financial support for the dialysis centers. In fact, the patient selection criteria were defined at each dialysis center and varied among the different communities allocating scarce dialysis places. A

1969 study of eighty-seven dialysis centers, sponsored by the Department of Health, Education, and Welfare, found a wide variety of selection processes and criteria.[24] Eight of the centers used lay committees in some stage of the selection process; most centers relied on physician committees or a single physician for selection; a few included nurses, social workers, and psychiatrists on their patient selection committees. The actual selection criteria also varied. Some centers relied on the patient's ability to pay; others selected patients on a first-come, first-serve basis; many other centers used implicit or explicit "social worth criteria," including family environment, employment record, availability of transportation, willingness to cooperate, ability to understand treatment, occupation, or future potential.[25] The different selection criteria reflected different values and commitments in the various communities.[26]

Again, the important point is not the justification for the actual criteria used in selecting patients, but the fact of local control.[27] Different localities funded dialysis to different degrees and devised their own ways of selecting among medically acceptable patients. These differences reflected the communities' different ethical values.

Such local control over resources and selection criteria only ended when dialysis was provided to all chronic renal failure patients by the federal government through the ESRD program. At one level this was a significant improvement, averting the premature deaths of thousands of people and eliminating the wrenching moral dilemmas surrounding patient selection. Still it constituted an important loss in the usurpation of local control, a loss rarely acknowledged. In Seattle, as in most other communities, the dialysis center had altered the very social structure. It "became a community-oriented social institution" that granted individuals a chance to demonstrate their commitment of mutual support, beyond family and friends, to fellow citizens.[28] And reciprocally, most dialysis centers, even those not directly funded or operated by the community, "felt an obligation to serve the residents of the immediately surrounding area. This responsibility [was] felt even at institutions of international reputation [such as the Mayo Clinic], which [drew] some of their patients from very far afield."[29] By eliminating the need for strong communal support for dialysis centers, federal funding of dialysis eliminated the necessity for this type of local decision-making and communal solidarity. Indeed, whatever would be decided at the local level was overridden by the federal government. To put it simply, full federal funding eliminated both the need for and the power of local decision-making, undermining any rationale for local community groups committed to such efforts.

A third example of local control over the allocation of resources can be noted in the area of organ transplantation. This control occurs at several different levels. First, individual states have decided whether to provide Medicaid coverage for heart, liver, and bone marrow transplants. Recently, Arizona and Oregon decided that organ transplants were not as important as other types of care that could be provided to many more citizens and tried to stop funding such transplants. One Arizona health care official justified the choice: "[We are] looking at the larger public good . . . For the cost of [a] bone marrow transplant, [the state] could [provide] medical coverage for a full year to an average of 1,065 children, or cover the births of more than 175 children." [30] Conversely, in July 1984 the state of Illinois guaranteed every one of its citizens, whether indigent or not, up to $200,000 in state funds to cover the costs of any organ transplant procedure, if the cost was not covered by other sources, such as private insurance. [31] Illinois clearly argued that such life-saving transplants were more urgent than other types of needed but underfunded medical care, such as well-baby visits, immunizations, and prenatal care for pregnant mothers.

Decisions about funding organ transplants are not just state-level decisions. Health maintenance organizations have also had to decide whether to provide organ transplants to their members as part of the normal benefits package, whether to charge individual members an added premium for the service, or whether to have no policy on transplants, leaving individuals who desire coverage to buy supplemental insurance outside the HMO. The Group Health Cooperative of Puget Sound engaged its membership in discussions of these very options. It found that most members were more committed to routine and preventive care than to organ transplants for the few. [32]

Individual hospitals have also made important choices about establishing and supporting organ transplant programs. For instance, after the first heart transplant, Stanford University committed resources to Dr. Norman Shumway's program to develop heart transplantation. It became one of the only centers in the entire world doing any heart transplants during the decade of the 1970s. And among its criteria for patient selection was the ability to pay. Conversely, the Massachusetts

General Hospital's board of trustees refused to permit heart transplantations in 1974 and reaffirmed this decision in 1980. Part of the rationale behind these decisions was that a heart transplant program "would commit costly and scarce resources to a procedure that at best would benefit a very few patients; these are the same resources that public demand has kept available for the benefit of many."[33]

Other institutions have made similar decisions in regard to other organ transplantation services. In the area of kidney transplants, Howard Hiatt notes that one Boston hospital decided to start a transplantation program despite the fact that four other hospitals in the city of Boston offered renal transplants. The rationale offered by this hospital had nothing to do with the allocation of resources, but focused on the need for transplantation services to ensure a high-quality education and training program for the surgical interns and residents at the hospital.[34]

This limited survey indicates that local control over critical health care issues is not the exception. Different communities have adopted different policies and justified them by appeal to different ethical ideals. The tradition of local control over health care policies is old and pervasive in the current health care system.

Finally, it is worth noting that many previous calls for reform had urged a single national health care program, whether by insurance or by a nationalized health care system. A national program, it was thought, would be the best way to make health care policies uniform and thereby secure equal access. This approach has been all but abandoned. As one health insurance official remarked, "the spirit of local initiative and voluntary effort in the health-care field was dampened by the spate of federal and state legislation in the 1960s and 1970s," but its importance has been recognized again in the last decade.[35] Indeed, recognizing the tradition of local control, recent reform proposals have urged retaining "our tradition of multiple pathways" with the adoption of many state or locally run programs rather than a single national scheme.[36]

Examples of Democratic Deliberations on Medical Policies

While local control over health policies is a dominant American tradition, the same is not true of communal deliberations on these issues. Most health policy decisions are made by select boards at hospitals and HMOs and by state regulatory agencies, "unfortunately, often with input only from health care professionals."[37] As just noted, for instance, it was the Massachusetts General Hospital's board of trustees who decided that heart transplants should not be performed in its institution. Generally, the health policy decisions have been made in a hierarchical and not a democratic manner.

While the need for expertise is often cited to justify the absence of democratic decision-making, this is not the complete explanation. Entrenched interests, especially those of administrators and physicians, have sometimes opposed communal deliberations on health care policies.[38] But the main explanation I have already noted: The contradictory institutional structures, especially financial and reimbursement schemes, preclude realization of this ideal by undermining the possibility of a stable pool of patients who would participate over a sustained period in democratic deliberations on health care policies.

Despite these obstacles, there is a minority tradition of democratic deliberation on health care policies, especially, but not exclusively, within the area of community medicine. As an Institute of Medicine study concluded:

> An outstanding, relatively constant, and important feature of community medicine as it has been practiced in this country since the early 1960s has been the formal involvement of community members in the governance of the practice . . . While the level of sophistication and degree of involvement of community members has varied significantly, the principle has been articulated in a variety of ways and written into regulation for most of the federal programs (community health centers, migrant health, Title X) that provide services for underserved populations . . . Community involvement in medical practices has attracted sufficient adherents and captured the loyalties of patients, administrators, and clinicians enough to remain a strong theme in community-oriented practices in the United States.[39]

Supporting this recognized principle are important instances of communal deliberations on health care policies.

One example occurs in the system for protecting human subjects and animals during medical research. All hospitals conducting federally funded research are required to have an institutional review board (IRB) to establish standards for protecting human research subjects and to review and approve research proposals using these standards.[40]

Membership on these committees must extend beyond hospital medical and nursing staff to include community or lay representatives with "sensitivity to such issues as community attitudes."[41] In addition to the institutional review boards, medical institutions receiving federal research funds are also required to have Institutional Animal Care and Use Committees to review "the care and treatment of animals in all animal study areas."[42] Like IRBs, they are also required to have community representatives to participate in their deliberations on and approval of research proposals.

Admittedly these committees are representative, not democratic, and most lay members are not elected, but selected by hospital officials. The absence of election stems from structural constraints: it is not clear who should constitute the citizens eligible to vote. Nevertheless, such committees were established to foster communal participation in defining acceptable standards for research on human subjects and animals. They provide a forum for communal review of and control over the treatment of people and animals by medical researchers. Thus while these committees are not perfect models of communal participation on health care policies, their establishment does constitute a clear attempt within the confines of the existing health care system to engage community members in deliberations on health care policies.

A second example can be found in the Group Health Cooperative of Puget Sound, Washington, an HMO with more than 350,000 members spread over twenty-five centers (excluding subsidiaries).[43] Its board of trustees is required to be a lay board, elected by the members.[44] Traditionally, the board has determined the range of services covered by the HMO. Unlike governing bodies of other HMOs, this board has developed mechanisms to foster communal deliberations. One is an annual meeting of the membership open to participation by all members. At this open meeting resolutions on policy matters are debated and voted on. Any member of the HMO or medical staff can collect signatures of members and submit a resolution for debate. Although the passed resolutions are not binding on the board, they create moments for communal deliberations and constitute tangible evidence of the members' judgments. A recent general meeting that discussed the controversial issue of eliminating abortion services to the HMO members produced a turnout of some 3,000 members for the discussion.

A second forum for communal deliberations at Group Health Co-operative occurs at each of the individual health centers. Each health center has a council composed of elected members. The council meets with the clinic's director and participates in setting the budget, consid-ering development issues, and reviewing quality-of-care issues. In ad-dition, members of these councils come together with council mem-bers from other centers in regional councils for joint policy planning.

A third forum for communal deliberation is the "town meetings" at the Group Health Cooperative's various centers.[45] These town meetings are not permanent institutions but have recently been used to discuss three important and controversial policy questions: whether the HMO should cover heart, liver, and other organ transplants, whether the HMO should grow, and whether the HMO should pro-vide care to people who are not insured. In the town meetings devoted to the question of transplant coverage, for instance, members of Group Health Cooperative's task force on organ transplantation made an informational presentation to members about the medical and fi-nancial aspects of organ transplantation. Then the members discussed the issue of transplantation, whether these procedures should be paid for by the HMO, and how funds should be collected. The entire pro-cess was geared toward exchanging information and discussing the issue to clarify ideas and positions; members did not vote on any pol-icy resolution. The task force who presented information and mod-erated the discussions summarized the opinions expressed for review by the board of trustees. Attendance at these town meetings was vol-untary. The process was repeated at five forums throughout the geo-graphic area covered by Group Health Cooperative and occurred over a two-month period. Such town meetings provide an opportunity for education and thus for educated communal discussions.

These institutional arrangements established by the Group Health Cooperative of Puget Sound represent an important model for com-munal deliberation of health policy matters confronting an HMO. While they do not grant the membership direct control over policy decisions, they do permit members to discuss critical issues confront-ing the HMO and to articulate their considered opinions in resolu-tions. The Group Health Cooperative's arrangements illustrate that such communal deliberations exist and are practically feasible within large medical institutions.

Another example comes from the original neighborhood health

centers begun in 1966 as part of President Johnson's War on Poverty. These centers, originally funded under the community action program of the Office of Economic Opportunity, were situated in poor urban and rural communities with the intention of coordinating health care and related community services. Early in the program the Department of Health, Education, and Welfare had developed plans to establish 1,000 such centers to serve 25 million people. Yet by 1978 there were "only" 125 centers serving over 1.5 million people.[46] The extensive plans were never realized in part because of changing and contradictory governmental policies for the centers, and in part because the Nixon and Ford administrations "downplayed the neighborhood health center model," reducing their funds, making long-term funding unpredictable, and curtailing implementation of services.[47] While the aims of the centers include accessible, high-quality primary care, this is not their "sole or perhaps even their main concern."[48] Instead one of their most important aims is to foster "intensive participation by and involvement of the population to be served, both in policy making and as employees."[49] Having this as a main objective of a large federal health care program is itself an important demonstration of the communal deliberation ideal in medical care.

One health center associated with Montefiore Hospital in the Bronx established four different forums for communal deliberations on the center's policies. The health center first formed three ad hoc advisory boards from local residents attending meetings. These covered the areas of medical care, training, and organization of a permanent community advisory board. These ad hoc boards did have an important influence on decisions. The "Committee on Medical Care decided whom the first satellite Health Center would serve, since it [could] provide service for only a fraction of the population . . . some 8,000 of the 45,000 [eligible] residents."[50] A 21-member neighborhood advisory board composed of community residents was elected. After a 21-session orientation intended to educated lay people on a health program, the board began organizing subcommittees to oversee various aspects of the health center.[51] The staff of the health center also held "an extensive series of dialogues with the residents of the community—more than 150 apartment meetings with small groups of people" and meetings with formal organizations in the area—to discover what aims the community had for the center and how the center could help the community members. Further, the center organized block health clubs to provide more permanent "liaison between community residents [and] the health center staff." Finally, since the health center also obtained many of its employees by training community members, these people provided "an important bridge . . . [for communicating] the needs of the community to the professionals." [52] The Montefiore program began in a run-down area of the Bronx where fewer than 10 percent of the population voted in national elections, where education was low, familiarity with health care took place in hospital clinics, and cynicism and apathy were rampant. And yet through these forums, the program was able to begin to generate community involvement by providing extensive opportunities for communal participation in defining the health care policies and practices of the center.

The Lee County (Arkansas) Cooperative Clinic provides another example. Opened in 1970, this clinic served the poor black residents of a southern rural county. As in the Montefiore-affiliated clinic, one level of community participation in health care decisions in Lee County comes from the fact that many of the clinic's employees are community members who were trained and supported in seeking additional formal education by the clinic. On a more formal basis, the clinic has a 14-member board elected by patients registered at the clinic. The board meets monthly, and the board's director follows the center's daily activities. As a clinic to serve poor blacks in a rural southern county, it became a focal point in conflicts between blacks and whites in the county. In combating the systematic impediments erected by the white residents of Lee county, the clinic provided an institutional structure to foster communal participation and solidarity: "In overcoming the opposition of local physicians, the county judge, white citizens, county health departments, and pharmacists, the black community [of Lee County] has developed a sense of strength and participation in the political process." [53]

Of course, not all neighborhood health centers were able to develop successful arrangements for communal participation in defining policies of the centers. And further, the neighborhood health center program has had much adverse publicity; it is often attacked along with the other Community Action Programs (CAPs) established during President Johnson's Great Society program as fostering more "misunderstanding" than actual democratic participation.[54] Yet such criticisms involve more guilt by association than substance. Indeed, as a prominent health economist put it, "a close examination of [the neighborhood health care] program shows it to be a surprisingly successful governmental health program . . . [T]he large majority [of neighborhood health centers] have survived, flourished, and attained considerable success as providers of high quality health care."[55] Indeed, even by the narrow measures of improved mortality and morbidity at competitive costs, and of reductions in hospitalization and inappropriate use of emergency room services for routine primary care, the neighborhood health centers are generally quite successful.[56] And, interestingly, those with more community participation have seemed more successful in many respects.[57] If there is any reason for the failure of these centers, it is less intrinsic than a consequence of the constantly changing policies from Washington and ultimately their abandonment by the federal government.

The final example comes from a recent project to implement concretely the "goal of broader public involvement in bioethical decision-making."[58] Beginning in 1983 and 1984, a newly founded organization, Oregon Health Decisions, began a three-step process of (1) training community leaders to organize and moderate discussions on health care issues, (2) holding hundreds of community meetings and symposia on ethical problems in health care with existing community groups, such as the Rotary Club and Chamber of Commerce, and (3) organizing general "town meetings" to discuss bioethical issues.[59] After these local meetings community representatives attended an Oregon "Citizens Health Care Parliament" in which resolutions on specific health care issues were introduced, debated, and voted on over a two-day period. These resolutions served to communicate back to the local meetings and to form the basis of lobbying efforts with health care organizations and state government. In practical terms, the project seemed to develop a consensus within Oregon on policies relating to terminating care and "death with dignity" and to prompt state legislation on the issue. In addition, Oregon Health Decisions initiated public discussions on the more complex problem of health care costs as part of its Oregon Health Priorities for the 1990s project. This project's ultimate aim is "to make specific recommendations to the Governor's Office and state legislature regarding the priority and approximate level of funding" among fifteen different state-supported programs.[60]

Beginning *de novo,* without a clear institutional mechanism or political authority for implementing ideas and sentiments, Oregon Health Decisions has encountered many difficulties. In some sense it suffers from being a democratic process devoid of power, making many citizens unwilling to expend the effort necessary for meaningful communal discussions. In addition, the parliament was less democratic and more representative since it was limited to fewer than 100 participants from the entire state. And furthermore, the "representatives" were not elected from the community meetings.[61] Yet, for all its difficulties, Oregon Health Decisions represents an important attempt to create an institution which can both educate the community on important health policy matters and engage them in discussions of policy options. And it seems to have strong appeal. Many other states have developed projects to foster community participation in health care policy formulation modeled on Oregon Health Decisions.

There are other components of the tradition that conflict with this vision, especially hierarchical decision-making by boards of trustees and medical boards removed from communal participation. But Oregon Health Decisions, like the other examples, shows the possibilities of fostering communal discussions on health care policies even without direct institutional avenues for implementing these decisions. The rapid spread of similar projects to many other states reveals a desire for institutionalization of local control over and communal participation in health care policy formulation. The main problems or constraints on developing such participation have been from institutional barriers—reimbursement schemes and bureaucratic inertia—that have made it quite difficult to create a stable, long-term patient constituency to participate in shaping their own medical care services. Further, existing forms of participation often consist of democratic deliberations without correlative power, undermining the motivation of people to participate on a sustained basis.

At a minimum, these examples illustrate that the liberal communitarian vision is not foreign to the existing system, although it may stress aspects that are not dominant in the system. But the question is whether these practices exist as aberrations of history or locality or whether, upon reflection, the values intimated in such examples are deemed valuable, to be cultivated and sustained by restructuring of the health care system.

Philosophical Plausibility of CHPs

Resolving Medical Ethical Dilemmas

In the area of medical ethics, liberal political philosophy has failed to realize its objective by failing to provide a framework for principled public deliberations on the issues of terminating medical treatments to incompetent patients and the just allocation of resources in medical care. Does the liberal communitarian vision provide such a framework? In other words, is the liberal communitarian vision a philosophically plausible alternative to liberal political philosophy?

In some sense I have already answered this challenge. In Chapters 3 and 4 I suggested that by appealing to specific conceptions of the good life, it would be possible to create a framework for addressing these medical ethical issues. And within the liberal communitarian vision, CHPs are granted the financial resources and political authority to deliberate on and formulate policies over the whole range of medical ethical issues by appeal to particular conceptions of the good life. For instance, we might imagine a CHP with members committed to the relational conception of the good life. This CHP would then consider what type of specific policies to have for terminating medical care and allocating resources by appeal to this conception. The members might agree to have a strict age limit, say 72, for the provision of medical services. Those under this age would receive all medically necessary treatments, but those 72 or over would not receive hospital admissions and the provision of all acute medical services, except inexpensive ones such as antibiotics. Conversely, there would be extensive home nursing and social services and devices to assist in daily living for those over 72. All patients in a persistent vegetative state would be denied all forms of medical treatments; primitive and receptive patients (see Table 3.1) might receive nursing care, while interactive patients would be eligible for acute medical services. The CHP might also contribute to a fund for research into new devices to assist the handicapped and might offer to test such devices for companies.[62] Clearly this CHP would have to address many other health issues, but its conception of the good life would guide deliberations on these matters.

Within the liberal communitarian vision we would expect different CHPs to espouse different conceptions of the good life and, therefore, to provide their members different types of medical services. An elderly community might espouse the physical conception, funding all life-saving treatments but leaving the cost of nursing home care and medical devices to individuals. A homosexual CHP might espouse the autonomous conception and decide to allocate its resources to outpatient drug treatments for AIDS patients aimed at forestalling life-threatening infections and tumors, but might decide that in-hospital life-saving treatments should not receive funding while hospice care would be supplied. This CHP might support a particular type of AIDS research and arrange to participate in studies of experimental therapies.

The philosophical plausibility of the liberal communitarian vision inheres in the creation of a framework for deliberation on medical ethical issues. In this framework individual CHPs can justify laws and policies governing these issues by appeal to their particular conception of the good life. Pluralism is protected because different CHPs can espouse different values.

Deliberation and Conceptions of the Good Life

This argument for the philosophical plausibility of liberal communitarianism might suggest that conceptions of the good life are mechanically applied to diverse medical ethical issues. It might appear that once CHP members espouse a particular conception of the good life, policies are deduced and little more need be discussed. Deliberation then would consist of discussing the technicalities of implementation and administration.

This image is misleading. As I argued in Chapter 5, conceptions of the good life are never settled and immutable; a conception embodies a picture of human life that is but a sketch in need of specification and refinement. These details are added in the process of deliberation, whether that deliberation is abstract, about the conception of the good life itself, or whether it focuses on a specific policy and implicates refinement of the conception of the good life. There will be a dialectical relationship between conceptions of the good life and particular ethical judgments; considerations of each may lead to reciprocal revisions. This can be made clearer by elaborating the role of deliberation in policy formulation.

In some CHPs, especially those created around preexisting and highly developed conceptions of the good life, many medical policies will already be specified in great detail. For instance, Orthodox Jews have fairly well developed views against the termination of care to incompetent patients, DNR, abortion, and euthanasia as well as clear priorities for certain types of medical services, with a high priority placed on reproductive services and life-sustaining interventions. Nevertheless, in the process of health care policymaking even such a CHP would have to develop even finer specifications of a fairly detailed and comprehensive conception of the good life. For example, the issue of heart transplants has created important debates about the precise method of defining death and whether harvesting of hearts in the presence of brain death is consistent with Jewish law and traditions. Similarly, the development of fetal tissue transplants for Parkinson's disease would confront an Orthodox Jewish CHP with the need to articulate a policy. But this would require considering many basic ethical questions and elaborating the CHP's conception of the good life. The community would have to consider whether the use of fetal tissue in human transplants is absolutely precluded; or whether tissue from spontaneous abortions is permissible but tissue from therapeutic abortions is prohibited by Jewish traditions; or whether transplantation of tissue to alter the functioning of a human brain is inconsistent with Jewish values; or whether the chance for a person to regain near-normal neurological functioning without altering higher brain functions is a higher good. The CHP members would have to deliberate on such questions, offering different answers to them, suggesting why one view would cohere better with Jewish traditions and understandings, and coming up with an authoritative policy to reflect their final position. Such a process of deliberation would be necessary for specifying policies to regulate many other medical interventions, such as genetic engineering for Tay-Sachs disease.

If CHPs created in communities that share a fairly detailed and well-articulated conception of the good life will need ongoing substantive deliberations on basic moral issues, then CHPs in which the members only agree on some broad moral principles and a few specific policies will need them even more. Indeed, we can expect that many CHPs will form among people who share some specific views on a handful of the most visible and controversial medical ethical issues, but have not explored other issues or elaborated more abstract moral positions. For instance, some people might form a CHP because they agree on the need to provide organ transplants to all people, to develop life-sustaining care for all people, to implement extensive antenatal genetic screening and abortions, to terminate all types of medical interventions including artificial nutrition for all permanently incompetent adults, to prohibit physician-assisted euthanasia but permit assisted suicide, and the like. Agreement on such specific policies would outline a very rough conception of the good life, the broad strokes of a picture. But clearly there is a myriad of other issues that such a CHP would have to confront in providing medical services to its citizen-members. The CHP members would have to decide in much more detail what services should be given high funding priority, whether to fund nursing home care, what type of compensation scheme to have for medical errors and predictable side-effects of certain treatments, what type of informed consent should exist for patients with mental disorders, whether a pregnant mother should be forced to receive certain treatments for her fetus, whether to purchase organs for transplantation, and so on. Devising specific policies on these and other issues would require discussing and refining the roughly sketched conception of the good life. The process of deliberation should make the isolated but important positions that formed the basis of the CHP cohere and should expand their application to less prominent issues. This process of deliberation would be more one of creating collective values than of interpreting existing ones.

One issue that such a CHP might address is what type of medical services to provide terminally ill but competent patients where there are no known medical interventions to prevent death, but where there are some palliative treatments. This issue arises in the case of patients with heart failure who are bed-bound and are not expected to survive for more than another year. Such patients may not qualify for heart transplants because they are over 60 years of age or have some complicating diseases.[63] It also arises for patients with idiopathic pulmonary fibrosis, a chronic progressive disorder of unknown cause that reduces the oxygen transfer capacity of the lung tissue. Currently the disease is fatal four to five years after onset despite therapy. Clearly the same situation arises for many cancer patients. What services should the CHP provide such patients? Should they be given every available medical intervention whether or not it has any effect on longevity? Should they be given medical interventions, such as antibiotics for infections, that might prolong survival for six months or longer? Should they be given hospice or home supportive care but no medical interventions? In answering such questions, the CHP would be making ethical judgments about the worth of certain kinds of terminal lives. It would also be elaborating the ends of medicine, what it means to ameliorate ill health. And clearly in considering such options the CHP would have to balance the costs for such care against using the resources for other medical services.

We can imagine several different positions that CHP members might advance. Some might think that patients afflicted with these chronic, progressive diseases, who have no hope of cure or even of prolongation of life, should receive no medical care. The advocates of this view might argue that a meaningful life requires the capacity to pursue normal human activities; when there is no chance of a functional life or returning a patient to some normal human activities, medical care is futile and should not be provided. Thus once a person has become afflicted with a disease for which there are no therapies and which leaves him bed-bound, he should receive no further medical interventions. Such patients should be able to receive supportive care at home or in a hospice, but no medical interventions. The advocates of this position might indicate that such a view is consistent with the CHP's policy of not providing treatments to even mildly mentally incompetent patients. They might suggest that patients with heart failure or terminal cancer are analogous because they may be considered "physically incompetent."

Other CHP members might argue that while such patients may not be able to engage in work or other physical activities, they are still competent and capable of engaging in meaningful human activities, especially being with their families. These human moments are worth preserving, especially for terminally ill patients. Hence medical care should be provided when it gives competent patients the chance to live a bit longer in the company of their family and friends. In this vein treatments for pneumonia or even surgical operations, say removal of a diseased gallbladder, might be provided. In support of their position, advocates might cite the CHP's policy of providing extensive life-support interventions and organ transplants even though in some cases almost half of all transplant patients do not survive a year.

Other CHP members might advance other positions. Given such initial positions and justifications, the CHP members would deliberate. They would listen to the arguments of those who held other positions; they would begin to refine their conceptions of a worthy human life and to assess their ideas by delineating their policy implications for other types of medical treatments. In addition, the members of the CHP would try to make the entire range of policies cohere within a single conception of the good life. For example, the advocates of one position might apply their conception to other instances of medical care such as dialysis or care for AIDS patients, seeing if the results support the CHP's policy proposals.

This process of deliberation would go on until one set of members persuaded the other of their position, or until they found some other conception and set of policies that more accurately captured their shared convictions. In the end there still might be some residual differences of vision and policy. Assuming the residua would be what I have called resolvable conflicts, then a policy might have to be adopted by a vote. But the issue would remain open for further discussion. And experience with the agreed-upon policy might reveal new considerations for CHP members to discuss or might form the basis for policy revisions. Of course, there is the possibility that some CHP members would find the residual differences, if there were any, fundamental. For instance, a member might find an unequivocal policy that absolutely refused to provide any medical care to mentally competent but debilitated patients too incompatible with his views of a worthy human life. And he might believe the CHP members were so settled in their position and so far beyond persuasion as to make modification of the policy almost impossible. A member in such a position might feel the need to leave. Such possibilities cannot be excluded. Nevertheless, it does not seem they will be frequent, since agreement on the most controversial basic ethical and policy issues will be what has brought the various CHP members together. And such deliberations will center on less controversial, and probably less fundamental, matters.

These brief examples reveal the ways in which conceptions of the good life will require development when informing the formulation of medical care policies within CHPs. They also suggest the indispensable role of communal deliberation in this process, both in the further specification of a conception of the good life and in relating a conception to particular policy issues.

The Liberal Communitarian Vision and Toleration

In the liberal communitarian vision pluralism is assured by the multiplicity of different communities pursuing different conceptions. Individual communities can espouse their own particular conception of the good life. Communities dedicated to a variety of aims are permitted in the liberal communitarian vision.

But the democratic ideal embodied in this vision is not neutral. At the least we can say that some conceptions of the good life, while not excluded by the liberal communitarian vision, do not share a commitment to the same ideals. The traditions and practices of these communities will discourage participation in the deliberative democratic processes and commitment to the ideals of liberal communitarianism. And for a polity committed to the liberal communitarian vision, the proliferation of such communities would be destructive. Commitment to the liberal communitarian vision then suggests there should be stronger support for some particular conceptions of the good life that cohere with and sustain the liberal communitarian ideals. This can be made clear by considering possible conceptions of the good life that some CHPs might espouse and their effect on liberal communitarian ideals.

For example, there might be a CHP committed to the principles of unfettered free market competition and to the minimal state with no redistributive powers or deliberative political institutions. It might be called "The Adam Smith CHP," and its members might include Milton Friedman, Robert Nozick, and Ronald Reagan, if they all retired to the same area of California. In this CHP each member would receive a cash refund for the voucher and obtain his health care in the market, through unaffiliated physicians and hospitals, using his own financial resources. Each CHP member's health care decisions would be individual and private. There would be no communal deliberations on policies; there would be no need for communal meetings. Indeed the CHP members would not really be members, for there would be no common political institution to be members of.

Clearly "The Adam Smith CHP" shares few of the ideals of the liberal communitarian vision. For instance, its conception of respect for freedom centers on respecting the individual's property rights and rejecting the role of political autonomy. Institutionally, this is demonstrated by the elimination of the structures of deliberation necessary for such political participation. Consequently, although the liberal communitarian vision would permit people to form such CHPs, their excessive flourishing would be detrimental to this vision. The members of such CHPs would not share the liberal communitarian ideals and would not support their perpetuation. Those committed to liberal communitarianism would permit but not endorse communities espousing the values of the "Adam Smith CHPs." Fortunately, it seems unlikely that there would be a proliferation of such "Adam Smith CHPs." While many people profess commitment to the free market in the abstract, few accept its value in the area of medical care.[64] Indeed, we are increasingly unwilling to see those with few resources suffer from diseases that can be cured or ameliorated by modern medicine. And this attitude is unlikely to be altered under CHPs.

Similarly, there might be a CHP committed to the principles of utilitarianism and the application of cost-benefit analysis to all areas of life. It might be called "The Jeremy Bentham CHP," and its members might include many prominent members of Wall Street, executives of major corporations, economists, and utilitarian philosophers. In this CHP all decisions about the provision of medical services and the termination of care would be subject to cost-benefit calculations. To do this the CHP might establish a cost-benefit review committee composed of health economists to evaluate all interventions, with the intention of ranking available services from the most to the least cost-effective. The purpose of the CHP then would provide only those services that passed a certain cost-benefit threshold. The CHP's communal meetings would be to inform the members of the cost-benefit calculations of new interventions.

Such a "Jeremy Bentham CHP" would not be committed to public deliberation on a common conception of the good life. The very activity of communal deliberation is quite inefficient. The time spent on education of the participants, discussions, and continual opportunities to reinvestigate settled policies is always excessive in comparison with hierarchical decision-making. And the benefits of such democratic deliberations, self-rule, self-development of the participants, and the establishment of a common life, are very hard to quantitate and do not lend themselves to assessment by cost-benefit calculations. For this reason a true utilitarian CHP would not give communal deliberations much importance. Furthermore, in the process of applying cost-benefit calculations to the various medical interventions there will be an inevitable reduction in the qualitative assessments of opportunities and human pursuits. Indeed, regardless of how expansive the notions of costs and benefits may be when conceived, the inevitable tendency of such calculations, especially within medical care, is to reduce these factors to easily quantified units, such as money, mortality, and return of economically productive functions. Using such analyses and their attendant scales of measurement will undermine the possibility of assessing medical services by their effects on qualitatively different opportunities. Indeed, over time such utilitarian analyses might undermine the meaning and possibility of appealing to such qualitative distinctions. And this would eliminate the significance of any public deliberation. Thus a "Jeremy Bentham CHP" would tend to undermine the values of the liberal communitarian vision by undermining both the very activity of communal deliberations and the content of such deliberations.

While such utilitarian CHPs would be permitted within the liberal communitarian vision, their proliferation could undermine the stability of the vision. Unlike the case of "Adam Smith CHPs," there is a strong tendency to favor such analyses, especially in efforts to contain medical costs. "Jeremy Bentham CHPs" might flourish just as cost-benefit analysis now flourishes.

In contrast, the ideals of some of the communities' particular conceptions of the good life will cohere better with the ideals of the liberal communitarian vision; that is, a commitment to liberal communitarianism is more consistent with some particular conceptions of the good life. The liberal communitarian vision places great value on communal deliberation aimed at political autonomy, self-development, and the establishment of a common life. Community members are committed to one another, to the community itself, and to the perpetuation of their common conceptions and ideals. Consequently, the flourishing of those particular conceptions of the good life, such as the relational conception, that affirm the importance of a common life, the obligations of one generation to serve posterity by educating them and granting them authority, sustains the liberal communitarian vision. The coincidence of values between liberal communitarianism and these particular conceptions of the good life means that in sustaining the community's particular vision, the community also strengthens the commitment to liberal communitarianism. Those committed to liberal communitarianism as an ideal should want to see such conceptions of the good life and their policies sustained.

The question then arises as to the limits of toleration. In a liberal communitarian vision can "Jeremy Bentham CHPs" be suppressed? Conversely, can other CHPs more conducive to the ideals of liberal communitarianism be differentially encouraged and supported? The acceptance of a plurality of conceptions of the good life does not mean toleration of any conception of the good life. Just as liberal political philosophy excludes those conceptions of the good life that conflict with justice, so too does liberal communitarianism. But the emphasis need not be on excluding and limiting CHPs that advocate conceptions of the good life hostile to liberal communitarianism. Instead extra support for those CHPs that espouse conceptions of the good life congenial to the liberal communitarian vision is possible. Such support might include additional funding or legal protections for CHPs which hold regular communal deliberations and organize other efforts to broaden the participation of their citizen-members in decision-making. We need not delve into the details of what such programs might be. The important point is that the justification for such interventions would appeal to the worthiness of the ideals embedded in the liberal communitarian vision, the worthiness of political autonomy, individual self-development, and the establishment of an ongoing communal life.

In this way the liberal communitarian vision is neither neutral nor necessarily autocratic. The flourishing of certain conceptions of the good life will therefore reinforce commitment to liberal communitarianism. Reciprocally creating institutions that embody the ideals of liberal communitarianism will tend to enhance the appeal of those conceptions of the good life that share its ideals. This is not to say that liberal communitarianism necessarily prohibits CHPs committed to conceptions of the good life which do not cohere with its ideals. But this vision can justify differential support of certain political institutions by appeal to the ideals embedded in liberal communitarianism.

Political Practicality of CHPs

No political ideal, including the liberal communitarian vision, should be evaluated by the probability of actual enactment. The vagaries of actual political decisions often depend upon contingencies unrelated to the merits of a vision. Nevertheless, my proposal raises many pressing practical questions that cannot simply be ignored. The answers to these practical questions may also dispel some conceptual reservations.

In considering the political practicality of the liberal communitarian vision, the constant temptation to apply criteria of efficiency evaluated through quantitative input and output variables, such as morbidity and mortality, must be restrained. The objective of the liberal communitarian vision, and of CHPs, is to institutionalize a political ideal to resolve medical ethical issues, including the issue of allocating medical resources. Realizing this objective cannot be achieved merely by monitoring statistical measures. While CHPs should improve the health of their citizen-members, what will count as good health will vary among CHPs and will frequently not correspond to the usual standards of longevity. In addition, other worthy ideals, especially democratic participation and control and the capacities they develop, cannot be statistically measured. Therefore, the practicality of CHPs must be evaluated by many measures.

I shall consider three major issues regarding the implementation of the liberal communitarian vision: the transition period, the actual provision of health care, and physician and community participation.

The Transition to CHPs

Obviously, switching from the current agglomeration of fee-for-service practice, HMOs, other forms of managed medical care, private health insurance involving many companies, federally funded Medicare, state-run Medicaid programs, and much uninsured care to a system of CHPs with federal and state oversight boards would entail enormous changes. But the sheer quantity of transformations should not condemn such a proposal as unrealistic. The structure of American medicine is in the midst of a fundamental transition. The final result is still undetermined. Indeed, as yet there is no clear objective, much a less a blueprint. In such an atmosphere, implementing a new scheme may be easier than it might first appear.

Furthermore, many changes are conducive to the introduction of CHPs. While health maintenance organizations (HMOs) have existed for many decades, they have grown from enrolling just 2 percent of Americans in 1970 to 4 percent in 1980 to 9 percent in 1986. And they continue to grow in excess of 20 percent per annum.[65] By the mid-1990s, it is estimated that almost 90 percent of health care services will occur within managed programs.[66] In addition, beginning with Medicare and diagnostic related groups (DRGs), there has been widespread introduction of prospective payments throughout the last decade. There has also been a transition from hospital-based, acute care toward outpatient treatments and surgical interventions as well as toward more long-term, chronic care. In the context of such changes, CHPs may not be so alien.

We might begin by imagining a biphasic implementation plan for CHPs. The first phase would be a deliberative phase, granting "start-up" funds for the planning and initial organization of a CHP to pre-existing community organizations or newly formed CHP planning groups. This would include discussing and formulating broad policy proposals to cover the most controversial aspects of medical services, contracting with existing medical institutions such as hospitals and physician practices, distributing information to potential CHP members, obtaining initial commitments for membership, and initiating communal discussions on the more specific policy details.

The second phase would be an implementation phase, beginning a year or so after the deliberative phase, in which CHPs would begin to provide health care. Vouchers would be given to people who demonstrated affiliation with a particular CHP. The vouchers could then be redeemed by the CHP at an oversight board by satisfying a few minimal requirements to ensure that the actual provision of health care services would occur.

Initially, the deliberative and implementation phases might be directed at four target groups. The first group would be the uninsured and those covered by Medicaid. As with the start of the neighborhood health care program, the CHPs might be organized by community groups, university departments of community medicine, and others already involved with the poor, unemployed, and underinsured. While such an approach seems desirable because it attacks the greatest need for health care services, it has also been criticized because it lacks effective cost control mechanisms and because it "does not provide a building block for a more universal structure."[67] No doubt providing medical care coverage to the uninsured first would require a net total increase in health care costs. And no doubt providing care to those now excluded would appear more of a "hand-out" program for society's "have-nots" than the first phase of a comprehensive scheme for all citizens.

These objections could be mitigated if three other groups were included for the initiation of CHPs. A second target group would be the elderly. Rather than provide Medicare, the federal government might offer inducements to permit elderly groups, such as retirement communities and associations, to create their own CHPs. Such a program might emulate recent efforts granting unions, corporations, and other organizations the opportunity to manage health care services for their retirees using Medicare funds.[68]

A third target group might be members of managed health care programs such as HMOs, union health care programs, preferred provider programs, and others. These managed programs are similar to CHPs, with the major differences being in size and decision-making and administrative structures. Consequently, in these managed programs the deliberative phase would involve breaking the enormous existing managed programs into smaller units and instituting democratic procedures for decision-making.[69]

A fourth target group might be any community organizations that want to begin a CHP for their members. There might be certain religious groups that would like to begin a CHP in order to implement their values in their own medical services. Similarly, there might be other community groups organized around neighborhoods or in small towns that would form CHPs in which the citizen-members determined health care policies for themselves.

As each of these groups began to operate CHPs, other citizens would be given the opportunity to join these CHPs with government-supplied vouchers. This would provide a chance for CHPs to broaden their membership and for individuals to join CHPs that implemented policies consistent with their views.

Such a two-step phase-in, aimed at several distinct groups which would be eager to form CHPs, would present several important advantages. First, the start-up funding of the deliberative phase would permit these groups to begin to debate the services and other health care policies they want to institute. There would be time to organize the initial aspects of such policies before the CHP was responsible for the actual health care of its citizen-members. Thus the funding of a deliberative phase would permit institutionalization of a democratic decision-making process. Second, by having the uninsured among the first target groups, CHPs will immediately fill health care needs. In addition, there will be the important effect of indirectly supporting institutions that have provided uncompensated care for these people, many of which are under extreme financial stress because of this generous care. Third, because the uninsured are combined with the elderly, middle-class citizens already in managed health care programs, and voluntary community groups, the program will not suffer the political stigma that afflicts public assistance programs. Indeed, by incorporating politically powerful groups concerned about health care issues, this phase-in plan for CHPs should ensure sustained support. Furthermore, by including diverse groups the CHP program will be a suitable foundation for a comprehensive system applicable to all citizens.

Of course, phasing in a program with these four target groups cannot ensure that all citizens will become members of a CHP. Creating CHPs for the uninsured, the elderly, and the members of existing managed programs even at best could only include half the United States population. Creating and organizing CHPs for the remaining portion of the population will require other steps. These might include the elimination of tax advantages for health insurance, inducements for the creation of work-site CHPs at individual factories and major office and governmental centers, inducements to physician group practices to create CHPs among their patients, and the like.[70] Given the tremendous increases in the number of HMOs and their enrollments, it seems probable that many people would be willing to create managed care programs.

The Provision of Medical Care through CHPs

Can a CHP organize the full range of health care services for its members? From purely supply-and-demand considerations, CHPs should have no difficulty attracting physicians. The impending surplus of physicians, as well as the tendency for many recent medical graduates to shun private practice for managed health care programs, should be favorable for CHPs. The avoidance of prepaid plans by physicians is no longer valid and is unlikely to recur.[71] Furthermore, while in the past community-based programs had to compete with the allure of lucrative private practice, in the future the alternatives for physicians will be fewer and less lucrative. In addition, studies of neighborhood health centers showed that those with more community participation in decision-making actually had an easier time retaining physicians.[72]

Second, CHPs should be able to contract with physicians and hospitals for services their staff physicians cannot provide. Many neighborhood health centers, HMOs, and other managed programs already supply the full range of medical care services to their members by contracting for specialized services their own physicians cannot provide. For example, the Watts Health Plan has entered into service contracts with four different medical groups to provide specific types of medical services beyond the capacities of their own staff physicians and "maintains contracts with six public and private hospitals and one nursing home" for all inpatient care.[73] The past difficulties that managed health care groups had in obtaining access to hospitals and obtaining hospital privileges for their staff physicians should not exist with the current oversupply of hospital beds and hospitals searching for a guarantee of patients.

Third, as all doctors know, many factors besides the existence of medical services can affect an individual's health, including housing, food, pollution, the location of medical clinics, and so forth. One of the common frustrations of current medical practice is the physician's limited ability to control and influence these other, "nonmedical" factors. They cannot be bought with a prescription at the pharmacy or ordered in a hospital like a chest X-ray. CHPs should alter this by enabling the community to provide related social services that can improve the health of its members. As community organizations with financial resources and a sizeable number of community members, CHPs will be better able to develop community initiatives. For instance, assuming the community wants to develop adolescent clinics in high schools with full contraceptive and prenatal services, it should be relatively easy for CHPs to do this, in part because the CHP and the school will serve the same community and in part because the CHP will be able to mobilize resources to provide a comprehensive service. This has been the experience of neighborhood health centers that have instituted clinics in schools.[74] Other neighborhood health centers have assisted their members by developing food markets with farmers to improve nutrition, by changing public transportation services for their handicapped members, and the like.[75]

Fourth, there is the perpetual problem of providing complex medical services to residents of rural communities. These problems are specific neither to CHPs nor to the American medical system. The CHP structure may provide resources to alleviate some of the difficulties. For example, a rural CHP might decide to establish an extensive network of nurse practitioners and other non-physician medical personnel to provide primary medical services, relying on fewer physicians. A rural CHP might be more willing and able to incur financial losses in maintaining a rural hospital with its primary care services than is currently possible. Further, there are the resources of a community collectively confronting a common problem. By bringing together a community with guaranteed funding for years in advance, a CHP can create options that individual people devoid of a large pool of resources and power do not have. This is especially true in the case of training local residents to provide some medical services in rural areas.

Fifth, having a community with guaranteed long-term funding should permit CHPs to develop and provide services that may not be offered or are offered only to a small extent within the current system. Thus a CHP should be able to fund the provision of more extensive nursing home care, home health services, and similar services that may not already exist.[76] In addition, it should be relatively easy for several CHPs to form joint enterprises to provide services that each of them wants but cannot afford individually.

Finally, it is worth noting that there is no reason to expect the costs of providing medical care services with CHPs to be higher than under the current system. HMOs are certainly cost-competitive with the fee-for-service sector, and because they can guarantee a certain number of patients to hospitals and other medical service providers, they can negotiate reduced rates for care. Similarly, studies of neighborhood health centers have shown them to be cost-competitive with the fee-for-service sector as well, and when their overall effect on improving health through changes in housing, education, and other related social institutions is measured, they reduce the use of hospitals and probably total health costs.[77] CHPs will have a strong incentive to make their services cost-effective because the amount and range of medical services that citizen-members can receive will depend upon the cost and use of these services.

Participation in CHPs

Will physicians participate in organizations in which non-physicians have a role in policy formulation? Will citizens participate in the democratic decision-making structures? Will CHPs degenerate into health care schemes indistinguishable from current HMOs? Can the polity do anything to sustain democratic deliberation within CHPs? These are important questions which focus on the stability of CHPs and whether they can realize the liberal communitarian ideal. Without an actual test of CHPs there can be no definitive answer, but there are some points worth considering.

In considering the likelihood of physician participation in and acceptance of CHPs, one can differentiate two areas in which the community might try to formulate policies. First, the community might try to set medical and professional standards, standards defining the appropriateness of certain diagnostic tests or the most effective therapies for certain diseases. Second, the community might formulate ethical policies, defining priorities among services, establishing guidelines for the treatment of incompetent patients, outlining the type of informed consent procedures to be instituted, and the like. The line distinguishing these two types of policies has not always been clear. Often physicians have objected if community groups or others discuss either type of decision. In the first area physicians do have expertise, and this is the proper province of their professional judgment. Physicians and physician organizations rightly object to attempts by non-physicians to formulate policies over these matters, whether explicitly or more subtly through reimbursement policies.

The second policy area does not include medical choices within the technical province of physicians. Decisions on the issues of allocating resources and care for incompetent patients are properly conceived of as communal decisions. It is precisely these types of policy choices that the community should be discussing. Like other CHP citizen-members, the medical staff of a CHP will have the opportunity to participate in communal discussion. Indeed, with their experience and expertise, physicians are the "guardians" of medical ethical issues and the community's representatives in doing the primary medical ethical work. In any community discussion, physicians' views should carry significant influence (see Chapter 1).

Distinguishing these types of choices and recognizing the legitimate communal control over policies in the second area should be welcomed by physicians. As they have grappled with medical ethical issues, especially the ones relating to the termination of care and the allocation of resources, physicians have increasingly recognized that such issues must be influenced by community values and, consequently, that communal decision-making is important. Indeed, in many cases physicians want more guidance from the community than they have received. And some have been frustrated because in the current system it is not clear who is responsible for providing such guidance: the legislature, the courts, professional associations, blue-ribbon commissions, or others. In this way CHPs could be seen as an improvement in providing physicians with an institutional structure responsible for addressing such ethical policies. The deliberations of CHPs should be viewed favorably by physicians because they will have an integral role in defining the policies rather than being issued policies from external regulatory bodies that have not consulted them.[78] In the current environment, which many physicians decry, CHPs would constitute an alternative more hospitable both to facilitating communal input on those matters where communal values are determinative and retaining professional control over those policy matters where the standards are properly defined by physicians.[79] As such, CHPs should constitute an important institutional arrangement that unites democratic deliberations with professional autonomy.

The question of whether community members will participate in CHP deliberations is fundamental. The ideal of communal participation has traditionally been tied to self-sufficient communities in which the deliberations have encompassed the entire range of social policies, from education and welfare to the common defense. In CHPs, however, deliberations will be limited to medical care. Even when those social policies related to health are included in deliberations, the influence of CHPs will still touch on a limited range of issues. This could undermine the citizenry's motivation to participate in the governing of CHPs, especially when the deliberations will be lengthy and extend over a long period of time. After all, who is willing to spend one night a month, let alone one night a week, for months on end just discussing health care issues?

Since everyone will eventually have to use the medical services pro-

vided and will have loved ones in need of these services, there are natural incentives for participation. In addition, within the last decade or
so there has been a dramatic increase in the public's interest in medical
issues. More than ever before, people are interested in all facets of
medicine, not just new technologies and therapies but also the ethical
issues of medical care. Since every CHP will have to confront and
establish policies on controversial medical ethical issues, there should
be a strong citizen interest. Whether these natural incentives and interests can be translated into active participation in actual policy formulation, whether they can make people leave the comforts of their
home once a month or so for health policy debates and discussions, is
an open question. And skepticism is the proper posture.

The answer to this question depends upon citizens' viewing moments of participation both as meaningful aspects of their self-
conception and as practically effective. Meaningful and important debates breed participation. Significantly, these two factors are related in
a typically Aristotelian fashion. The existence of meaningful participation will encourage people to participate actively and consider such
participation an indispensable facet of their lives. In large part, how
people value participation in democratic deliberation depends upon
the significance of its content and whether it is effective. Conversely,
the experience and habit of participation in meaningful communal deliberations will perpetuate meaningful debates and participation.
Consequently, the extent of participation in CHPs depends upon the
suitability of structures for this participation, the commitment of the
CHPs and their leading members to foster such democratic discussions, and the efficacy of such deliberations in shaping CHP policies.
With institutions promoting meaningful and effective communal deliberations, citizens will tend to view participation as a part of their
lives.

Unfortunately, the recent past has not prepared most people for
such opportunities. Voting is too passive and indirect to engender the
commitment necessary for democratic deliberations. The turnouts
show how many of us remain passive in this simple but almost vacuous act of participation. The paucity of town meetings, industrial
democracy, or other forms of self-governing institutions within our
society means that only a small minority has grown up with a strong
experience and tradition of actual participation in governing institutions of any size. Few of us understand or have been trained to partic-

ipate in the sustained, long-term meetings, discussions, and arguments necessary for democratic self-government. Few of us have any experience with the political commitment and the style of ongoing discussions constitutive of democratic self-government. Furthermore, almost everyone in the United States has grown up in a medical care system characterized by hierarchical decision-making, with few or no opportunities for communal participation. Hence, we cannot expect immediate, widespread communal participation with the introduction of CHPs. We cannot test the success of CHPs in fulfilling the liberal communitarian ideal of democratic deliberations on public policies by the turnouts in the first few years after their establishment. Developing the experience and tradition of actual participation in policy debates takes time.

As a result, CHPs will require sustained efforts to foster participation. Realistic expectations and policies should be based on this fact. It will mean developing different types of forums for participation, educating the CHP members on the issues and the procedures of democratic deliberations, and ensuring that the discussions are meaningful, that they produce policies that affect the lives of the CHP members. In addition, widening the range of issues and policies to be considered will also be important since the more significant the decisions, the greater will be the interest in participation. Such efforts will require investment of funds. They require extensive investments of time and energy both in their creation and in their actual operation. Thus in addition to the voucher for medical care services there should be separate funds for the support of CHP projects facilitating democratic participation. The federal oversight board might set aside, say, 1 percent of all funds for medical services in a separate "deliberation fund" to be allocated to those CHPs that institute structures for significant communal participation in deliberations and policy formulation. Those CHPs, like "The Adam Smith CHP," that do not create such institutional structures should not receive such funds. Conversely, those CHPs that face greater barriers to facilitating such participation, rural CHPs for example, might receive a higher proportion of the "deliberation funds."

Even with this investment in deliberative institutions, there is no guarantee that people will participate in the deliberations at CHPs. While, in the extreme, people can be forced to attend communal meetings, they cannot be forced to reflect and to discuss their views

on medical care issues. Even with the best of efforts at fostering participation in effective policy formulation, there is no insurance against
consumerism. The best that can be provided is the opportunity for
deliberations.

> We can recognize rights, we can distribute power or at least the oc-
> casions of power, but we cannot guarantee the prideful activity that
> rights and occasions make possible. Democratic politics, once we
> have overthrown every wrongful dominance, is a standing invita-
> tion to act in public and know oneself a citizen . . . But there is no
> way to make sure that you or I, or anyone, will seize the opportu-
> nity. This, I suppose, is the secular version of Locke's proposition
> that no one can be forced to be saved.[80]

But before pessimism about communal participation in CHPs
overtakes us, we should recall the historical experience of democratic
participation. Even in the quintessential instance of democratic deliberations, New England town meetings in the eighteenth and nine-
teenth centuries, only an average of 25 percent of citizens routinely
turned out. Participation swelled to more than half of the eligible citizens only during crises. These are modest levels of regular participation. Yet this seems to be the degree of participation that elicited
Tocqueville's tremendous admiration and was fundamental to the average American's unique commitment and self-respect as a free and
equal citizen of a self-ruling polity. Indeed, with our perception of
political participation shaped by the act of voting, we may place too
much emphasis on the quantifying of participation in any particular
town meeting. We may forget the way such a forum may affect other
aspects of communal life and instigate deliberations which extend
outside of the actual town meetings into more informal but influential
settings. The experience of participation in the decision-making of
neighborhood health centers and health maintenance organizations
that have developed communal meetings for policy decisions is consistent with the historical record. There is a low but constant level of
regular participation that increases dramatically when the community
confronts controversial decisions.[81] Sustained efforts at attracting
people, using a variety of forums and coordinating with preexisting
organizations, can increase participation.[82]

Extensive communal participation in CHPs will depend upon both
the commitment of citizens to shaping the institutions in which they

live and the significance and quality of the participation. Since most people have not had the opportunity to participate in such democratic institutions, we cannot expect extensive participation initially. But we can establish and financially support institutions that encourage communal participation. Such efforts will not guarantee participation, and some of them might well fail. But history and experience suggest there are no inherent practical barriers to realizing the liberal communitarian vision. It is worth the attempt, especially since the current system has proved itself impotent in the face of pressing medical ethical issues.

Objections Considered

Providing a framework for rational deliberation on controversial medical ethical issues requires invoking a political philosophy that rejects the ideal of neutrality. I have outlined the conceptual structure of such a political philosophy: liberal communitarianism. In developing its implications for a reconstructed medical care system I have tried to show that this vision is justifiable, philosophically plausible, and politically practical. No doubt this outline has raised many objections. In this section I shall consider six potential objections.

Freedom of Practice

The first objection focuses on the effect of CHPs on the physician's freedom to practice. CHPs would be organized around conceptions of the good life. Consequently, it is argued, the affiliations of individuals and physicians would depend on their conception of the good life, and they might be forced to switch CHPs depending upon their moral values. For instance, a physician might be practicing in a CHP, completely agreeing with its policies. Subsequently an issue, such as whether the CHP ought to permit euthanasia, might arise in which the physician might disagree with the position adopted by the CHP members and would find it unethical to continue practicing within the CHP. But why should a physician's professional affiliations and site of practice depend upon his moral convictions?

Currently physicians change their professional affiliations because of considerations of salary, prestige, power, geographic location, cultural and recreational amenities, and a myriad of other factors. Our society certainly does not prohibit—or even frown upon—the influence of such factors on a physician's decision about where and under what circumstances to practice. That some find it objectionable for physicians to have to choose where to practice on the basis of moral ideals demonstrates the extent to which we have ignored moral considerations in justifying our choices among professional, residential, and other affiliations. Indeed, while these critics are content to let materialistic, climatic, recreational, and other interests influence such choices, they object when moral values do.

The liberal communitarian vision opposes this tendency. In this view, a physician would not be denied his citizenship or professional certification because of his conception of the good life; a physician would not be forced to choose between being an American or not, or practicing or not, depending on his moral convictions. Instead the choice would be about the community in which he lives and practices and the conception of the good life that should guide his interpretation of the ideal of medicine. And since there would be a diverse number of CHPs espousing different conceptions of the good life, presumably the physician would find at least one CHP with ethical ideals that he shared. In addition, a physician would never be forced to leave a CHP because he disagreed with its policies. In a liberal communitarian vision the community cannot ostracize a citizen. He would have the option of remaining within the CHP, raising the issue again for communal deliberations, and trying to persuade his fellow CHP members to his position. He would even have the option of civil disobedience against the CHP's policies. The physician would leave only when he felt the conflict was what I have called fundamental. Practically this may be more difficult for a physician in a rural area, but certainly in an urban community it should be relatively easy for a physician to find a compatible CHP.

This is not to minimize the significance of the choice among CHPs. In the ideal, CHPs would form the basis for distinctive communities that would establish a whole range of local policies in areas from education to housing to transportation, based on the members' particular conception of the good life. In this ideal, the physician's choice among CHPs is not merely a choice about location or salaries, but a choice about different ideals and ways of life, about the community's ultimate commitments. It seems perfectly ethical that these ideals should form the basis of a person's affiliations and attachments. Indeed, we should be surprised if they did not. We would find a person for whom moral ideals did not influence his affiliations and attachments unreflective.

Finally, this objection seems to assume that within the current system the affiliations and attachments of physicians are independent of moral ideals. But, for example, there are physicians who refuse to perform abortions and to be affiliated with hospitals that do. Similarly, some physicians refuse to practice in hospitals that do not permit the termination of artificial nutrition and hydration for incompetent patients. Some physicians leave hospitals that refuse to initiate certain services, such as organ transplantation, because they think the hospital is denying people urgent services. And physicians may decide not to practice at some HMOs because they deem their cost control incentive structure coercive and unethical. Indeed, in many ways moral ideals already influence physicians' professional affiliations. CHPs would simply make these ideals more central. But they would not make such ethical ideals the basis of national citizenship or professional certification.

The Justice of the Liberal Communitarian Vision

A second objection is directed against the fact that members of different CHPs would be entitled to different basic medical services. Since different CHPs would espouse different conceptions of the good life, they would guarantee their members different medical care services, violating the principle of equal access. One person would be entitled to a bone marrow transplant, but his neighbor with the identical affliction, affiliated with another CHP, might not be able to receive such a transplant. According to these critics, this is unfair. Why should the medical services a person receives depend upon the particular CHP he happens to belong to? Justice requires that all citizens be treated equally and have access to the same basic medical services.[83]

This objection misconstrues justice. As I demonstrated in Chapter 4, there is no way for a polity to balance or weigh the demands for the various goods without invoking a conception of the good life; determining the medical services that citizens should be guaranteed by the polity as a matter of justice must be informed by a conception of the good life. This claim can be made consistent with the claim of pluralism only by permitting different political communities to formulate policies based on their particular conception of the good life. Thus, these two claims imply that within any particular political community, all citizens should be treated equally and should be entitled to access to the same basic medical services as determined by that polity's conception of the good life, but between communities there will be different views of what is just and therefore of what constitutes basic medical services.[84] The precise entitlements of justice will not be universal, but will vary among communities based on their conceptions of the good life.

Finally, an objection should not compare the guarantees for any single medical intervention, but for the entire medical care system espoused by each CHP. Different CHPs would have different ways of life, ideals, traditions, and practices, and the different entitlements would reflect these different ways of life. The scheme of medical services constitutes a whole because together they reflect and sustain the conception of the good life. Thus the relational CHP that denies life-saving treatments to those over 70 years of age guarantees them nursing home care and better therapies for chronic diseases. The denial of one service and the guarantee of the others are intertwined in realizing a single vision of human life. It is a distortion to compare specific services such as organ transplants without comparing the collection of services and how they are connected into a whole. What differs among CHPs is entire schemes of medical care services because these correspond to different conceptions of the good life.

The fairness of the liberal communitarian arrangement inheres in the fact that the citizens of a particular CHP are guaranteed those services that fulfill their avowed conception of the good life. And no individual can be forced to espouse a particular conception of the good life. If a person placed great importance on access to all organ transplant services, then he could join a CHP which offered such guarantees. Justice is not realized by comparing entitlements to individual services, but by respecting the community's particular conception of the good life expressed in its distribution of goods.

Total Medical Resources and the Good

A third objection has to do with the value of the voucher. In the CHP system the value of the vouchers might be established on the basis of the current proportion of the GNP being spent on medical care. Annual increases would reflect the consumer price index. But why, it is objected, should the value of the voucher reflect the proportion of the GNP we currently spend on medical care? Should we allocate more of society's resources to medical care? Should we allocate less? How was the current distribution of resources at the political level determined? If the current distribution at the political level relies on an implicit conception of the good life, which conception is it? How is this particular conception adopted and justified? And how does using one conception of the good life cohere with the acknowledgment of pluralism in society?[85]

The health care system implied by liberal communitarianism does not force all CHPs to spend a particular sum of money on medical care services. In the liberal communitarian vision, CHPs could tax their members for additional medical care resources or, conversely, rebate some of the voucher money to their members. CHPs would not be forced to allocate to medical care a socially defined quantum of resources. Whatever the value of the voucher, the tax and rebate options would permit each individual CHP to define the urgency of medical services for itself and to adjust the resources committed to medical services in light of this determination.

This response does not, however, completely answer the objection. The basic value of the voucher must assume some conception of the good life. Indeed, as I have argued, just as it is necessary to appeal to a conception of the good life to weigh claims among medical services at the medical level of distribution, so it is possible to weigh claims for social services at the political level only by appeal to a conception of the good life. There is no way of determining how much of the GNP to spend on medicine while adhering to the ideal of neutrality. The conception of the good life that should inform the political distribution of resources would derive from the partial conception of the good life contained in the liberal communitarian ideal. This conception of the good life, centering on a citizen's participation in democratic deliberations to formulate a community's policy, defines a good for the determination of the distribution of resources at the political level. It establishes priorities among those available medical care services. So the collection of medical services that cure or ameliorate diseases, permitting an individual to participate in communal deliberations and the community to perpetuate itself, should provide a basis for defining the value of the voucher. This again indicates that the liberal communitarian ideal is not neutral but serves as the justification for public

policies. And yet it would permit pluralism by leaving individual
CHPs—even poor CHPs—to provide their own medical allocation of
resources within the limit set at the political level. That is, even within
a defined total quantity of resources, a CHP would decide which particular medical services should receive priority. This would permit the
CHPs to express their values in the priorities of services they provide.[86]

Discrimination in CHPs

A fourth objection attacks CHP membership procedures as potentially legitimating discrimination. In many cases the membership criteria might rely on age, sex, religious affiliation, and the like. A lesbian community, for instance, might want to exclude men from their
CHP because they are committed to escaping male domination and
its distorting effects on female relationships and support structures.
This lesbian CHP may even want to exclude a man willing to live by
such feminist views and the health care policies they justify. Similarly,
a white community might exclude blacks and other minorities based
on its view of the importance of pure races. Or, more likely, the same
community might disguise its real racist views by offering a more
tolerable conception of the good life that produced the same effect of
excluding minorities. To sanction membership selection based on
such criteria would be to permit invidious discrimination based on
race, sex, religion, and the like. In liberal communitarianism, communities could easily justify racism, sexism, or ageism by appealing
to their particular values.

In response it might be argued that a community might want to
exclude from membership individuals who would willingly abide by
the community's policies but did not espouse its conception of the
good life because such members might undermine its character. Having non-believing members of a community is analogous to having
silent, considerate non-participants in a religious service. They do not
overtly disturb or interrupt the religious service. Nevertheless, because their presence does not contribute to it, they "flatten" the religious service by creating a dead space and thereby detract from it.
Similarly, non-believing members do not perpetuate the community's
traditions; they do not articulate and specify the community's ideals;
they do not sustain the community's activities. Their non-contribu-
tion to the community's distinctive character is not benign but a de-

traction. For this reason many communities may not want to accept such respectful but non-believing people as members. The exclusion of respectful non-believers is necessary to sustain communities. This is a position the liberal communitarian vision should endorse even when it means that the communities may exclude individuals from membership on the basis of age, sex, religion, and the like.

Sanctioning such exclusions from CHPs, however, would not deny those excluded either citizenship or the rights to form and participate in their own CHP. There is no possibility of permanently denying the excluded political rights for participation. In this sense, whatever a particular CHP might do, even if it tried to exclude minorities on the basis of racist motives, this would be distinctly different from the attempts to deny blacks civil rights before the 1960s. In the case of blacks, the exclusion was of those who believed in the American ideal of equality and yet were denied political membership. Conversely, in the case of CHPs, those who are excluded from particular CHPs are non-believers who want membership.

Of course, not every exclusion on the basis of age, sex, religion, and the like would be permissible. The justification for such exclusions as well as the correspondence between the justification and actual practices must be examined. To be legitimate, the exclusions must be necessary to sustain a community's commitment to a particular conception of the good life. Thus a Hispanic community might reject non-Hispanic applicants either because they want to perpetuate their particular traditions and culture or for racist reasons. The first would be permitted and the second prohibited. Even in the first case, however, the claims of the community would have to be tested by its actual practices. If traditions and cultural activities were neither observed nor celebrated, then the justification for exclusions based on race might be factitious and therefore prohibited. Clearly some of the judgments involved, such as determining whether a community actually celebrates a particular culture and respects its traditions, will be difficult and open to interpretation. But there is no escape from such difficult moral judgments.

But, it might be asked, on what basis could the liberal communitarian vision prohibit communities that rejected applicants for discriminatory or racist reasons? Is the liberal communitarian vision not committed to permitting racist CHPs because they are just pursuing their own, albeit racist, conception of the good life?

There is a difference between communities that espouse a conception of the good life, excluding those who do not similarly espouse the ideal, and communities that espouse a conception of the good life in which the ideal is exclusion. The difference is between a conception of the good life with an internal, positive ideal and a conception of the good life based on the opposition to and denigration of others. While the first view will oppose some conceptions of the good life, it has its own ideals that can be characterized without counter-defining them against the ideals of others. The content of the second is provided only in opposition to others. This second form becomes discriminatory when it aims not merely at separation but at denigration and domination of the groups it opposes. In its discriminatory form it conflicts with the respect for the freedom and equality of citizens that is essential for deliberation. Without commitment to this respect, there is no chance of realizing the liberal communitarian vision or any democratic political vision. The liberal communitarian vision need not sanction racism when it permits communities to reject applicants for membership on the basis of conceptions of the good life which may overlap with age, sex, religion, and the like.

The Absence of Pluralism

The fifth objection focuses on whether the liberal communitarian vision actually affirms pluralism. The liberal communitarian ideal is one of deliberative democracy in which the citizens participate in formulating their own conception of the good life and policies. Deliberative democracy then becomes a common element in all conceptions of the good life. The liberal communitarian polity may justify strong incentives against the formation of "non-deliberative" communities, such as "The Adam Smith CHP," and in the extreme, critics argue, might actually prohibit them by appealing to the ideal of deliberation. In this way, it is claimed, the liberal communitarian ideal is not pluralistic but, because it aims to impose democratic deliberation on all, coercive and autocratic.

In response, it should be recognized that commitment to pluralism does not mean relativism. Pluralism does not imply permitting all possible conceptions of the good life to be pursued. To permit all possible conceptions of the good life to flourish is an absurd standard that even liberal political philosophy rejects. Nevertheless, the liberal communitarian ideal is compatible with many worthy conceptions of the good life, from particular religions to moral liberalism.

More important, the liberal communitarian ideal is not a comprehensive ideal. It provides an ideal for only one facet of life; many other facets are left for individuals and communities to define. In this sense, the liberal communitarian ideal does not provide a conception "of what is of value in human life . . . that [is] to inform much of our non-political conduct (in the limit our life as a whole)."[87] As I argued in Chapter 5, to make politics all of life would be to make life one-dimensional. Liberal communitarianism is against this and recognizes other worthy ideals and goods, from solitude and love to art and philosophy, that cannot be (fully) realized in public life. Indeed, by its very nature liberal communitarianism can only make opportunities for democratic deliberation possible; citizens are always permitted to refuse to exercise these opportunities and to stay away pursuing these other goods. To provide a common element to all acceptable conceptions of the good life is not to foist a comprehensive view on all.

Finally, realizing both the claim of pluralism and the possibility of having an ethical framework for principled deliberation on controversial public matters requires political structures that provide citizens the opportunity to debate about fundamental values and conceptions of the good life. If this is to be a real opportunity, if this debate is not to be empty, there must be substantial citizen participation. After all, providing citizens the opportunity to debate about values without a forum, without other participants, and without the power to affect policy is not providing a genuine opportunity. These considerations imply that any polity committed to pluralism will also have to be committed to the structures of democratic deliberation as an ideal. And liberal communitarianism is one framework that permits the justification of laws and policies by appeal to conceptions of the good life and also permits pluralism. Indeed, any political philosophy which affirms pluralism will have to adopt principles similar to those found in liberal communitarianism.

Excessive Pluralism

The sixth objection is the obverse of the fifth and focuses on the question of whether the liberal communitarian ideal is too pluralistic. According to these critics, the liberal communitarian vision seems to permit almost every CHP flavor, from "The Adam Smith CHP" to "The Jeremy Bentham CHP" to "The Moral Majority CHP." There seems to be no real commitment to CHPs that create deliberative structures for their members. Further, because there is no geographic basis for dividing into CHPs, because individuals are permitted to leave and join other CHPs, there seems no real incentive for people to be committed to a particular CHP. A young individual may join a CHP espousing the relational conception because it provides more services to younger people. But as this individual ages he might experience a medical "conversion" and want to join a CHP committed to the physical conception to obtain more life-sustaining care as an elderly person. This provides such an individual the best of both worlds without commitment to either. Similarly, certain citizens may be prone to conversions and request changes in CHPs precisely when their health status changes. By having this variety there is a tendency for people to shop around, choosing CHPs not by any commitment to a conception of the good life but by consumerist preferences for more services and fewer commitments. In this way, it is charged, the liberal communitarian vision seems nothing more than a form of libertarianism, similar to Nozick's utopia.[88]

To use geographic criteria to determine CHP membership in contemporary society will probably not be compatible with the liberal communitarian vision. Contemporary neighborhoods tend not to reflect any shared religious, cultural, or philosophical conceptions among the residents. Indeed, probably the only shared traits among neighborhood residents are socioeconomic class, income, and wealth. This implies that using geography as a basis for CHPs will force people who espouse incommensurable conceptions of the good life to deliberate and formulate policies. Inevitably the policies will offend individuals whose conceptions of the good life conflict with the policies. And if the conceptions of the good life are truly incommensurable, then we should not expect compromise positions. The inevitable result will be less deliberation and more conflict resolved only by ballot box power.

Further, under the CHP scheme, it must be admitted that medical conversions might occur; there is no guarantee against such consumerism. And the right of exit must be respected as an integral element of political autonomy. But the right of exit does not mean that a person has the right to join a CHP that provides the very service he desires. A person experiencing a medical conversion might want to join a CHP that provides services for his particular ailment, but there is no right to be admitted to such a CHP. And there is no requirement that the desired CHP should admit the medical convert. Such converts will take their chances.

We must recognize that the possibility of such conversions is greater with a consumerist attitude toward medical care. It may be that the restrictions on switching CHPs and the incentives for creating deliberative structures are too weak to obstruct the path of this consumerism. The liberal communitarian vision, which emphasizes medical care not as a consumer item but as an element in a larger conception of the good life, militates against such conversions. To the extent that this vision becomes stronger through CHPs, the tendency to conversions will be reduced. But since most Americans do not have any experience of participation in deliberative democratic institutions, this option may well require strong promotion at least initially, until citizens gain experience. There is nothing to prohibit altering the incentive structure to promote stronger commitments to deliberative structures over consumerist ones. More funds could be given to those CHPs that establish deliberative institutions; a tax could be placed on rebated health care vouchers; additional restrictions on receiving a voucher to switch CHPs could be implemented; restrictions on certain activities that conflict with deliberative institutions could be instituted; and, in the extreme, non-deliberative CHPs could be prohibited. Such interventions may be necessary. Indeed, if anything this objection seems to argue for such programs that discourage consumerist attitudes and promote the liberal communitarian vision.

These last two objections, accusing the liberal communitarian vision of being both too pluralistic and not pluralistic enough, both too communitarian and not communitarian enough, may actually illuminate a virtue of the vision. This vision recognizes two requirements for a political philosophy: the claim of pluralism and the need for a conception of the good life to inform any framework for public deliberation on political issues. These requirements are in tension, and institutional structures that satisfy both requirements will display this tension. But there is no magical way to evade or avoid it. From the isolated perspective of either requirement, the final political scheme may appear flawed. And yet this flaw only shows that the tension is being accommodated.

But if we are to err on one side rather than the other, it should be toward more incentives for deliberative institutions. As I have noted, our polity has few of these institutions and people have little experience with them. On the other hand, the structures promoting consumerism, especially the economic market, are very strong. To provide a genuine opportunity for participation in deliberative democratic institutions, we must build up these institutions, the citizenry's experience with them, and traditions of participation in them. This will require active, possibly even vigorous, promotion of them.

Medical Ethics for the Physician

Coming to the end of this book, readers may have an ill-defined but nagging sense of dissatisfaction. Indeed many people, especially practicing physicians, may find themselves even more pessimistic about solving medical ethical dilemmas than before they began reading. For if my claims are valid and the resolution of major ethical dilemmas in medical practice requires reconceiving the political values that inform discussions in medical ethics, then what help are these insights for those who must live and practice today? I may have offered a vision that "may be true in theory but does not apply in practice," at least in the political world in which we live and physicians practice. Therefore, some may charge me with offering a wonderful, (possibly) even practical ideal that is completely irrelevant and useless to Dr. Wolf, Andrew's physician, or to a physician taking care of a patient like Karen Quinlan or even to a citizen wanting to know what medical care he should be entitled to. This work, critics may claim, does nothing to alleviate the ill effects and costs that arise out of the irresolution of contemporary medical ethics created by liberalism. Do the claims advanced in this book provide us, physicians and citizens, with help in making health care decisions in the circumstances under which we live and practice?[1]

My initial response is a negative piece of advice, more a warning about what to avoid or renounce than what to embrace. Attempts to address the issues of terminating care for incompetent patients and the allocation of medical resources by invoking rights will be futile. Appeals to the right to refuse treatment and the right to equal access will not help us determine what treatments incompetents should receive or what basic medical services citizens should receive as a matter of justice. Rights are merely procedures; by themselves they do not indicate what substantive ethical decisions should be made. They seem to satisfy us by offering the illusion of resolution, while leaving the actual ethical dilemmas unexamined. Thus we should ignore the attempts to discuss medical ethical issues in the language of rights and abstain from efforts to extend such rights.[2]

This admonition against the language of rights intimates a companion warning: The political conception of medical ethics suggests that there will be no easy answers, no set of specified "ethical principles and rules [that can be applied] to illuminate and resolve specific moral problems."[3] The hope, especially harbored by busy practitioners confronted by an increasing number of ethical questions, of having three or four simple and fixed general principles to help resolve most questions by deductive reasoning is illusory. It is not that medical ethical questions present uniquely difficult dilemmas or involve poorly elaborated ethical principles; rather, the problem is that medical ethical questions are real ethical questions that invoke basic ethical conceptions and require dialectical moral deliberation. And this is no easy deductive reasoning process beginning with a few principles.

This brings us to the first aspect of positive advice: Medicine should be viewed more as a unique moral enterprise engaging us—both physicians and patients—in interpreting our shared values for guidance concerning the ends of life. Among the normal circumstances of life, it is only in the practice of medicine that we are required to confront the meaning of human frailty and finitude and the many entwined ethical questions. To practice medicine and to answer these questions requires specifying and balancing the ends of medicine. And this, in turn, entails an interpretation of fundamental political conceptions, a preliminary answer to the ethical question, and a dialectical process of qualifying and refining our understanding of the basic ethical conceptions as well as our resolution of the questions. In this way, the practice of medicine is as much painstaking moral deliberation as it is biomedical technology and clinical judgment. And physicians, as the guardians of medical ethics entrusted with providing to society the preliminary ethical understanding in areas related to their practice, increasingly must view the practice of medicine as a moral endeavor, an attempt to articulate shared ethical values and their practical implications for health care.

The second positive contribution this book can offer physicians is establishing the goal of pursing medicine as a moral enterprise by offering models for moral deliberations. The moral arguments presented in the detailed considerations of the issues of terminating care and allocating medical resources—the analysis of the basic conceptions, their relationship to conceptions of the good life, and their different implications for medical practices—are not merely arguments about the deficiencies of liberalism as related to medicine, they are also typical ways of deliberating on the medical ethical questions. The examples presented in Chapters 3 and 4 reveal three important steps in the process of moral deliberation on medical ethical questions confronting physicians. First, these examples define some of the fundamental medical ethical questions that need to be addressed; they also implicitly and explicitly show what types of questions are peripheral and need to be bracketed. Second, they indicate how to begin moral deliberations on these questions by illuminating the basic ethical conceptions and values that should be considered. Third, they indicate the outlines of certain prominent conceptions of the good life and the relationship between these conceptions and different types of health care decisions. By demonstrating these three steps in the process of moral deliberation on two separate medical ethical questions, this work should help physicians and patients engage the moral aspects of medical practice.

These first two positive pieces of advice should not be disdained either by physicians or by patients as further impositions on their autonomy. Instead they should be seen as an attempt to minimize the economic and merely technical aspects of the physician-patient relationship by reclaiming the traits that make this a relationship between friends, albeit friends who have differences of knowledge, need, and vulnerability.[4] By stressing the practice of medicine as an enterprise suffused with moral deliberation, this work should provide a justification for preserving and enriching the best aspects of the traditional physician-patient relationship so threatened by contemporary circumstances. The hope is to encourage physicians not to renounce the traditions of medical practice, but rather to begin articulating the moral vision embedded in their current practices as the basis of their moral deliberations with patients and others on health care decisions.

Obviously rules, financial pressures, and legal barriers are being imposed by outsiders, such as insurance companies and government bureaucrats, to discourage moral deliberations in the practice of medicine. There can be no expectation that initially the view expressed here will be widely endorsed and the barriers to it promptly dissolved.

This is a long-term process. And this brings us to the third positive contribution of this book: it is a call for physicians to begin developing the institutional structures necessary for increased democratic deliberations on medical ethical questions.

Moral deliberations on medical ethical questions and the substantive conceptions of the good life necessary to address these questions do not spontaneously occur; they require institutional structures and, to engage people, they need to affect policies. Such structures could be established within and by existing medical care institutions, especially since these institutions need to develop policies for the resolution of the ethical dilemmas we have been examining. For example, physicians who work in and administer managed health care plans could begin establishing various meetings between physicians and patients on medical ethical issues. They could institute periodic educational and deliberative meetings on specific medical ethical issues confronting the health care plan or the larger society. They might let health care plan members consider whether all members should be required to discuss advance care documents or organ donation cards with their physicians. Such efforts might be applicable to all types of managed health care programs, including health maintenance organizations, union and corporation programs, and health care programs provided in retirement communities. Thus, to sustain the moral element of medical practice, it is incumbent upon physicians to begin creating institutional arrangements conducive to the discussion of shared values and health practices between physicians and patients. Again, because most of us have not been in the habit of engaging in democratic deliberations, we cannot expect these discussions to be well attended, informed, or efficient right away. These endeavors must be initiated for the long run with the intention of cultivating habits and developing shared ideals through deliberations, not with the hope of immediate changes in behavior or policy.

Finally, this book offers not just procedural assistance to the practicing physician, but also the embryonic elements of a substantive conception of the good life that could inform health care decisions. The ideals of the liberal communitarian vision form a distinct, although not comprehensive, conception of the good life. In Chapter 5 I sketched some of its basic features. People aspire to be members of a community by participating in its political deliberations. Through such participation, citizens can realize political autonomy, that is, living under conditions they legislate. They also can realize certain capacities, such as the capacity for responsibility and moral reflection. And finally, through their participation in communal deliberations citizens become bound to the larger community, seeing their own interests in its common interest. In this way they transcend their individual existence to become part of an ongoing community with a posterity.

We might call the conception of the good life underlying the liberal communitarian vision the deliberative conception. This conception, I believe, is intimated not only in the American culture but also in the best aspects of the traditions of medical practice. I should emphasize that this conception of the good life is incomplete and requires elaboration by other specific ideals and traditions. Therefore, different particular communities may espouse ideals which are consistent with those of liberal communitarianism and yet result in diverse ways of life with different practices, laws, and policies. Nevertheless, this deliberative conception informs a distinct framework in which to address medical ethical issues. For instance, in the area of the physician-patient relationship, it suggests that patient autonomy understood as control over medical interventions should be de-emphasized. Instead the physician–patient relationship is a deliberative interaction in which the physician and patient articulate, as friends, worthy ideals to be realized through medical care. Similarly, in the area of selecting medical interventions, the deliberative conception suggests that certain capacities are necessary for a worthy and meaningful life. Without the potential capacities for engaging in deliberations, one is not a full person. In addition, the deliberative conception of the good life suggests a principled way of determining basic medical services to be provided to citizens. Such services should ensure the continuance of the common life as well as the possibility for individuals to realize the capacities of self-development unique to political participation.

This is merely a sketchy outline from which the detailed picture of this deliberative conception of the good life must be drawn and its implications for medical ethical issues more completely developed. Such elaboration will have to await a future study. But this deliberative conception can begin the ongoing process of specifying a conception of the good life in light of actual ethical judgments, including judgments about medical ethical issues. And it is to this process that we should now commit ourselves.

Notes

Introduction

1. This case is adapted and modified from *Evans* v. *Bellevue Hospital* (Wirth) (no. 16536/87 New York Supreme Court, N.Y. County, July 27, 1987) (Sandifer J.), N.Y.L.J. July 28, 1987, at 11 col. 1.
2. In this book I use the terms "moral" and "ethical" interchangeably. Some authors, such as Bernard Williams, *Ethics and the Limits of Philosophy* (Cambridge, Mass.: Harvard University Press, 1986), distinguish the moral and the ethical. I am sympathetic to this distinction, yet in this book I will not adhere to it.
3. Thomas Nagel, *Mortal Questions* (New York: Cambridge University Press, 1979).
4. "Ethics Committees Double since '83: Survey," *Hospitals,* November 1, 1985, p. 64.
5. The National Commission for the Protection of Human Subjects of Biomedical and Behavioral Research, *The Belmont Report: Ethical Principles and Guidelines for the Protection of Human Subjects of Research* (Washington, D.C.: U.S. Government Printing Office, 1979).
6. President's Commission for the Study of Ethical Problems in Medicine and Biomedical and Behavioral Research, *Deciding to Forego Life-Sustaining Treatment* (Washington, D.C.: U.S. Government Printing Office, 1983). The Commission published many other reports which I do not list here.
7. One typical example is The Massachusetts Task Force on Organ Transplantation, *Report of the Massachusetts Task Force on Organ Transplantation* (Boston: Department of Public Health, 1984).
8. David Hilfiker, "Allowing the Debilitated to Die: Facing Our Ethical Choices," *New England Journal of Medicine* 308 (1983), 716–719.
9. Alan A. Stone, "Law's Influence on Medicine and Medical Ethics," *New England Journal of Medicine* 312 (1985), 309–312.

1. The Political Conception of Medical Ethics

1. Ruth Macklin, *Mortal Choices: Bioethics in Today's World* (New York: Pantheon, 1987), pp. 7–8.
2. See, for example, Howard P. Lewis, "Machine Medicine and Its Rela-

tion to the Fatally Ill," *Journal of the American Medical Association* 206 (1968), 387–388; John Joakim Skillman, "Ethical Dilemmas in the Care of the Critically Ill," in J. J. Skillman, ed., *Intensive Care* (Boston: Little, Brown, 1979).

3. See, for instance, Henry J. Aaron and William B. Schwartz, *The Painful Prescription: Rationing Hospital Care* (Washington, D.C.: The Brookings Institution, 1984).

4. See, for example, *In re Kathleen Farrell,* 108 N.J. 335 (1987); George J. Annas, "Reconciling *Quinlan* and *Saikewicz:* Decision Making for the Terminally Ill Incompetent," *American Journal of Law and Medicine* 4 (1979), 367–396; Daniel G. Suber and William J. Tabor, "Withholding of Life-Sustaining Treatment from the Terminally Ill, Incompetent Patient: Who Decides? Part I," *Journal of the American Medical Association* 248 (1982), 2250–51; and John R. Ball, "Withholding Treatment: A Legal Perspective," *Journal of the American Geriatric Society* 32 (1984), 528–530.

5. Norman Fost, "Ethical Issues in the Treatment of Critically Ill Newborns," *Pediatric Annals* 10 (1981), 383–389.

6. Terry A. Travis, Russel Noyes, and Dennis R. Brightwell, "The Attitudes of Physicians toward Prolongation of Life," *International Journal of Psychiatry in Medicine* 5 (1974), 17–26.

7. Richard A. McCormick, "To Save or Let Die: The Dilemmas of Modern Medicine," *Journal of the American Medical Association* 229 (1974), 172–176.

8. Tomas J. Silber, "Introduction: Bioethics and the Pediatrician," *Pediatric Annals* 10 (1981), 381–382.

9. Morris B. Abram, "Ethics and the New Medicine," *New York Times Magazine,* June 5, 1983, p. 69.

10. Gerald R. Winslow, *Triage and Justice* (Berkeley, Calif.: University of California Press, 1982), p. 12.

11. Daniel Callahan, "Shattuck Lecture—Contemporary Biomedical Ethics," *New England Journal of Medicine* 302 (1980), 1228–33.

12. Joseph Fletcher, *Morals and Medicine* (Princeton, N.J.: Princeton University Press, 1954).

13. Immanuel Jakobovits, *Jewish Medical Ethics* (New York: Bloch, 1959).

14. Pope Pius XII, "The Prolongation of Life," reprinted in S. J. Reiser, A. J. Dyck, and W. J. Curran, eds., *Ethics in Medicine: Historical Perspectives and Contemporary Concerns* (Cambridge, Mass.: MIT Press, 1977), pp. 501–504.

15. Henry K. Beecher, "Ethics and Clinical Research," *New England Journal of Medicine* 274 (1966), 1354–60.

16. Ad Hoc Committee of the Harvard Medical School to Examine the

Definition of Brain Death, "A Definition of Irreversible Coma," *Journal of the American Medical Association* 205 (1968), 337–340.

17. Among the earliest commentaries on the ethics of reproductive technologies was Leon R. Kass, "Babies by Means of In Vitro Fertilization: Unethical Experiments on the Unborn?" *New England Journal of Medicine* 285 (1971), 1174–79, and "Making Babies: The New Biology and the 'Old' Morality," *The Public Interest* 26 (Winter 1972), 18–56.

18. For this view see Robert M. Veatch, *A Theory of Medical Ethics* (New York: Basic Books, 1981).

19. The notion that technology can resolve many of the ethical dilemmas created by technology has been popularized by Lewis Thomas's rhetoric if not his precise ideas. He often argues that "half-way" technologies actually create ethical dilemmas, while genuine technologies can resolve them. One example he often notes is how dialysis is only a partial technology which creates a problem of allocating resources, while the polio vaccine is a genuine technology that is cheap and solves the problem of allocating resources. For attack on this idea see Larry R. Churchill, *Rationing Health Care in America: Perceptions and Principles of Justice* (Notre Dame, Ind.: University of Notre Dame Press, 1987), pp. 16–19.

20. Peter Singer, "'Bioethics': The Case of the Fetus," *New York Review of Books,* August 5, 1976, pp. 1–4.

21. Austin Flint, "Medical Ethics and Etiquette: Commentaries on the National Code of Ethics," *New York Medical Journal,* March 17, 1883, p. 286.

22. Dr. Austin Flint distinguished medical ethics from medical etiquette quite well when he wrote: "The rules of conduct adapted to the peculiarities of medicine constitute medical ethics. These rules have a moral weight. Medical etiquette, on the other hand, consists of the forms to be observed in professional intercourse. Those are conventional." Austin Flint, "Medical Ethics and Etiquette," March 17, 1883, p. 286. Clearly when the Hippocratic oath and other codes advise on the absolute prohibition against abortion or euthanasia, or on the need to avoid sexual intercourse with a patient, or on the need for confidentiality, they are dealing with medical ethics, not etiquette.

23. Kenneth J. Ryan, "Tradition and Change in the Teaching of Bioethics: Observations from the Field," *Harvard Medical Alumni Bulletin* 60 (Summer 1986), 25–27.

24. Paul Starr, *The Social Transformation of American Medicine* (New York: Basic Books, 1982), similarly claims that "the professional's judgment and advice are oriented toward a set of substantive values, such as health" (p. 15). And James Luther Adams, "The Social Import of the Professions: Address to the 21st Biennial Meeting of the American As-

sociation of Theological Schools" (Boston, June 1958), claims that there is a "historic idea that a professional man does not work primarily for economic success but for the general welfare" (p. 9), which is certainly a moral end.

25. James Luther Adams, "The Social Import of the Professions," p. 3.

26. Leon Kass, *Toward A More Natural Science* (New York: Free Press, 1985), makes a similar point about the devotion required of professionals when he writes that a profession is an activity "in service to some high good, which . . . is capable of calling forth devotion, because it is both good and high." He also argues that the professional devotes himself to his particular clients: "The teacher devotes himself to assisting the learning the young . . . the lawyer devotes himself to rectifying injustice for his client"(p. 215).

27. We can imagine, for instance, that a lawyer might have to lie to secure the acquittal of an innocent client, or that a physician might have to lie to obtain life-saving medications for a poor patient. Such conflicts of devotion require the balancing of the ends of a profession. As I shall argue, this requires going beyond the profession's ends to political philosophy.

28. See Dennis F. Thompson, *Political Ethics and Public Office* (Cambridge, Mass.: Harvard University Press, 1987), chap. 6.

29. Of course, clients do not always come voluntarily; sometimes, as children or as incompetent or mentally ill adults, they are brought by others. But we want to say that, in the counterfactual case in which they understood their condition, they would have voluntarily brought themselves to the professional.

30. If these abstract comments on the ethical dimension of a profession are valid, they might be useful in understanding the nature of ethics in other professions. For instance, the claim about every profession having a defined client may help explain our uncertainty about characterizing business as a profession. We, and businessmen, are unclear about who constitutes the client of business. Is it the shareholders? The managers? The workers? The customers? The larger community? Each of these have been proposed, but none has been agreed on. Agreement on the client of business, and therefore agreement on who should receive the businessman's devotion, is part of the necessary requirements for business to become a full-fledged profession. Furthermore, if a profession is other-directed, then the businessman's client cannot be the managers; for then it would be the case that businessmen pursued their own economic gain instead of serving others. But these are thoughts for another place.

31. Much of what follows has been informed by Leon Kass, *Toward A More Natural Science*.

32. This contrast between the physician and the public health professional has an interesting parallel with individualism and utilitarianism. The public health professional adopts a utilitarian perspective, primarily aiming to maximize health over the entire community regardless of the effect on particular individuals. By contrast, the physician adopts a more individualist perspective, primarily aiming to promote the health of particular individuals regardless of the consequence for the entire community. This distinction is only approximate, since the public health professional has a secondary interest in the health of individuals and the physician is also interested in the community's health.

33. See, for example, "The Art" in W. H. S. Jones, ed., *Hippocrates,* The Loeb Classical Library (Cambridge, Mass.: Harvard University Press, 1923); Darrel W. Amundsen, "The Physician's Obligation to Prolong Life: A Medical Duty without Classical Roots," *Hastings Center Report* 8 (August 1978), 23–30; and Jacob Bigelow, "Self Limited Diseases: Address to the Massachusetts Medical Society, May 27, 1835" in *Nature in Disease* (Boston: Ticknor and Fields, 1854).

34. See, for example, Winslow, *Triage and Justice;* Louis Cohn-Haft, "The Public Physicians of Ancient Greece," *Smith College Studies in History* 42 (1956), 40; and Stuart Hinds, "On the Relation of Medical Triage to World Famine: An Historical Survey," in G. R. Lucas and T. W. Ogletree, eds., *Lifeboat Ethics: The Moral Dilemmas of World Hunger* (New York: Harper and Row, 1976).

35. This also makes clear that the physician's professional role is not all-encompassing. The physician is also a citizen and may be called upon to do things *qua* citizen.

36. For an elaboration see Ezekiel J. Emanuel, "Do Physicians Have an Obligation to Treat Patients with AIDS?" *New England Journal of Medicine* 318 (1988), 1686–90.

37. For instance, the first AMA Code of Medical Ethics, written in 1847, stated that the physician's second duty was to keep the patient's information confidential except when required to testify in a court of law. See American Medical Association, *First Code of Medical Ethics,* reprinted in Reiser, Dyck, and Curran, eds., *Ethics in Medicine,* pp. 26–33.

38. Eric J. Cassell, "The Nature of Suffering and the Goals of Medicine," *New England Journal of Medicine* 306 (1982), 639–645.

39. This is the view of political philosophy that is modeled on Aristotle's method of always looking to what the few and the many say about political questions and then synthesizing their responses into an ideal theory. It is the procedure followed by most political philosophers in the tradition, from Locke, Kant, and the American founders, down to Rawls. It may be thought that there is another tradition of political phi-

losophy, the tradition which invents political values. See Michael Walzer, *Interpretation and Social Criticism* (Cambridge, Mass.: Harvard University Press, 1987), chap. 1. Whether invention is a model found in Plato, Hobbes, and others is an open question. It is not clear whether their expression of "new" political values is actually inventing political values or offering an interpretation of inchoate existing values.

40. This conception of political philosophy is consistent with the one expressed by John Rawls, "Justice as Fairness: Political not Metaphysical," *Philosophy and Public Affairs* 14 (1985), 223–251, as well as by Michael J. Sandel, "The Procedural Republic and the Unencumbered Self," *Political Theory* 12 (1984), 81–96. While there are differences in their views, especially as political philosophy relates to moral philosophy, it does not affect the issue presented here.

41. See Daniel Callahan, *Setting Limits* (New York: Simon and Schuster, 1987) and *What Kind of Life* (New York: Simon and Schuster, 1990); Norman Daniels, *Just Health Care* (New York: Cambridge University Press, 1985); and President's Commission for the Study of Ethical Problems in Medicine and Biomedical and Behavioral Research, *Making Health Care Decisions,* vol. 1 (Washington, D.C.: U.S. Government Printing Office, 1982) and *Deciding to Forego Life-Sustaining Treatment* (Washington, D.C.: U.S. Government Printing Office, 1983).

42. See Kass, *Toward a More Natural Science,* chap. 9; Edmund D. Pellegrino, "Toward a Reconstruction of Medical Morality: The Primacy of the Act of Profession and the Fact of Illness," *Journal of Medicine and Philosophy* 4 (1979), 32–56; and Mark Siegler, "Clinical Ethics and Clinical Medicine," *Archives of Internal Medicine* 139 (1979), 914–915.

43. Leon Kass, *Toward A More Natural Science,* does argue that "medicine [has] never been a completely autonomous profession" (p. 225), but he does not indicate the precise relationship between it and the political sphere. And he does argue that medicine as a profession should be self-governing. In his work the metaphor of separation is dominant but not exclusive. Attributing this view to him, therefore, is slightly inaccurate, but it serves to illustrate a distinction I am making.

44. See Tom L. Beauchamp and James F. Childress, *Principles of Biomedical Ethics,* 3rd ed. (New York: Oxford University Press, 1989); Veatch, *A Theory of Medical Ethics;* Samuel Gorovitz, *Doctors' Dilemmas* (New York: Oxford University Press, 1982); and H. Tristram Engelhardt, *The Foundations of Bioethics* (New York: Oxford University Press, 1986).

45. Beauchamp and Childress, *Principles of Biomedical Ethics,* pp. 9–10.

46. David Luban, *Lawyers and Justice* (Princeton, N.J.: Princeton University Press, 1988), chaps. 6–8. Probably because of the dominance of the applied ethics approach, there does not seem to be an advocate of this view

within medical ethics. I include it here to clarify my position on professional ethics.

47. This term was initially inspired by Luban, *Lawyers and Justice,* chap. 7. However, as will become clear, my use of it differs from Luban's because he thinks it suggests that professionals have complete control over their role morality. This I reject.

48. Rawls, "Justice as Fairness," pp. 226–231.

49. John Rawls, "Kantian Constructivism in Moral Theory," *Journal of Philosophy* 77 (1980), 561.

50. Rawls, "Justice as Fairness," p. 230.

51. John Rawls, "Social Unity and Primary Goods," in B. Williams and A. Sen, eds., *Utilitarianism and Beyond* (New York: Cambridge University Press, 1982), p. 168.

2. The Nature of Liberal Political Philosophy

1. Ronald Dworkin, *A Matter of Principle* (Cambridge, Mass.: Harvard University Press, 1985), p. 4.

2. See Charles E. Larmore, *Patterns of Moral Complexity* (New York: Cambridge University Press, 1987), pp. 42–50.

3. John Rawls, "The Priority of the Right and Ideas of the Good" (unpublished manuscript, August 24, 1987), p. 14.

4. Dworkin, *A Matter of Principle,* p. 191. This is one of those places in which we can see Dworkin adopting a liberalism which is hostile to the moral liberalism he seemed to adopt in arguing for state support of the arts. But the view expressed here seems more naturally congenial to his true position, although given the apparent conflicts among his positions one can never be sure what his true position really is.

5. This dichotomy is borrowed from John Rawls, "Justice as Fairness: Political not Metaphysical," *Philosophy and Public Affairs* 14 (1985), 223–251. I use slightly different terms from his, but the grounds of the distinctions are the same.

6. Amy Gutmann, "Children, Paternalism, and Education: A Liberal Argument," *Philosophy and Public Affairs* 9 (1980), 338–358. Subsequently in *Democratic Education* (Princeton, N.J.: Princeton University Press, 1987) Gutmann shifts away from this position, but the justification quoted here is a typical moral liberal view.

7. See Dworkin, *A Matter of Principle,* chap. 11, in which he argues that state subsidy of art is justified when it enhances "a rich cultural structure, one that multiplies distinct possibilities or opportunities of value" (p. 229).

8. See George Kateb, "Democratic Individuality and the Claims of Politics," *Political Theory* 23 (1984), 331–360.

9. This term was initially used in John Rawls, "The Idea of an Overlapping Consensus," *Oxford Journal of Legal Studies* 7 (1987), 1–25.

10. The influence of political liberalism is fairly clear. Explicitly, Rawls's theory of justice has had a profound effect on how justice in medical ethics is approached. Similarly, the notion of autonomy and neutrality has dominated thinking about medical ethics. See, for example, President's Commission for the Study of Ethical Problems in Medicine and Biomedical and Behavioral Research, *Making Health Care Decisions,* vol. 1 (Washington, D.C.: U.S. Government Printing Office, 1982), chap. 2, and *Deciding to Forego Life-Sustaining Treatment* (Washington, D.C.: U.S. Government Printing Office, 1983), chap. 2.

11. Frequently medical ethicists erroneously believe that a mechanical application of Rawls's two principles of justice to the distribution of health care resources is possible. The consequences are usually at odds with the theory more fully understood. See Samuel Gorovitz, *Doctors' Dilemmas* (New York: Oxford University Press, 1982) and Robert M. Veatch, *A Theory of Medical Ethics* (New York: Basic Books, 1981) for this error, and Norman Daniels, *Just Health Care* (New York: Cambridge University Press, 1985) for the more comprehensive approach to political liberalism and just health care.

12. The seven tenets outlined here are merely an adaptation of Rawls's own outline of his philosophy as being "built up from six fundamental intuitive ideas." However, as anyone familiar with Rawls's work will recognize, my outline leaves out two ideas commonly thought to be critical to understanding Rawls, the original position and the veil of ignorance. Not only do I believe these ideas are completely dispensable to understanding political liberalism, I think they have lead to more confusion than elucidation and should be passed over.

13. John Rawls, "Kantian Constructivism in Moral Theory," *Journal of Philosophy* 77 (1980), 536.

14. John Rawls, *A Theory of Justice* (Cambridge, Mass.: Harvard University Press, 1971), p. 579.

15. Rawls, "Justice as Fairness," p. 225.

16. See Rawls, "Kantian Constructivism in Moral Theory," pp. 560–564; "Justice as Fairness," pp. 226–231; and "The Idea of an Overlapping Consensus," pp. 1–25.

17. Rawls, *A Theory of Justice,* p. 7.

18. In "Kantian Constructivism in Moral Theory" Rawls claims that both the principles of justice and the notion of primary goods "rest upon a particular conception of the person."

19. Rawls, "Justice as Fairness," p. 233.
20. Fair equality of opportunity is stronger than simple equality of opportunity because it requires not just elimination of overt discrimination but programs to ensure that social disadvantages are compensated for, permitting children with the same talents and motivation the same chance of success. Practically, this may require heavy investment in education and other programs to support poorer children.
21. Rawls, "Kantian Constructivism in Moral Theory," p. 526.
22. John Rawls, "Social Unity and Primary Goods," in B. Williams and A. Sen, eds., *Utilitarianism and Beyond* (New York: Cambridge University Press, 1982), p. 162.
23. This presentation should make clear that political liberalism recognizes "spheres of justice." (See Michael Walzer, *Spheres of Justice,* New York: Basic Books, 1983.) There are three different principles of distribution in the public sphere related to different goods. The principles are different in part because the goods—rights, opportunities, and income—have different social significance because of how they are related to a conception of the person. Furthermore, completely excluded from this scheme are the distributions made in the private sphere. The social distributions of "private" goods will have their own principles of distribution which need not bear any relationship to the political principles. Thus scientific associations might distribute honors and awards which might be based not on equality or the difference principle but on merit or contribution. Hence political liberalism has a complex view of distributions which includes at least four different "spheres" of justice.

3. Terminating Medical Care for Incompetent Patients

1. *In re Quinlan,* 70 N.J. 10 (1976).
2. *In re Quinlan,* 137 N.J. Super. 227 (Ch. Div. 1975).
3. *In re Quinlan,* 137 N.J. Super. 227 (Ch. Div. 1975).
4. For terminating care cases raising similar criminal issues, see *Barber* v. *Superior Court,* 195 Cal. Rptr. 484 (1983) and *Satz* v. *Perlmutter,* 379 So.2d 359 (1980).
5. *In re Colyer,* 99 Wn.2d 114, 121 (1983). See also Martha Minow, "Beyond State Intervention in the Family: For Baby Jane Doe," *University of Michigan Journal of Law Reform* 18 (1985), 952: "I maintain instead that some degree of state intervention always exists. The argument is not simply that the state always has power to assess its own power to intervene, although it is worth noting how this latent state power casts a shadow over parental decision making. But expressing more than this latent power, the state always intervenes because it allocates power over

the medical care decision, whether it carves out a sphere of parental autonomy or instead permits strangers or state officials to challenge and supplant parental decisions."

6. Others have offered somewhat different classifications. See, for example, Sidney H. Wanzer, S. James Adelstein, Ronald E. Cranford, Daniel D. Federman, Edward D. Hook, Charles G. Moertel, Peter Safar, Alan Stone, Helen B. Taussig, and Jan van Eys, "The Physician's Responsibility toward Hopelessly Ill Patients," *New England Journal of Medicine* 310 (1984), 955–959, and Daniel Callahan, *Setting Limits* (New York: Simon and Schuster, 1987), pp. 180–185.

7. See Barbara J. McNeil, Ralph Weichselbaum, and Stephen G. Pauker, "Speech and Survival: Tradeoffs between Quality and Quantity of Life in Laryngeal Cancer," *New England Journal of Medicine* 305 (1981), 982–987. Similar issues arise in prostatectomies; see Floyd J. Fowler, John E. Wennberg, Robert P. Timothy, Michael J. Barry, Albert G. Mulley, and Daniel Hanley, "Symptom Status and Quality of Life Following Prostatectomy," *Journal of the American Medical Association* 259 (1988), 3018–22.

8. This is the case of *Lane* v. *Candura,* 6 Mass. App. Ct. 377 (1978). Over the objections of her daughter, the patient refused amputation.

9. See William Osler, *The Principles and Practice of Medicine,* 3rd ed. (New York: D. Appleton and Co., 1898), p. 108. Significantly, Osler justifies his judgment by arguing that death by pneumonia is "an acute, short, not often painful illness, [in which] the old man escapes those 'cold gradations of decay' so distressing to himself and to his friends."

10. See *Bouvia* v. *Superior Court,* 225 Cal. Rptr. 297 (1986), and "Quadriplegic Chooses Job Search over Death," *American Medical News,* February 2, 1990, p. 6.

11. David Hilfiker, "Allowing the Debilitated to Die: Facing Our Ethical Choices," *New England Journal of Medicine* 308 (1983), 716–719.

12. One qualification of my study: In outlining the ethical issues involved in terminating medical services to patients, I did not mention the issue of cost and the allocation of resources. The cost of maintaining a patient such as Karen Quinlan on a respirator, with artificial nutrition and hydration and competent nursing care, is about $160,000 per year. This amount is not inconsiderable and raises important questions concerning the just allocation of medical resources. Nevertheless, in this chapter I shall set aside such questions. Instead, at first, we should try to disentangle the medical ethical questions concerning the allocation of resources and those concerning the determination of medical interventions. We should try to consider what should be done for patients such

as Karen Quinlan as if there were no problems of cost or justice, focusing on the ends of medicine and other human ends besides justice. Indeed, once we have explored these ethical issues we may find that the matter of allocation of resources is not actually important, or that its importance is circumscribed to particular situations.

13. John Rawls, "Social Unity and Primary Goods," in B. Williams and A. Sen, eds., *Utilitarianism and Beyond* (New York: Cambridge University Press, 1982), p. 165.

14. Laurence H. Tribe, *American Constitutional Law,* 2nd ed. (Mineola, N.Y.: Foundation Press, 1988), p. 1308.

15. *Griswold* v. *Connecticut,* 381 U.S. 479 (1965).

16. *Pratt* v. *Davis,* 118 Ill. App. 161 (1905). See also *In re Eichner* (Brother Fox), 52 N.Y.2d 363 (1981), where the New York Court of Appeals claims: "Neither do we reach that question [whether the right to refuse treatment is guaranteed by the Constitutional right of privacy] in this case because the relief granted to the petitioner, Eichner, is adequately supported by common-law principles."

17. *Schloendorff* v. *Society of N.Y. Hospital,* 211 N.Y. 125 (1914).

18. President's Commission for the Study of Ethical Problems in Medicine and Biomedical and Behavioral Research, *Deciding to Forego Life-Sustaining Treatment* (Washington, D.C.: U.S. Government Printing Office, 1983), p. 44.

19. *Superintendent of Belchertown State School* v. *Saikewicz,* 373 Mass. 728, 735 (1977).

20. George J. Annas and Leonard H. Glantz, "The Right of Elderly Patients to Refuse Life-sustaining Treatment," *Milbank Quarterly* 64, supp. 2 (1986), 95–162.

21. See Ezekiel J. Emanuel, "A Review of the Ethical and Legal Aspects of Terminating Medical Care," *American Journal of Medicine* 84 (1988), 291–301.

22. *In re Peter,* 108 N.J. 365 (1987).

23. *Cruzan* v. *Director, Missouri Department of Health,* 110 .S. Ct. 2841 (1990).

24. See Ronald Dworkin, "Autonomy and the Demented Self," *Milbank Quarterly* 64, supp. 2 (1986), 4–16.

25. *Cruzan* v. *Director, Missouri Department of Health,* 110 S. Ct. 2841 (1990) (Justice Brennan's dissent). Interestingly, all the cases cited by Justice Brennan in support of the incompetent patient's right to refuse medical care dealt with patients who had some decision-making capacity and therefore some capacity for self-determination, such as children, mentally disturbed individuals, and so forth. None of the precedents cited

concerned patients who completely lacked self-determination in the way that patients in a persistent vegetative state do.

26. *Superintendent of Belchertown State School* v. *Saikewicz,* 373 Mass. 728, 738 (1977).

27. See, for example, Los Angeles County Medical Association and Los Angeles County Bar Association, *Principles and Guidelines concerning the Foregoing of Life-Sustaining Treatment for Adult Patients* (1985), and Ad Hoc Committee on Medical Ethics, *American College of Physicians' Ethics Manual* (Philadelphia: American College of Physicians, 1984) and Massachusetts Medical Society Resolution (July 17, 1985).

28. President's Commission for the Study of Ethical Problems in Medicine and Biomedical and Behavioral Research, *Deciding to Forego Life-Sustaining Treatment,* p. 132.

29. Tribe, *American Constitutional Law,* p. 1368. See also "The Tragic Choice: Termination of Care for Patients in a Permanent Vegetative State," *New York University Law Review* 51 (1976), 285, 293.

30. *In re Quinlan,* 70 N.J. 10 (1976).

31. *Cruzan* v. *Director, Missouri Department of Health,* 110 S. Ct. 2841 (1990).

32. Annas and Glantz, "The Right of Elderly Patients to Refuse Life-sustaining Treatment," p. 104. What is so strange about this quote and the whole approach in this article is that the authors assume such patients already have rights—moral rights—which courts are merely recognizing as legal rights. But this assumption needs to be justified.

33. Michael Walzer, *Spheres of Justice* (New York: Basic Books, 1983), p. xv, argues that proliferating rights is not the only way to guarantee human respect. The values we think we can achieve by rights, he argues, can be realized in other ways through our "shared conceptions of social goods."

34. Annas and Glantz, "The Right of Elderly Patients to Refuse Life-sustaining Treatment," p. 105.

35. See Raymond S. Duff, "Guidelines for Deciding the Care of Critically Ill or Dying Patients," *Pediatrics* 64 (1979), 17–23; Wanzer et al., "The Physician's Responsibility toward Hopelessly Ill Patients"; Los Angeles County Medical Association and Los Angeles County Bar Association, *Principles and Guidelines Concerning the Foregoing of Life-Sustaining Treatment for Adult Patients* (1985); Ad Hoc Committee on Medical Ethics, *American College of Physicians' Ethics Manual;* Richard A. McCormick and Robert Veatch, "The Preservation of Life and Self-Determination," *Theological Studies* 41 (1981), 390–396; Allen Buchanan, "Medical Paternalism or Legal Imperialism: Not the Only Alternatives for Handling

Saikewicz-type Cases," *American Journal of Law and Medicine* 5 (1979), 97–117; *In re Spring,* 380 Mass. 629 (1979); *Bowen* v. *American Hospital Association et. al.,* 106 U.S. 2102 (1986); and President's Commission for the Study of Ethical Problems in Medicine and Biomedical and Behavioral Research, *Deciding to Forego Life-Sustaining Treatment.*

36. See *In re Conroy,* 98 N.J. 321 (1985), and Hilfiker, "Allowing the Debilitated to Die."

37. Richard F. Uhlmann, Robert A. Pearlman, and Kevin C. Cain, "Physicians' and Spouses' Prediction of Elderly Patients' Resuscitation Preferences," *Journal of Gerontology* 43 (1988), M115–M121, and Nancy R. Zweibel and Christine K. Cassel, "Treatment Choices at the End of Life: A Comparison of Decisions by Older Patients and Their Physician-Selected Proxies," *The Gerontologist* 29 (1989), 615–621.

38. *New York Times,* January 14, 1985, p. A1.

39. *Lane* v. *Candura,* 6 Mass. App. Ct. 377 (1978).

40. John La Puma, David L. Schiedermayer, Stephen Toulmin, Steven H. Miles, and Jane A. McAtee, "The Standard of Care: A Case Report and Ethical Analysis," *Annals of Internal Medicine* 108 (1988), 121–124.

41. See, for example, J. Brant, "Last Rights: An Analysis of Refusal and Withholding Treatment Cases," *Missouri Law Review* 46 (1981), 337–370; John A. Gustafson, "Mongolism, Parental Desires and the Right to Life," *Perspectives in Biology and Medicine* 16 (1973), 529–557; Charles Krauthammer, "What to do about 'Baby Doe,'" *The New Republic,* September 2, 1985, pp. 16–21; and John A. Robertson and Norman Fost, "Passive Euthanasia of Defective Newborn Infants: Legal Considerations," *Journal of Pediatrics* 88 (1976), 883–889.

42. An interesting case in which a family clearly became emotionally exhausted and then, without any change in the patient's physical or mental condition, asked to terminate care, is *In re Spring,* 380 Mass. 629 (1980). For cases in which parents' interests may conflict with those of their children, see *Custody of a Minor,* 379 N.E.2d 1053 (1978) and *In re Phillip B.,* 156 Cal. Rptr. 48 (1979). For commentary on Phillip B., see Minow, "Beyond State Intervention in the Family."

43. *In re Storar,* 52 N.Y.2d 363 (1981).

44. Arnold S. Relman, "The Saikewicz Decision: A Medical Viewpoint," *American Journal of Law and Medicine* 4 (1978), 233–242.

45. *Barber* v. *Superior Court,* 147 Cal. App. 3d 1006 (1983). See also *In re Dinnerstein,* 380 N.E. 2d 134 (1978).

46. Charles Baron, "The Case for the Courts," *Journal of the American Geriatric Society* 32 (1984), 734–738; Charles L. Baron, "Medical Paternalism and the Rule of Law: A Reply to Dr. Relman," *American Journal of*

Law and Medicine 4 (1979), 337–365; and Allen Buchanan, "Medical Paternalism or Legal Imperialism: Not the Only Alternatives for Handling Saikewicz-type Cases."

47. See, for example, Baron, "The Case for the Courts" and "Medical Paternalism and the Rule of Law."
48. *Superintendent of Belchertown State School* v. *Saikewicz,* 373 Mass. 728 (1977).
49. See *In re Spring,* 380 Mass. 629 (1979).
50. *Custody of a Minor,* 385 Mass. 697 (1982).
51. See *In re Quinlan,* 70 N.J. 10 (1976); *Barber* v. *Superior Court,* 147 Cal. App. 3d 1006 (1983); and *In re Conroy,* 98 N.J. 321 (1985).
52. *In re Conroy,* 98 N.J. 321 (1985).
53. John D. Arras, "Toward an Ethic of Ambiguity," *Hastings Center Report* 14 (1984), 25.
54. Paul A. Freund, "Mongoloids and 'Mercy killing,'" in S. J. Reiser, A. J. Dyck, and W. J. Curran, eds., *Ethics in Medicine: Historical Perspectives and Contemporary Concerns* (Cambridge, Mass.: MIT Press, 1977), pp. 536–539.
55. Ronald Dworkin, *A Matter of Principle* (Cambridge, Mass.: Harvard University Press, 1985), p. 34.
56. See H. Tristram Engelhardt, *The Foundations of Bioethics* (New York: Oxford University Press, 1986), pp. 248, 307; Robert Weir, *Selective Nontreatment of Handicapped Newborns* (New York: Oxford University Press, 1984), p. 212; and James J. McCartney, "The Development of the Doctrine of Ordinary and Extraordinary Means of Preserving Life in Catholic Moral Theology before the Karen Quinlan Case," *Linacre Quarterly* 47 (1980), 215–224.
57. Gerald Kelly, *Medico-Moral Problems* (St. Louis: The Catholic Hospital Association, 1958), p. 129.
58. Paul Ramsey, *Ethics at the Edges of Life* (New Haven, Conn.: Yale University Press, 1978), pp. 145–227.
59. Robert M. Veatch, *Death, Dying, and the Biological Revolution* (New Haven, Conn.: Yale University Press, 1976), pp. 105–114.
60. President's Commission for the Study of Ethical Problems in Medicine and Biomedical and Behavioral Research, *Deciding to Forego Life-Sustaining Treatment,* pp. 87–89.
61. Ibid.
62. Weir, *Selective Nontreatment of Handicapped Newborns,* pp. 211–215, 233–238.
63. Allen Buchanan argues that a judgment about what factors should constitute extraordinary care is not "a technological or even a clinical, but rather a moral decision." "Medical Paternalism," *Philosophy and Public*

Affairs 7 (1978), 370–390. Buchanan believes that the ordinary/extraordinary distinction merely serves to perpetuate medical paternalism. This conclusion seems dubious, especially since the distinction has found more favor among lawyers, bioethicists, theologians, and others not known for their support of medical paternalism.

64. See Ramsey, *Ethics at the Edges of Life,* chap. 5.

65. See Raymond S. Duff, "Counseling Families and Deciding Care of Severely Defective Children: A Way of Coping with 'Medical Vietnam,'" *Pediatrics* 67 (1981), 315–320.

66. President's Commission for the Study of Ethical Problems in Medicine and Biomedical and Behavioral Research, *Deciding to Forego Life-Sustaining Treatment,* p. 88.

67. Ibid., p. 83.

68. A. Martin Waldman, "Medical Ethics and the Hopelessly Ill Child," *Journal of Pediatrics* 88 (1976), 890–892.

69. President's Commission for the Study of Ethical Problems in Medicine and Biomedical and Behavioral Research, *Deciding to Forego Life-Sustaining Treatment,* p. 83.

70. *In re Conroy,* 98 N.J. 321, 338–339 (1985).

71. *In re Conroy,* 98 N.J. 321 (1985). See also *Brophy* v. *New England Sinai Hospital,* 398 Mass. 417 (1986); *Barber* v. *Superior Court,* 147 Cal. App. 3d 1006 (1983); Ramsey, *Ethics at the Edges of Life,* chap. 5; and President's Commission for the Study of Ethical Problems in Medicine and Biomedical and Behavioral Research, *Deciding to Forego Life-Sustaining Treatment,* p. 83.

72. *In re Jobes,* 108 N.J. 394 (1987) (concurring opinion by Justice Handler). Justice Handler writes: "No one would fail to characterize the extensive treatment that serves to keep her in a biologically-viable condition as extraordinary and heroic." And at other points he states that Ms. Jobes is receiving "massive, extraordinary medical and health care measures." See also *John F. Kennedy Hospital* v. *Bludworth,* 452 So. 2d 921 (1984); *New York Times,* January 14, 1985, p. A1; David T. Watts and Christine K. Cassel, "Extraordinary Nutrition Support: A Case Study and Ethical Analysis," *Journal of the American Geriatrics Society* 32 (1984), 237–242; and Joanne Lynn, ed., *By No Extraordinary Means* (Bloomington, Ind.: Indiana University Press, 1986).

73. See, for example, *Superintendent of Belchertown State School* v. *Saikewicz,* 373 Mass. 728 (1977), and John A. Robertson, "Organ Donation by Incompetents and Substituted Judgment Doctrine," *Columbia Law Review* 76 (1976), 48–78 for a brief history of the substituted judgment doctrines in other areas of the law.

74. *In re Mary Moe,* 385 Mass. 555 (1982).

75. President's Commission for the Study of Ethical Problems in Medicine and Biomedical and Behavioral Research, *Deciding to Forego Life-Sustaining Treatment*, p. 132.

76. *Superintendent of Belchertown State School* v. *Saikewicz*, 373 Mass. 728 (1977).

77. *In re Mary Moe*, 385 Mass. 555, 565 (1982), quoting from *In re Carson*, 39 Misc. 2d 544, 545 (N.Y. Sup. Ct. 1962). The *Moe* case involved the question of sterilizing a 26-year-old girl who functioned at the mental level of a 4-year-old.

78. *In re Quinlan*, 70 N.J. 10 (1976).

79. *Superintendent of Belchertown State School* v. *Saikewicz*, 373 Mass. 728 (1977).

80. *In re Mary Moe*, 385 Mass. 555 (1982).

81. *In re Dinnerstein*, 380 N.E. 2d 134 (1978) and *In re Spring*, 380 Mass. 629 (1980).

82. *Custody of a Minor*, 379 N.E. 1053 (1978). This case involved a 2-year-old child suffering from acute lymphocytic leukemia. The parents did not want to give him conventional chemotherapy, even though this is one of the cancers in which there is a real possibility of a cure with chemotherapy. The issue before the court was whether to force the child to have the treatments against the wishes of the parents. In the case the court argues: "In a case like this one, involving a child who is incompetent by reason of his tender years, we think that the substituted judgment doctrine is consistent with the 'best interests of the child' test." The court sanctioned the use of the substituted judgment analysis.

83. President's Commission for the Study of Ethical Problems in Medicine and Biomedical and Behavioral Research, *Deciding to Forego Life-Sustaining Treatment*, p. 136.

84. *In re Conroy*, 98 N.J. 321, 360 (1985).

85. *In re Jobes*, 108 N.J. 394 (1987).

86. *In re Guardianship of Barry*, 445 So.2d 365, 366 (1984).

87. See Annas and Glantz, "The Right of Elderly Patients to Refuse Life-sustaining Treatment," p. 106, who "strongly agree that the substituted judgment test is the primary and preferred test."

88. *Superintendent of Belchertown State School* v. *Saikewicz*, 373 Mass. 728 (1977).

89. *In re Mary Moe*, 385 Mass. 555, 566 (1982).

90. See the President's Commission for the Study of Ethical Problems in Medicine and Biomedical and Behavioral Research, *Deciding to Forego Life-Sustaining Treatment*, p. 133. The Commission argues that "the substituted judgment standard can be used only if a patient was once capable of developing views relevant to the matter at hand." The Com-

mission, however, never quite extends the point to see that in the limiting case where one is really certain about an incompetent individual's wish, there is then no real substituted judgment.

91. Judge Nolan dissenting in *In re Mary Moe,* 385 Mass. 555, 573 (1982). See also the commentary of Arthur J. Dyck, "Ethical Aspects of Care for the Dying Incompetent," *Journal of the American Geriatrics Society* 32 (1984), 661–664.

92. Thomas G. Gutheil and Paul S. Appelbaum, "Substituted Judgment: Best Interests in Disguise," *Hastings Center Report* 13 (1983), 8–11.

93. *In re John Storar,* 52 N.Y.2d 363, 380 (1981). See also Paul Ramsey, "The *Saikewicz* Precedent: What's Good for an Incompetent Patient?" *Hastings Center Report* 8 (1978), 36.

94. "Live or Let Die: Who Decides an Incompetent's Fate? *In re Storar* and *In re Eichner,*" *Brigham Young University Law Review* 64 (1982), 387–400.

95. See *In re Estate of Longeway,* 123 Ill. 2d 33 (1988) (dissenting opinion of Judge Ward).

96. *In re Jobes,* 108 N.J. 394 (1987) (J. Handler's concurring opinion).

97. *In re Earle Spring,* 380 Mass. 629 (1979).

98. Minow, "Beyond State Intervention in the Family," p. 973.

99. Steven R. Steiber, "Right to Die: Public Balks at Deciding for Others," *Hospitals,* March 5, 1987, p. 72.

100. Uhlmann, Pearlman, and Cain, "Physicians' and Spouses' Predictions of Elderly Patients' Resuscitation Preferences," and Zweibel and Cassel, "Treatment Choices at the End of Life."

101. See Michael J. Sandel, *Liberalism and the Limits of Justice* (New York: Cambridge University Press, 1982), conclusion.

102. See, for example, Sean M. Dunphy, "Deciding the Fate of Incompetent Patients: What Roles Should Doctor and Judge Play?" *Massachusetts Medicine* (July/August 1986), 32–36. In 1986 a Massachusetts judge argued for the substituted judgment standard even in cases where the patient has been incompetent since birth; and again in 1987 the New Jersey Supreme Court invoked this standard in *In re Jobes,* 108 N.J. 394 (1987).

103. Note "Live or Let Die: Who Decides an Incompetent's Fate? *In re Storar* and *In re Eichner,*" which suggests that "the need for the fiction of substituted judgment seems to arise out of a desire to accord the incompetent the dignity to which society believes every human being is entitled." Again on this view we seem to find the ethical problem of according dignity by way of rights.

104. *Barber v. Superior Court,* 147 Cal. App. 3d 1006, 1019 (1983).

105. Annas and Glantz, "The Right of Elderly Patients to Refuse Life-sustaining Treatment," p. 109.

106. George J. Annas, "Reconciling *Quinlan* and *Saikewicz:* Decision Mak-

ing for the Terminally Ill Incompetent," *American Journal of Law and Medicine* 4 (1979), 377.

107. Richard A. McCormick and Robert Veatch, "The Preservation of Life and Self-Determination," p. 391.

108. *Custody of a Minor* (Chad Green), 379 N.E.2d 1053, 1065 (1978).

109. *In re Jobes,* 108 N.J. 394 (J. Handler's concurring opinion, 1987), where Justice Handler argues: "[T]he courts must develop some variation of [the best interests] approach to deal with the extreme cases where subjective approaches seeking individual self-determination are unavailing."

110. See President's Commission for the Study of Ethical Problems in Medicine and Biomedical and Behavioral Research, *Deciding to Forego Life-Sustaining Treatment,* pp. 134–136; *In re Conroy,* 98 N.J. 321 (1985); and *Barber* v. *Superior Court,* 147 Cal.App.3d 1006 (1983).

111. See *In re Hamlin,* 102 Wn.2d 810 (1984).

112. See Arras, "Toward an Ethic of Ambiguity," pp. 25–31, and Ruth Macklin, *Mortal Choices* (New York: Pantheon, 1987), chaps. 7 and 8.

113. Allen Buchanan and Dan W. Brock, "Deciding for Others," *Milbank Quarterly* 64, supp. 2 (1986), 28.

114. This claim suggests that any commentator who uses the best interests standard will implicitly have a *personal* quality-of-life judgment despite his vociferous objections. Paul Ramsey objects to quality-of-life judgments. Yet he argues that children suffering from Lesch-Nyhan syndrome (a fatal genetic disorder resulting in bizarre behavior including self-mutilation) can be denied medical treatments because there is no cure or effective means to relieve the pain of children with this disorder and their lives are too painful and burdensome. Clearly this assumes a *personal* quality-of-life assessment about life with Lesch-Nyhan syndrome. See Ramsey, *Ethics and the Edges of Life,* chaps. 5 and 6.

115. President's Commission for the Study of Ethical Problems in Medicine and Biomedical and Behavioral Research, *Deciding to Forego Life-Sustaining Treatment,* p. 135.

116. A. R. Jonsen, R. H. Phibbs, W. H. Tooley, and M. J. Garland, "Critical Issues in Newborn Intensive Care: A Conference Report and Policy Proposal," *Pediatrics* 55 (1975), 756–765.

117. Engelhardt, *The Foundations of Bioethics,* p. 231.

118. *In re Conroy,* 98 N.J. 321 (1985).

119. Earle E. Shelp, *Born to Die?* (New York: Free Press, 1986), pp. 127–128.

120. See Henry K. Beecher, "Pain in Men Wounded in Battle," *Annals of Surgery* 123 (1946), 96–105; Ronald Melzack, "Measurement of the Dimensions of Pain Experience," in B. Bromm, ed., *Pain Measurement in Man: Neurophysiological Correlates of Pain* (New York: Elsevier, 1984); and H.

Mersky and F. G. Spear, *Pain: Psychological and Psychiatric Aspects* (London: Bailliere, Tindall and Cassell, 1967).
121. *In re Conroy,* 98 N.J. 321, 393–394 (1985).
122. It should be noted here that liberals who accept the ideal of neutrality might have a different view of whether there is an objective view of the best life. They might simply express skepticism about it and deny its possibility, or they might affirm that there are many different, equally good ways to live.
123. Rawls, "Social Unity and Primary Goods," p. 170.
124. This is not the only justification for informed consent. But for the purposes of this section, I simply articulate the justification provided through a liberal political philosophy.
125. President's Commission for the Study of Ethical Problems in Medicine and Biomedical and Behavioral Research, *Deciding to Forego Life-Sustaining Treatment,* p. 43.
126. *In re Jobes,* 108 N.J. 394 (1987) (concurring opinion of Justice Handler).
127. John A. Robertson, "Involuntary Euthanasia of Defective Newborns: A Legal Analysis," *Stanford Law Review* 27 (1975), 254.
128. Chambers, "Advocates for the Right to Life," *New York Times Magazine,* December 16, 1984, p. 94. See also Nat Hentoff, "The Awful Privacy of Baby Doe," *Atlantic Monthly,* January 1985, pp. 54–62.
129. See, for example, Immanuel Jakobovits, *Jewish Medical Ethics* (New York: Bloch, 1959), chaps. 3, 4, 5, and 11, and J. David Bleich, *Judaism and Healing: Halakhic Perspectives* (New York: Ktav, 1981), chaps. 3, 24, and 25.
130. See Freund, "Mongoloids and 'Mercy Killing.'"
131. Franklin H. Epstein, "No, It's Our Duty to Keep Patients Alive," *Medical Economics,* April 2, 1973, pp. 97–114; "The Role of the Physician in the Prolongation of Life," in F. J. Ingelfinger, A. S. Relman, and M. Finland, eds., *Controversies in Internal Medicine,* vol. 2 (Philadelphia: Saunders, 1974), pp. 103–109; and "Responsibility of the Physician in the Preservation of Life," *Archives of Internal Medicine* 139 (1979), 919–920. See also Allen Jay, "The Judge Ordered Me to Kill My Patient," *Medical Economics,* August 10, 1987, pp. 120–124, and Samuel C. Bukantz, "Life-and-Death Decisions," *Hospital Practice* 13 (April 15, 1986), 17, 20.
132. Hentoff, "The Awful Privacy of Baby Doe."
133. *In re John Storar,* 52 N.Y.2d 363, 380–382 (1981). The court suggests no grounds could be given for adducing death preferable to life.
134. *Federal Register* 49 (1984), 1622–54. I say "possibly" here because the "Baby Doe" rules do contain the notion that treatment can be withheld if it is merely "prolonging the dying process" or if it is "futile." These

qualifications may only be to pacify the political opposition and may not reflect the true intentions of those within the Reagan administration who probably had more of a physical conception.

135. Krauthammer, "What to Do about 'Baby Doe,'" p. 19.

136. Carson Strong, "The Tiniest Newborns," *Hastings Center Report* 13 (1983), 14–19.

137. John Stuart Mill, "Remarks on Bentham's Philosophy," in *The Collected Works of John Stuart Mill*, vol. 10, ed. J. M. Robson (Toronto: Toronto University Press, 1969), pp. 5–18.

138. Richard A. McCormick, "To Save or Let Die: The Dilemma of Modern Medicine," *Journal of the American Medical Association* 229 (1974), 172–176.

139. Ibid.

140. Arras, "Toward an Ethic of Ambiguity," p. 32.

141. See Daniel Callahan, *Setting Limits* (New York: Simon and Schuster, 1987), pp. 174–193, and Arras, "Toward an Ethic of Ambiguity."

142. Some commentators suggest that when a patient is incompetent, "physicians and family members [can] not refer to the moral principle of autonomy to guide their resolution of the nutrition question [deciding whether to withhold intravenous nutrition]." Rebecca S. Dresser and Eugene V. Boisaubin, "Ethics, Law, and Nutritional Support," *Archives of Internal Medicine* 145 (1985), 122–1124. But clearly the principle of autonomy might be useful in the case of incompetent patients precisely in defining their good—that is, any treatment which did not return them to full autonomy would be deemed without benefit.

143. Wanzer et al., "The Physician's Responsibility toward Hopelessly Ill Patients."

144. President's Commission for the Study of Ethical Problems in Medicine and Biomedical and Behavioral Research, *Deciding to Forego Life-Sustaining Treatment*, p. 135.

145. *In re Dinnerstein*, 380 N.E.2d 134, 138 (1978).

146. *Custody of a Minor*, 379 N.E.2d 1053, 1055 (1978).

147. John Lorber, "Spina Bifida Cystica: Results of Treatment of 270 Consecutive Cases with Criteria for Selection for the Future," *Archives of Disease in Childhood* 47 (1972), 854–873.

148. See, for example, Guido Calabresi and Philip Bobbitt, *Tragic Choices* (New York: W. W. Norton, 1978), p. 184, and Henry J. Aaron and William B. Schwartz, *The Painful Prescription: Rationing Hospital Care* (Washington, D.C.: The Brookings Institution, 1984), pp. 29–37.

149. Peter Singer, *Practical Ethics* (New York: Cambridge University Press, 1979), p. 134.

150. See Michael Tooley, "Abortion and Infanticide," *Philosophy and Public*

Affairs 2 (1972), 37–65, and Jonathan Glover, *Causing Death and Saving Lives* (New York: Penguin, 1977), chap. 12.

151. This, in short, is Peter Singer's argument in *Practical Ethics,* chap. 4.
152. *In re Conroy,* 98 N.J. 321, 334 (1985).
153. See Callahan, *Setting Limits,* p. 191.
154. John Rawls, "Justice as Fairness: Political not Metaphysical," *Philosophy and Public Affairs* 114 (1985), 223–251.
155. President's Commission for the Study of Ethical Problems in Medicine and Biomedical and Behavioral Research, *Deciding to Forego Life-Sustaining Treatment,* p. 128.
156. When Rawls argues for the liberal state as a social union of social unions, it is important to note that these smaller social unions are provided no special legal recognition nor any special financial support. If they flourish, they do so on the basis of private decisions, not public commitments. See John Rawls, *A Theory of Justice* (Cambridge, Mass.: Harvard University Press, 1971), section 79.
157. *Barber* v. *Superior Court,* 147 Cal. App. 3d 1006, 1019 (1983). See also Joanne Lynn and James F. Childress, "Must Patients Always Be Given Food and Water?" *Hastings Center Report* 13 (1983), 17–21, who argue that "there is now widespread consensus that sometimes a patient is best served by not undertaking or continuing certain treatments that would sustain life, especially if these entail substantial suffering."
158. Bukantz, "Life-and-Death Decisions."
159. President's Commission for the Study of Ethical Problems in Medicine and Biomedical and Behavioral Research, *Deciding to Forego Life-Sustaining Treatment,* p. 3.
160. *In re Conroy,* 98 N.J. 321, 368 (1985).
161. However, this willingness of courts to permit the termination of care may be more apparent than real. In many of the most important legal cases—Saikewicz, Storar, Dinnerstein, Barber, Conroy—the patients had died before the court rendered its decision. And while the cases were not declared moot because of the public importance and likely recurrence of the situations, courts often qualify their judgments by arguing that "the reach of this decision does not extend beyond the particular facts presented in the case before us." *Satz* v. *Perlmutter,* 379 So.2d 359, 360 (1980). In addition, many of the decisions establish very stringent procedural requirements for terminating care that are often very difficult to carry out in actuality.
162. Hilfiker, "Allowing the Debilitated to Die."
163. See, for example, the claim that the "social commitment of the physician is to prolong life and relieve suffering" in the Judicial Council of the American Medical Association, *Current Opinions* (Chicago: Ameri-

can Medical Association, 1984), p. 11. And I noted previously that the President's Commission argued that, if uncertain, physicians should "err, if at all, in favor of preserving life."

164. Two recent surveys of physicians seem to suggest that physicians are very aggressive about treating aged, terminally ill, and debilitated patients even with artificial nutrition and fluids. See Kenneth C. Micetich, Patricia H. Steinecker, and David C. Thomasma, "Are Intravenous Fluids Morally Required for a Dying Patient?" *Archives of Internal Medicine* 143 (1983), 975–978, and Mary E. Charlson, Fredric L. Sax, Ronald MacKenzie, Suzanne D. Fields, Robert L. Braham, and R. Gordon Douglas, "Resuscitation: How Do We Decide?" *Journal of the American Medical Association* 255 (1986), 1316–1322.

165. Wanzer et al., "The Physician's Responsibility toward Hopelessly Ill Patients."

166. For an excellent case in which physicians recommend restraint in using medical interventions but offer no public justification, just their opinion, see Wanzer et al., "The Physician's Responsibility toward Hopelessly Ill Patients."

167. The only shared framework that can be appealed to is futility. Physicians are willing to forswear an intervention, such as resuscitation, that does not save any lives whatsoever.

168. Quoted in Richard D. Lamm, "Long Time Dying," *The New Republic,* August 27, 1984, p. 20.

169. Robert Stinson and Peggy Stinson, *The Long Dying of Baby Andrew* (Boston: Atlantic Monthly Press, 1983), p. 341.

170. See, for example, *Evans* v. *Bellevue Hospital* (Wirth) (no. 16536/87 New York Supreme Court, N.Y. County, July 27, 1987) (Sandifer J.), N.Y.L.J. July 28, 1987, at 11 col. 1., and E. R. W. Fox, "Nora's Living Will," *Western Journal of Medicine* 146 (1987), 118.

171. *New York Times,* December 24, 1985, p. A8.

172. *New York Times,* December 22, 1985, p. A20. See also the case of a father who held hospital workers at gunpoint while he disconnected his comatose son from a respirator. The police came to arrest him, and he stated: "I'll only hurt you if you try to plug my baby back in." He was charged with murder. *Washington Post,* April 27, 1989, p. A8.

173. *New York Times,* August 9, 1985, p. A10. See also *New York Times,* August 8, 1985, p. C22, for the review of a television show about the case.

174. *New York Times,* February 6, 1982, p. A7.

175. *New York Times,* February 21, 1983, p. B4.

176. Steiber, "Right to Die: Public Balks at Deciding for Others."

177. Other examples of matters of the quality of common life might include whether the community should support art and what kinds of art; what

subjects with what texts the community should teach in primary and secondary schools; whether the community should provide teenagers with sex education in schools; whether the community should provide maternity leave and day care; whether the community should permit surrogate motherhood; whether the community should permit the privatization of governmental services; what environmental policy the community should adopt; whether the community should permit prostitution or gambling; how the community should care for the mentally ill; whether the community should enact "blue" laws restricting commerce; or whether the community should restrict the construction of chain department stores and discount houses to protect small stores and their neighborhoods.

178. See Bernard Williams, *Ethics and the Limits of Philosophy* (Cambridge, Mass.: Harvard University Press, 1986).

4. The Just Distribution of Medical Resources

1. As I noted in Chapter 2, although Rawls himself has never published on the issue of just health care, he takes the issue seriously because a theory of justice must be able to guide public deliberations on the fair distribution of scarce resources, including medical resources.

2. I use the terms "distribution" and "allocation" interchangeably in this chapter. Occasionally the terms are distinguished, with distribution referring to the disbursement of goods by rules and procedures of a system in which individuals produce the goods and are enmeshed in ongoing relationships, while allocation refers to the disbursement of goods to specific individuals who do not produce the goods and have no further relationship. In this sense, allocation refers to a kind of rationing. In this chapter both terms will refer to the former conception. See John Rawls, *A Theory of Justice* (Cambridge, Mass.: Harvard University Press, 1971), p. 88.

3. Shep Glazer, Testimony before House Ways and Means Committee, 92nd Congress, National Health Insurance Proposals, Part 7 (November 3, 1971), pp. 1524–46 (72-H781–8.10). Although Glazer's efforts were important because they took place before a particularly powerful member of Congress, Wilbur Mills, he was not the first person to dialyze himself before members of Congress; at least two other individuals did a similar thing in the mid-1960s. See Richard A. Rettig, *Valuing Lives: The Policy Debate on Patient Care Financing for Victims of End-Stage Renal Disease* (Santa Monica, Calif.: Rand Corporation, 1976), pp. 34–35.

4. *Congressional Record,* September 30, 1972, p. 33004.

5. *Background Information of Kidney Disease Benefits under Medicare.* Report to Subcommittee on Health of the Committee on Ways and Means, U.S. House of Representatives (Washington, D.C.: U.S. Government Printing Office, June 24, 1975).

6. Glazer, Testimony before House Ways and Means Committee, pp. 1538–39.

7. *Congressional Record,* September 30, 1972, pp. 33003–8.

8. Health Care Financing Administration, *End Stage Disease Program Quarterly Statistical Summary,* April 17, 1987.

9. Roger W. Evans, Christopher R. Blagg, and Fred A. Bryan, "Implications for Health Care Policy: A Social and Demographic Profile of Hemodialysis Patients in the United States," *Journal of the American Medical Association* 245 (1981), 487–491.

10. Health Care Financing Administration, *End Stage Renal Disease Patient Profile Tables* (Washington, D.C.: U.S. Government Printing Office, 1985).

11. Diane M. Carlson, William J. Johnson, and Carl M. Kjellstrand, "Functional Status of Patients with End-Stage Renal Disease," *Mayo Clinic Proceedings* 62 (1987), 338–344.

12. Evans, Blagg, and Bryan, "Implications for Health Care Policy."

13. Figures calculated using *Health: United States, 1985* (Washington, D.C.: U.S. Government Printing Office, December 1985) and data from the "End-Stage Renal Disease Program Quarterly Statistical Summary," Office of Statistics and Data Management, Bureau of Data Management and Strategy, Health Care Financing Administration (1987).

14. Helen Laxenby, Katharine R. Levit, and Daniel R. Waldo, "National Health Expenditures, 1985," *Health Care Financing Review* 7 (September 1986), 1–31.

15. Congressional Budget Office, *Changing the Structure of Medicare Benefits: Issues and Options* (Washington, D.C.: U.S. Government Printing Office, 1983).

16. Mary O'Neil Mundinger, "Health Service Funding Cuts and the Declining Health of the Poor," *New England Journal of Medicine* 313 (1985), 44–47.

17. David A. Ansell and Robert L. Schiff, "Patient Dumping: Status, Implications, and Policy Recommendations," *Journal of the American Medical Association* 257 (1987), 1500–2.

18. Mundinger, "Health Service Funding Cuts and the Declining Health of the Poor."

19. See Maureen Hack and Avory A. Fanaroff, "Changes in the Delivery Room Care of the Extremely Small Infant (<750g): Effects on Morbidity and Outcome," *New England Journal of Medicine* 314 (1986), 660–664,

and Michael H. Boyle, George W. Torrance, John C. Sinclair, and Sargent P. Horwood, "Economic Evaluation of Neonatal Intensive Care of Very-Low-Birth-Weight Infants," *New England Journal of Medicine* 308 (1983), 1330–37.

20. See Ann M. Hardy, "Planning for the Health Care Needs of Patients with AIDS," *Journal of the American Medical Association* 256 (1986), 3140, and *New York Times,* May 29, 1987, p. A1.

21. President's Commission for the Study of Ethical Problems in Medicine and Biomedical and Behavioral Research, *Securing Access to Health Care,* vol. 1 (Washington, D.C.: U.S. Government Printing Office, 1983), p. 3.

22. With important differences, the typology offered here is similar to one suggested by H. Tristram Engelhardt, *The Foundations of Bioethics* (New York: Oxford University Press, 1986), pp. 344–348.

23. "The importance of the microallocative level [in Britain] is directly attributable to the macroallocative patterns that have emerged. If sufficient resources had been provided to treat virtually all ESRD [End Stage Renal Disease] patients, as in the United States, the microallocative decision as to whether to treat would have long since faded away, like the background in an old snapshot. Because such resources have not been made available [in Britain]—because, indeed, a condition of hyperscarcity has prevailed from the outset—the microallocative decision has retained immense significance and continues to raise a number of rather disturbing issues." Thomas Halper, "Life and Death in a Welfare State: End-stage Renal Disease in the United Kingdom," *Milbank Memorial Fund Quarterly* 63 (1985), 52–93. Technically, microallocative choices might not have been so severe even with very scarce total health care resources, if, at the medical level of distribution, the British had concluded that dialysis was very important and devoted a large proportion of the health care budget to this treatment while reducing other services.

24. For instance, the application of cost-benefit analysis to medical interventions is recommended by David Blumenthal, Penny Feldman, and Richard Zeckhauser, "Misuse of Technology: A Symptom, Not the Disease," in B. J. McNeil and E. G. Cravalho, eds., *Critical Issues in Medical Technology* (Boston: Auburn House, 1982), while elimination of unnecessary care to ensure wider access to care is recommended by Albert L. Siu, Frank A. Sonnenberg, Willard G. Manning, George A. Goldberg, Ellyn S. Bloomfield, Joseph P. Newhouse, and Robert H. Brook, "Inappropriate Use of Hospitals in a Randomized Trial of Health Insurance Plans," *New England Journal of Medicine* 315 (1986), 1259–66; Kathi J. Kemper, "Medically Inappropriate Hospital Use in a

Pediatric Population," *New England Journal of Medicine* 318 (1988), 1033–37; and Albert L. Siu and Robert H. Brooks, "Allocating Health Care Resources: How Can We Ensure Access to Essential Care?" in E. Ginzberg, ed., *Medicine and Society* (Boulder, Colo.: Westview Press, 1987).

25. William B. Schwartz, "The Inevitable Failure of Current Cost-Containment Strategies: Why They Can Provide only Temporary Relief," *Journal of the American Medical Association* 257 (1987), 2220–24.

26. Rashi Fein, *Medical Care, Medical Costs* (Cambridge, Mass.: Harvard University Press, 1986), p. 194.

27. Ohio Health and Old Age Insurance Commission, *Health, Health Insurance, Old Age Pensions* (Columbus, Ohio: February 1919), quoted in Paul Starr, "Medical Care and the Pursuit of Equality in America," in President's Commission for the Study of Ethical Problems in Medicine and Biomedical and Behavioral Research, *Securing Access to Health Care,* vol. 2 (Washington, D.C.: U.S. Government Printing Office, 1983), p. 9.

28. President's Commission on the Health Needs of the Nation, *Building America's Health,* vol. 1 (Washington, D.C.: U.S. Government Printing Office, 1952), p. 3.

29. Stuart Altman and Robert Blendon, Introduction, in S. H. Altman and R. Blendon, eds., *Medical Technology: The Culprit behind Health Care Costs?* (Washington, D.C.: Department of Health, Education, and Welfare, 1979), p. 1.

30. Amy Gutmann, "For and Against Equal Access to Health Care," *Milbank Memorial Fund Quarterly* 59 (1981), 542–560.

31. Norman Daniels, *Just Health Care* (New York: Cambridge University Press, 1985), p. 74.

32. Leon Kass, *Toward a More Natural Science* (New York: Free Press, 1985), p. 174.

33. David Gauthier, "Unequal Need: A Problem of Equity in Access to Health Care," in President's Commission for the Study of Ethical Problems in Medicine and Biomedical and Behavioral Research, *Securing Access to Health Care,* vol. 2, pp. 179–205. See also Christopher Boorse, "On the Distinction between Disease and Illness," *Philosophy and Public Affairs* 5 (1975), 49–68, and "Health as a Theoretical Concept," *Philosophy of Science* 44 (1977), 542–573; and Daniels, *Just Health Care,* pp. 26–32.

34. David E. Rogers, Linda H. Aiken, and Robert J. Blendon, *Personal Medical Care: Its Adaptation to the 1980s* (Washington, D.C.: Institute of Medicine, 1980), quoted in President's Commission for the Study of Ethical Problems in Medicine and Biomedical and Behavioral Research, *Securing Access to Health Care,* vol. 1, pp. 52–53.

35. Leighton E. Cluff, "Chronic Disease, Function and the Quality of Care," *Journal of Chronic Disease* 34 (1981), 299–304.

36. Robert M. Veatch, *A Theory of Medical Ethics* (New York: Basic Books, 1981), p. 275. See also Gauthier, "Unequal Need," vol. 2, p. 195.

37. Siu and Brook, "Allocating Health Care Resources."

38. Engelhardt, *The Foundations of Bioethics,* pp. 164–185. See also Thomas S. Szaz, *The Myth of Mental Illness* (New York: Harper and Row, 1974), and Peter Sedgwick, "Illness—Mental and Otherwise," *Hastings Center Studies* 1 (1973), 30–37.

39. Robert M. Veatch, "What is a 'Just' Health Care Delivery?" in R. M. Veatch and R. Branson, eds., *Ethics and Health Policy* (Cambridge, Mass.: Ballinger, 1976), p. 141.

40. Siu and Brook, "Allocating Health Care Resources."

41. Daniel Callahan, "Biomedical Progress and the Limits of Human Health," in Veatch and Branson, eds., *Ethics and Health Policy,* pp. 162–163.

42. President's Commission for the Study of Ethical Problems in Medicine and Biomedical and Behavioral Research, *Securing Access to Health Care,* vol. 1, p. 19.

43. A. A. Scitovsky and A. M. Capron, "Medical Care at the End of Life: The Interaction of Economics and Ethics," *Annual Review of Public Health* 7 (1986), 59–75.

44. Advocates of the principle of equal access might respond to these objections by claiming that if society cannot afford to give everyone a treatment, then, according to equal access, no one should get it. See Amy Gutmann, "For and Against Equal Access to Health Care," pp. 542–560. But when dialysis or organ transplants or any other scarce resource cannot be given to all, our society's response has not been to deny it to all. Instead, our response has been to provide what can be provided on an equal basis without factors other than medical need determining which patients should be considered for the care. The equal access principle, elaborated by Gutmann, conflicts with our considered moral judgments. Furthermore, even this stronger view of the equal access principle fails to provide a principled mechanism for deciding *what* services to provide; it just claims some limit will exist when we cannot afford the added care. But which services will be cut? Presumably it makes a difference, from the point of view of justice, which services are guaranteed and which left to individual discretion.

45. Veatch, "What is a 'Just' Health Care Delivery?" p. 142. In a later work, *A Theory of Medical Ethics,* Veatch backs away from his strong position by arguing that society "would rather arbitrarily set some fixed amount of the total [social] resources for health care"(p. 275). He then argues

that "presumably the arbitrary choice would fall" within the 5 to 10 percent of the GNP which he claims "every nation currently spends" on health care. Why Veatch thinks arbitrary determinations of the distribution of social resources are just is not clear. Nor is it clear why the distributive schemes of other nations should serve as a standard of justice.

46. Robert M. Veatch, "DRGs and the Ethical Reallocation of Resources," *Hastings Center Report* 16 (1986), 32–40.
47. See T. M. Scanlon, "Preference and Urgency," *Journal of Philosophy* 72 (1975), 655–669.
48. Ibid., p. 663.
49. Charles Fried, "Equality and Rights in Medical Care," *Hastings Center Report* 6 (1976), 29–34.
50. Michael Walzer, *Spheres of Justice* (New York: Basic Books, 1983), p. 88.
51. See Alain C. Enthoven, *Health Plan: The Only Practical Solution to the Soaring Cost of Medical Care* (Reading, Mass.: Addison-Wesley, 1980), p. 127, and PL 93–222, Health Maintenance Organization Act of 1973.
52. Howard H. Hiatt, *America's Health in the Balance* (New York: Harper and Row, 1987), p. 213.
53. Allan Gibbard, "The Prospective Pareto Principle and Equity of Access to Health Care," *Milbank Memorial Fund Quarterly* 60 (1982), 399–428.
54. President's Commission for the Study of Ethical Problems in Medicine and Biomedical and Behavioral Research, *Securing Access to Health Care*, vol. 1, p. 20.
55. Daniels, *Just Health Care*, p. 74.
56. President's Commission on the Health Needs of the Nation, *Building America's Health*, vol. 1, pp. 43–44. The Commission specified this list in urging the adoption of extensive "prepayment" schemes to pay for health services, not unlike health insurance or HMOs.
57. P.L. 93–222, December 29, 1973.
58. Enthoven, *Health Plan*, p. 127.
59. Karen Davis, *National Health Insurance: Benefits, Costs, and Consequences* (Washington, D.C.: Brookings Institution, 1975), p. 173.
60. Hiatt, *America's Health in the Balance*, p. 214.
61. See, for instance, Brian Abel-Smith, "Minimum Adequate Levels of Personal Health Care: History and Justification," *Milbank Memorial Fund Quarterly* 56 (1978), 1–21, and Charles Fried, "Equality and Rights in Medical Care," *Hastings Center Report*.
62. President's Commission for the Study of Ethical Problems in Medicine and Biomedical and Behavioral Research, *Securing Access to Health Care*, vol. 1, p. 42.
63. Fein, *Medical Care, Medical Costs*, p. 132.

64. *Current Opinions of the Council on Ethical and Judicial Affairs of the American Medical Association 1986* (Chicago: American Medical Association, 1986), p. 3.

65. John P. Bunker and Byron W. Brown, "The Physician-Patient as an Informed Consumer of Surgical Services," *New England Journal of Medicine* 290 (1974), 1051–55. It is also important to note that the federal government as well as organized medicine recognize the absence of clear clinical criteria for many interventions and are trying to study ways of creating such criteria. At the very least, then, we would be unable to use such criteria today, and using them would require significant additional research.

66. President's Commission for the Study of Ethical Problems in Medicine and Biomedical and Behavioral Research, *Securing Access to Health Care,* vol. 1, p. 19.

67. Enthoven, *Health Plan,* p. 128.

68. See a similar argument offered by Daniels, *Just Health Care,* pp. 20–22.

69. Enthoven, *Health Plan,* appendix.

70. Scanlon, "Preference and Urgency," p. 668.

71. Hiatt, *America's Health in the Balance,* p. 213. Similarly, Enthoven suggests using a list because we "need some agreed on, uniform definition of 'all the care you need' that is applicable to all." Enthoven, *Health Plan,* p. 128.

72. John Rawls, "Justice as Fairness: Political not Metaphysical," *Philosophy and Public Affairs* 14 (1985), 236, n. 19.

73. It is also worth noting that while the President's Commission and Davis were articulating *comprehensive* medical care, the Congress and Dean Hiatt were issuing *basic* health care lists.

74. Lazenby, Levit, and Waldo, "National Health Expenditures, 1985," pp. 1–31.

75. "Oregon Plan to Rank Services Rapped as Cutting Benefits," *American Medical News,* February 16, 1990, p. 3.

76. We might distinguish cosmetic surgery from plastic surgery because the former merely changes appearances whereas the latter aims at remedying a natural or created defect. In this sense we probably do consider plastic surgery basic medical care. See Kass, *Toward a More Natural Science,* chap. 6.

77. Daniels, *Just Health Care,* p. 42.

78. This has been the usual application of Rawls to health care. See, for instance, Veatch, *A Theory of Medical Ethics,* pp. 261–264, and Gauthier, "Unequal Need."

79. Daniels, *Just Health Care,* p. 31.

80. Ibid., pp. 33–34. It is important to note that the notion of opportunity

Daniels employs is broader than the one generally used in public life. Opportunity is usually not conceived as the opportunity to choose and to pursue any reasonable conception of the good life, but as the opportunity to obtain jobs and offices. It is this more limited notion of opportunity that provides the justification for establishing affirmative action plans. Further, Daniels argues that the objective of health care should be to preserve or to restore an individual's opportunity to choose and pursue the *full* range of conceptions of the good life that his talents and skills make available. While individuals may have already chosen a particular conception of the good life, pursued education, and developed skills to realize it, the polity must avoid making judgments about the access to medical services based on the individual's choices of conception of the good life; using the normal opportunity range "keeps facts about an individual's particular ends from unduly influencing *social* decisions. We do not want to be in the business, I believe, of deciding who gets what medical services on the basis of occupation or other results of prior individual choices of a similar sort."

81. Rawls, *A Theory of Justice,* sections 12–14, 17.
82. See Gary Wills, *Nixon Agonistes: The Crisis of the Self-Made Man* (Boston: Houghton Mifflin, 1969), pp. 223–224.
83. Daniels, *Just Health Care,* p. 41.
84. Ibid., p. 79.
85. It is worth noting that Daniels' account may help us understand why our society seems to place more importance on life-saving technologies than any other aspect of medical care, for instance, the tendency to support liver and heart transplants over funding programs such as prenatal care. We should support care for those afflictions "which involve a greater curtailment of an individual's share of the normal opportunity range." Dying is certainly the greatest curtailment of opportunity a person can have, and it takes no special or complex calculation of social benefits to see that saving lives by medical care will greatly increase those individuals' opportunities. Claims to fund other types of care which may increase the opportunity of those already alive are complex and, initially, seem less pressing than saving a life.
86. It is worth noting two important political implications of Daniels' view. First, if, upon reflection, citizens of a polity find themselves agreeing that the moral function of medical care is to guarantee fair equality of opportunity, then they have a strong indication that this is the correct interpretation of the ideal of equal opportunity for their polity. In this way a theory of just health care is not just an application of principles of justice to health care; it is an integral part of a general theory of justice. Second, Daniels' account seems consistent with other philosophical ac-

counts of the moral importance of functional limitations. In exploring the moral dimensions of the concept of well-being, the economist Amartya Sen argues that it cannot be reduced to utility and that "the primary feature of well-being can be seen in terms of how a person can 'function.'" Amartya Sen, "Well-Being, Agency and Freedom: The Dewey Lectures, 1984," *Journal of Philosophy* 82 (1985), 169–221. According to Sen, it is important to examine not just a person's well-being, but also his or her "freedom to achieve well-being . . . or well-being freedom." Sen does not develop these ideas as they relate to medical care or in the way they might create social obligations to provide for health care, but the idea of well-being freedom is similar to Daniels' concept of the ability to pursue the normal opportunity range. And thus Daniels' explanation of the moral importance of health care in preserving a person's normal functions and thereby his opportunity range is probably the way to develop Sen's concepts for health care.

87. Daniels, *Just Health Care*, pp. 31–32.

88. In answer to this point, it might be thought that aiming at preserving an individual's normal opportunity might impose a limit on medical treatments based on age. After an individual reaches a normal life span, we might conclude that society has provided sufficient care to fulfill the claims of fair equality of opportunity and that the individual is not entitled, as a matter of justice, to additional health care. Daniels examines whether such an age-based standard is consistent with his account and cautiously concludes that it *might* be. Since health care for those over 65 years of age accounts for 29 percent of the health care budget, it would seem that such a limit based on age might impose significant limits on health care expenditures. Without going into this issue in detail, we must wonder whether invoking such an age-based standard is acceptable. First, it is highly controversial whether we have, or can have, any clear notion of a "normal life span." Daniels suggests we might have a rule which prevented anyone over 70 from getting high-technology, high-cost medical services. But why is 70 the measure of a normal life span? Clearly what is average cannot be normal. And since it is now not unexpected, or that extraordinary, for people to live functional, active lives into their nineties, why is this not "normal"? Further, there seems no scientific way of defining a natural life span with any precision, or defining one that is not liable to changes in medical care. After all, with improvements in medicine the average life span has increased, and so has the functioning of the elderly. Similar improvements seem possible in the future consistent with our body's function. Second, is not defining a set age as a limit on normal opportunities to impose a conception of the good life on people? Some individuals may view their continued

existence for as many years as possible as supremely important, among the most important things to them. To impose an age-based standard which sets some arbitrary age as the ground for receiving care would seem to be overriding their conceptions of a meaningful life. This would seem to contravene liberal injunctions.

89. Daniels, *Just Health Care*, pp. 52–55.

90. The kind of information that this hypothetical deliberator is deprived of depends upon the question being asked. More information is withheld when the deliberator is articulating abstract principles of justice, but less information is withheld when he is deliberating on the application of these principles of justice to laws and policies. See Rawls, *A Theory of Justice*, section 31.

91. Daniels, *Just Health Care*, p. 54, uses the metaphor of "weighing," while Rawls, "Citizen's Needs and Primary Goods" (manuscript, October 17, 1986) uses the metaphor of "striking a balance between" the various claims on society's resources.

92. For the source and full justification of these limitations, see Rawls, *A Theory of Justice*, section 31.

93. Ibid., p. 136.

94. This approach is used by Daniels, *Just Health Care*, chap. 5, and in *Am I My Parents' Keeper? An Essay on Justice between the Young and the Old* (New York: Oxford University Press, 1987), chap. 4, under the heading of the prudent deliberator; by Rawls, "Citizens' Needs and Primary Goods"; by Gauthier, "Unequal Need," pp. 179–205; by Ronald Green in "Health Care and Justice in Contract Theory Perspective," in Veatch and Branson, eds., *Ethics and Health Policy*. A similar hypothetical choice situation is used by Ronald Dworkin, "What is Equality? Part 2: Equality of Resources," *Philosophy and Public Affairs* 10 (1981), 283–345. Dworkin examines a hypothetical auction and the development of social insurance to compensate people for handicaps including ill health.

95. Relying on intuitions in this process of weighing the various demands is an objection that Rawls raises against utilitarian and related "mixed conceptions" of justice. He claims that these conceptions of justice rely on "intuitionistic features" when they recommend that a variety of ends—"greater average well-being and a more equal distribution [of wealth]"—be considered in the design of social institutions because the conceptions are vague on how to fulfill these ends, leaving the weighing to unguided judgment. Rawls claims these "intuitionistic features" are not "a decisive objection" to such utilitarian and mixed conceptions of justice, but the avoidance of such features is, he claims, an advantage of his two principles. And so in pursuing the substance of the liberal legislator's deliberations we are just trying to see if Rawls's claims for his

theory stand up to his own standards. See Rawls, *A Theory of Justice,* sections 7 and 49.

96. The option is an adaptation of Daniel Callahan, *Setting Limits.* I have modified Callahan's proposed alternatives. In *Setting Limits* he suggests that life-saving technology be restricted at an age between "the late 70s to early 80s." Unfortunately, his scheme then offers no real alternatives since in essence it calls for more allocation of resources for the treatment of chronic diseases and support services. The minimal resources saved by the restriction on life-saving care to those over 80 would hardly contribute to these additional services. This seems to be something he grudgingly recognizes: "It may well be that reforms of the sweeping kind implied in these widely voiced criticisms [of chronic medical and nursing care] could more than consume in the short run any savings generated by inhibitions of the kind I am proposing in the development and use of [life-saving] medical technology" (p. 147). At this point Callahan changes the justification of his reforms from saving resources. But this admission seems to suggest that if we are looking for a scheme to save resources, we need stiffer—more realistic—criteria. This is what I have done in modifying Callahan's scheme. This should retain his idea if not his details.

97. In *Just Health Care* Norman Daniels shies away from specifying the concrete policies which are entailed by his theory. Thus, I have had to do this for him. The result may not be precisely to his liking, but scheme 3 does seem consistent with his view. It is a schematized version of liberalism in health care.

98. We of course must assume that without life-saving technologies, older people would actually live fewer years. For if it turned out that the average age in scheme 2 was the same as in scheme 1, then the life-extending technologies would be futile and there would be no argument about which scheme should be selected.

99. This is certainly what Daniel Callahan, one of the principal defenders of scheme 2, thinks should be the outcome of adopting it. See *Setting Limits,* pp. 143–144.

100. Rawls suggests that the liberal legislator should adopt the "least well off" standard, which evaluates competing schemes based on how well off they make the least advantaged. But this seems wrong because it makes medical care subject to the difference principle. Once we accept the idea that medical care should be viewed as part of the institutions that guarantee fair equality of opportunity, once we accept Daniels' argument—and this seems more akin to the intention of Rawls's position—then the distribution of medical resources should be governed not by the difference principle, but by the need to ensure fair equality of

opportunity. On this view the "least well off" standard has no role to play in judging alternative medical service schemes. But even if we did adopt the difference principle for the allocation of health care resources, most of the arguments raised against weighing the opportunity criteria would apply to specifying the difference principle.

101. Daniels, *Just Health Care*, p. 35. This standard is repeated in Daniels, *Am I My Parents' Keeper?*, p. 112. Daniels does not actually suggest that this quantitative standard should help guide the liberal legislator, but he does offer it as a "crude measure" of the importance of health care needs and services. His view is complicated because at other points he departs from this quantitative scale by suggesting that "the justification for meeting one set of needs rather than another is that it is *more important* to do so, in view of effects on opportunity" (*Am I My Parents' Keeper?*, p. 128, emphasis added). There is an ambiguity in the phrase "more important." It could mean more important because quantitatively more opportunities are guaranteed, or it could mean that more qualitatively important opportunities are guaranteed. If the latter is the case, then the assessment is not quantitative but qualitative. Such ambiguities crop up often in Daniels' account. But the quantitative view seems more congenial to his overall presentation, which is why I have adopted it here.

102. Daniels, *Just Health Care*, p. 50.

103. Clearly this overstates the truth. Not every individual actually recognizes this, since utilitarians and most economists argue that goods are commensurable, defined in terms of happiness produced or a utility function. The point is that this commensurability is something that those who defend liberal philosophy—Rawls, Dworkin, and others—do not accept.

104. Having always thought that blindness and the inability to read books would be the worst disability, I was surprised to hear an elderly lady who was losing both her sight and her hearing say that losing her hearing was the more distressing because it removed her from the activities around her. Others might have judged the losses differently.

105. Daniels, *Just Health Care*, p. 35.

106. Daniels, *Am I My Parents' Keeper?*, p. 115.

107. This is exactly the point Rawls makes when he writes of utilitarianism: "The striking feature of the utilitarian feature of justice is that it does not matter, except indirectly, how this sum of satisfactions is distributed among individuals any more than it matters, except indirectly, how one man distributes his satisfactions over time. The correct distribution in either case is that which yields the maximum fulfillment . . . Thus there is no reason in principle why the greater gains of some should not compensate for the lesser losses of others" (*A Theory of Justice*, p. 26).

108. Daniels, *Just Health Care,* pp. 50–52 and chap. 5.

109. We might extend this objection to Rawls's principles of justice and primary goods. The high ranking of opportunities to pursue jobs and careers in Rawls's own principles seems unjustified, and any justification would seem to have to invoke a conception of the good life to explain why these opportunities are the most important ones.

110. John Lorber, "Spina Bifida Cystica: Results of Treatment of 270 Consecutive Cases with Criteria for Selection for the Future," *Archives of Childhood Diseases* 47 (1972), 854–873.

111. This approach is widely advocated, as in Ronald Dworkin, "What Is Equality? Part 2: Equality of Resources." While Dworkin does not suggest that the average assessment is to be used by the liberal legislator, this view arises while he is attempting to determine what types of social insurance schemes might be adopted in a just society committed to equality of resources to compensate people who have handicaps and medical needs. Similarly, T. M. Scanlon, in "Preference and Urgency," argues that it is most reasonable to have an objective notion of well-being that is used to decide what claims on resources are most urgent, and that this objective standard will result from a "consensus in the society on the relevant values."

112. Dworkin, "What is Equality? Part 2: Equality of Resources," p. 299.

113. Scanlon, "Preference and Urgency," p. 663.

114. President's Commission for the Study of Ethical Problems in Medicine and Biomedical and Behavioral Research, *Deciding to Forego Life-Sustaining Treatment* (Washington, D.C.: U.S. Government Printing Office, 1983), p. 43.

115. Actually the liberal legislator's choice is more complex than the individual patient's, not only because he must weigh all the potential medical services which might be available, but also because he must consider research projects and therefore the type of medical services available in the future.

116. Dworkin defends the reasonable person's assessment as "better than nothing," a "second best" alternative, no "worse, in principle, than the alternatives." But what is the basis of such a claim? Our original standard for assessment was (1) a practical scheme which (2) satisfied liberal principles of pluralism and neutrality and (3) the principles of justice. We have yet to find a conception of just health care that satisfies all three requirements. But do we view those that are impractical and those that violate liberal principles as equally flawed? And if different conceptions violate the liberal principles, how do we assess which is *less* flawed? If there is a violation of principle, is this not enough to reject the conception outright? The point here is not to deny that there might be reason-

able and just schemes of basic medical services, but to deny that we can define such schemes and justify them while respecting liberal principles. If this claim is true then we are not arguing about which scheme is less flawed, but about the fundamental defects of liberal principles in health care. And thus what is second best in a liberal view may be perfectly justifiable by rejecting liberal principles.

117. Such a compromise scheme might be better than unresolved disagreement. This may be what Dworkin has in mind when he suggests that a scheme would be "better than nothing," or what Scanlon has in mind when he suggests that one scheme will be "under the circumstances, the best available standard of justification that is mutually acceptable to people whose preferences diverge." See Scanlon, "Preference and Urgency," p. 668.

118. Matilda White Riley and John W. Riley, "Longevity and Social Structure: The Added Years," *Daedalus* 115 (Winter 1986), 51–75.

119. Thomas Nagel, "Death," in *Mortal Questions* (New York: Cambridge University Press, 1979).

120. See, for example, John K. Iglehart, "Transplantation: The Problem of Limited Resources," *New England Journal of Medicine* 309 (1983), 123–128, and Hiatt, *America's Health in the Balance.*

121. Callahan, *Setting Limits,* p. 43.

122. See, for example, Callahan, *Setting Limits;* Kass, *Toward a More Natural Science,* chap. 6; and Richard Lamm, *New York Times,* February 19, 1987, p. A31, and *American College of Physicians Observer,* March 1988, p. 6.

123. See, for example, Daniels, *Just Health Care,* and Sidney H. Wanzer, S. James Adelstein, Ronald E. Cranford, Daniel D. Federman, Edward D. Hook, Charles G. Moertel, Peter Safar, Alan Stone, Helen B. Taussig, and Jan van Eys, "The Physician's Responsibility toward Hopelessly Ill Patients," *New England Journal of Medicine* 310 (1984), 955–959.

124. See Blumenthal, Feldman, and Zeckhauser, "Misuse of Technology"; Thomas Schelling, "Standards for Adequate Minimum Personal Health Services," *Milbank Memorial Fund Quarterly* 57 (1979), 212–233; Alexander Leaf, "The Doctor's Dilemma—And Society's Too," *New England Journal of Medicine* 310 (1984), 718–721; Carl J. Schramm, "Can We Solve the Hospital-Cost Problem in Our Democracy?", *New England Journal of Medicine* 311 (1984), 729–732; Allan Gibbard, "The Prospective Pareto Principle and Equity of Access to Health Care," *Milbank Memorial Fund Quarterly* 60 (1982), 399–428; Gauthier, "Unequal Need"; and Helga Kuhse and Peter Singer, *Should the Baby Live?* (New York: Oxford University Press, 1985), pp. 164–169.

125. Gibbard, "The Prospective Pareto Principle and Equity of Access to Health Care."

126. Aaron and Schwartz, *The Painful Prescription,* and Thomas Halper, "Life and Death in a Welfare State: End-stage Renal Disease in the United Kingdom," *Milbank Memorial Fund Quarterly* 63 (1985), 52–93.

127. See Leaf, "The Doctor's Dilemma—And Society's Too"; John C. Moskop, "The Moral Limits to Federal Funding for Kidney Disease," *Hastings Center Report* 17 (1987), 11–15; and E. Lovell Becker, "Finite Resources and Medical Triage," *American Journal of Medicine* 66 (1979), 549–550.

128. Alexander Leaf, "The MGH Trustees Say No to Heart Transplants," *New England Journal of Medicine* 302 (1980), 1087–88.

129. Daniel Callahan, *American Medical News,* February 19, 1988, p. 34. See also Callahan, *Setting Limits,* chap. 2.

130. Rawls, "Justice as Fairness," pp. 245–246.

131. Rawls, "Citizens' Needs and Primary Goods." See also Daniels, *Just Health Care,* p. 54.

132. This appears to be the practical analogue of the problems of deliberation in the original position behind the veil of ignorance. See Michael J. Sandel, *Liberalism and the Limits of Justice* (New York: Cambridge University Press, 1982), pp. 122–132.

133. The list of those who endorse democratic procedures on this matter includes President's Commission for the Study of Ethical Problems in Medicine and Biomedical and Behavioral Research, *Securing Access to Health Care,* vol. 1, p. 42; Walzer, *Spheres of Justice,* p. 90; Fein, *Medical Care, Medical Costs,* pp. 195–196; and Rawls, *A Theory of Justice,* p. 201, who suggests that when the deliberations of the liberal legislator are indeterminate, we should turn to democratic procedures.

134. Gutmann, "For and Against Equal Access to Health Care," p. 557.

135. Dr. Seuss, *The Sneetches and Other Stories* (New York: Random House, 1961), pp. 3–25.

136. See John Rawls, "The Idea of an Overlapping Consensus," *Oxford Journal of Legal Studies* 7 (1987), 12, and Charles E. Larmore, *Patterns of Moral Complexity* (New York: Cambridge University Press, 1987), pp. 50–55.

137. Rawls, *A Theory of Justice,* p. 201. See also Rawls's discussion of majority rule in section 54.

138. President's Commission for the Study of Ethical Problems in Medicine and Biomedical and Behavioral Research, *Securing Access to Health Care,* vol. 1, p. 42.

139. See, for instance, Daniels, *Just Health Care,* and President's Commission

for the Study of Ethical Problems in Medicine and Biomedical and Behavioral Research, *Securing Access to Health Care,* vol. 1, both of whom are completely silent on what these democratic political procedures are and why they are justified.

140. Dennis F. Thompson, *Political Ethics and Public Office* (Cambridge, Mass.: Harvard University Press, 1987), p. 3. This should not be taken as Thompson's view; instead, it is the view he opposes.

141. Rawls, "Citizens' Needs and Primary Goods."

142. Rawls, *A Theory of Justice,* p. 359.

143. Ronald Dworkin, *Taking Rights Seriously* (Cambridge, Mass.: Harvard University Press, 1978), chap. 11.

144. Rawls, *A Theory of Justice,* p. 201.

145. "Oregon Legislators Face Up to the Hard Job of 'Playing God,'" *Washington Post National Weekly Edition,* February 15–21, 1988, p. 33, and "Lobby to Seek Ariz. State Funding for Transplants," *American Medical News,* December 4, 1987, p. 34.

146. Richard Lamm, "We Can't Afford the Health Plan," *New York Times,* February 19, 1987, p. A31.

147. Callahan, *What Kind of Life,* p. 30.

148. Daniels, *Just Health Care,* p. 44, n. 2.

149. Rawls, "Social Unity and Primary Goods," p. 163.

150. The analysis of justice in health care and the problem of weighing suggests that the weighing problem is not limited to comparing different primary goods. In fact, this problem arises, as it were, within primary goods. Each primary good is not a single, univocal entity; each primary good is actually plural, a composite of many incommensurable goods. As I have argued, there is no such thing as opportunity; there are only diverse opportunities. And these opportunities are incommensurable. Considerations of justice will require not just weighing diverse primary goods, but weighing diverse goods collected within the rubric of a single primary good.

151. Rawls, *A Theory of Justice,* p. 318.

152. Rawls, "Social Unity and Primary Goods," pp. 162–163, writes: "In this paper, however, I shall, for the most part, take the two principles of justice in what I shall call their 'simplest form': that is part a) of the second principle (the 'difference principle') directs that the basic structure be arranged so that the life-time expectations of the least advantaged, estimated in terms of income and wealth, are so great as possible given fixed background institutions that secure the equal basic liberties and establish fair equality of opportunity. This simplest form serves as an example of the use of primary goods to make interpersonal comparisons; it ignores, however, the primary goods under c) and e) and hence

avoids the problem of defining an index" (emphasis added).

153. Rawls, "Citizens' Needs and Primary Goods."

5. The Liberal Communitarian Vision

1. This belief in the existence of only two types of ethical theories is one of the foundations of applied ethics. Through applied ethics, this dichotomy has infected many areas of medical ethics. Indeed the constant tendency in medical ethics to divide all ethical considerations according to the principles of autonomy and beneficence reflects this vision of ethical theories. Some prominent books that do this include Samuel Gorovitz, *Doctors' Dilemmas* (New York: Oxford University Press, 1982); Tom Beauchamp and James Childress, *Principles of Biomedical Ethics,* 3rd ed. (New York: Oxford University Press, 1989); and H. Tristram Engelhardt, *The Foundations of Bioethics* (New York: Oxford University Press, 1986). This tendency and its problems are not limited to medical ethics or other forms of applied ethics. One can find it among philosophers who do not write on medical ethics, for example, J. L. Mackie, *Ethics* (New York: Penguin, 1977).

2. For a start, see the collection of essays in Bernard Williams and Amartya Sen, eds., *Utilitarianism and Beyond* (New York: Cambridge University Press, 1982).

3. For expression of this view of the situated self, see Michael J. Sandel, *Liberalism and the Limits of Justice* (New York: Cambridge University Press, 1982); Hannah Arendt, *The Human Condition* (Chicago: University of Chicago Press, 1958); Charles Taylor, "What Is Human Agency?" in *Human Agency and Language: Philosophical Papers I* (New York: Cambridge University Press, 1985); and Alasdair MacIntyre, *After Virtue* (South Bend, Ind.: University of Notre Dame Press, 1981).

4. For an illuminating metaphorical representation of this relationship of attached distance see Hannah Arendt, *Between Past and Future* (New York: Viking Press, 1965), Preface.

5. This view is not dissimilar from that found in Rawls when he elaborates the good of the social union; see John Rawls, *A Theory of Justice* (Cambridge, Mass.: Harvard University Press, 1971), section 79.

6. See Charles E. Larmore, *Patterns of Moral Complexity* (New York: Cambridge University Press, 1987), pp. 50–51.

7. Clearly the liberal communitarian vision is found in some of the works of Aristotle, Rousseau, Tocqueville, and many early American writers, especially those who valued the New England town meeting. Indeed, something like this aspiration toward being part of a people which aims

to secure certain traditions and ideals for the future can be found in the preamble to the Constitution, which is expressed in the voice of a people aiming to secure a union dedicated to certain ideals for itself and posterity.

8. On the conception of the good life for democratic individuality, see George Kateb, "Democratic Individuality and the Claims of Politics," *Political Theory* 12 (1984), 331–360.

9. It has been claimed that communitarianism has a view of a settled and established conception of the good life. See Amy Gutmann, "Communitarian Critics of Liberalism," *Philosophy and Public Affairs* 14 (1985), 308–322.

10. See *New York Times,* February 10, 1990, p. 11.

11. MacIntyre, *After Virtue,* p. 206.

12. Clearly the emphasis on deliberation reflects the acceptance of the dialectical nature of political philosophy. The applied ethics view of ethics is more akin to seeing conceptions of the good life as settled and fixed, ready to be applied to cases.

13. Ronald Dworkin, *Taking Rights Seriously* (Cambridge, Mass.: Harvard University Press, 1978), chaps. 2 and 3.

14. Ronald Dworkin, *A Matter of Principle* (Cambridge, Mass.: Harvard University Press, 1985), p. 217.

15. This group is a derived and revised form of distinctions made by Donald W. Keim, "Participation in Contemporary Democratic Theories," Peter Bachrach, "Interest, Participation, and Democratic Theory," and Jane J. Mansbridge, "The Limits of Friendship," all in J. R. Pennock and J. W. Chapman, eds., *Nomos XVI: Participation in Politics* (New York: Lieber–Atherton, 1975). Similarly, Benjamin Barber, *Strong Democracy* (Berkeley, Calif.: University of California Press, 1984), delineates "nine functions of strong democratic talk" which include "1) The articulation of interests; bargaining and exchange. 2) Persuasion. 3) Agenda-setting. 4) Exploring mutuality. 5) Affiliation and affection. 6) Maintaining autonomy. 7) Witness and self-expression. 8) Reformulation and reconceptualization. 9) Community-building as the creation of public interests, common goods, and active citizens." These nine functions are an elaboration of the three objectives I outline.

16. For a related but not communitarian view on the effects of democratic institutions on ordinary individuals, see Kateb, "Democratic Individuality and the Claims of Politics."

17. John Rawls, "The Priority of Right and Ideas of the Good" (manuscript, August 24, 1987).

18. Rawls, for instance, indicates that his theory of justice is not universalist. It is applicable to societies with a democratic culture where the po-

litical ideal is one of social cooperation among free and equal citizens. Even this revision is clearly unbounded to any particular country.

19. Michael Walzer, *Obligations: Essays on Disobedience, War, and Citizenship* (Cambridge, Mass.: Harvard University Press, 1970), p. 233.

20. On this point see George Kateb, "Comments on David Braybrooke's 'The Meaning of Participation and of Demands for It,'" in Pennock and Chapman, eds., *Nomos XVI.*

21. Michael Walzer, *Spheres of Justice* (New York: Basic Books, 1983), p. 310.

22. This view is shared by John Rawls, "The Basic Liberties and Their Priority," *Tanner Lectures on Human Values,* vol. 3 (Salt Lake City, Utah: University of Utah Press, 1982), p. 9, and by Walzer, *Spheres of Justice.*

23. See, for example, Barber, *Strong Democracy,* pp. 148–150.

24. See Walzer, *Spheres of Justice:* "The restraint of exit replaces commitment with coercion. So far as the coerced members are concerned, there is no longer a community worth defending" (p. 39).

25. John Rawls, "Kantian Constructivism and Moral Theory: The Dewey Lectures 1980," *Journal of Philosophy* 77 (1980), 526. See also Rawls, "The Basic Liberties and Their Priority."

26. Keim, "Participation in Contemporary Democratic Theories," p. 32.

27. Robert A. Dahl, *After the Revolution?* (New Haven, Conn.: Yale University Press, 1970), p. 80.

28. Barber, *Strong Democracy,* pp. 269–270. See also Dahl, *After the Revolution?,* p. 70.

29. See Jane J. Mansbridge, *Beyond Adversary Democracy* (New York: Basic Books, 1980).

30. Dahl, *After the Revolution?,* p. 69.

31. U.S. Bureau of the Census, *Statistical Abstracts of the United States: 1987,* 107th ed. (Washington, D.C.: U.S. Government Printing Office, 1986), and American Hospital Association, *Hospital Statistics 1986* (Chicago: American Hospital Association, 1986).

32. Barber, *Strong Democracy,* p. 262.

33. See Rawls, *A Theory of Justice,* section 79.

34. This is a common criticism clearly articulated by Amy Gutmann, "Communitarian Critics of Liberalism."

6. A Liberal Communitarian Vision of Health Care

1. Rashi Fein, *Medical Care, Medical Costs* (Cambridge, Mass.: Harvard University Press, 1987), p. 197. Similarly, in devising a model system for the delivery of health care, Howard H. Hiatt, *America's Health in the*

Balance (New York: Harper and Row, 1987), chap. 12, aims to make as few changes in the existing health care system as possible.

2. The notion and term of a reconstructive ideal are taken from Dennis F. Thompson, *The Democratic Citizen* (New York: Cambridge University Press, 1970), pp. 47–51.

3. The proposal for decentralized health care programs, each making major administrative, distributive, and health care decisions, is akin to other recent reform proposals in health care. The specific scheme outlined here, however, goes beyond these other proposals in the magnitude of decentralization. One reform proposal is for each unit to be defined by states; see Fein, *Medical Care, Medical Costs,* chap. 11. Another proposal aims to have units of between 500,000 and 3 million people with budgets of $3.5 billion; see Hiatt, *America's Health in the Balance,* chap. 12.

4. The aim of democratizing such decisions stands in contrast to at least one recent alternative model. While this alternative assumes "a large number of lay and professional groups willing to work hard to bring about improvements in health care arrangements," its regional administrative and decision-making body is composed of five members "including two presidential and three gubernatorial appointees." The rhetoric of consulting representative groups is maintained, while the actual decisions are highly centralized in a small group not accountable to the people and not mandated to implement democratic procedures in the decision-making process. And in fact the suggested method of evaluating such health care arrangements does not include how well they embody the views of the patients, but is limited to improvements in typical health care indices. See Hiatt, *America's Health in the Balance,* chap. 12.

5. *The InterStudy Edge* (Excelsior, Minn.: InterStudy, Spring 1987), p. 3. The actual number of newly formed HMOs is slightly larger, but about fifty HMOs were eliminated because of consolidation with other HMOs.

6. Office of the Actuary, Health Care Financing Administration, "National Health Expenditures, 1986–2000," *Health Care Financing Review* 8 (September 1987), 1–35.

7. Fein, *Medical Care, Medical Costs,* pp. 203–206.

8. It is worth noting that this is already a problem among countries. Indeed, one of the complaints organized medicine has about comparing the American and Canadian health care systems is that while the United States pioneers medical innovations, the Canadians use these innovations without having paid for their development. Such a "free rider" problem is not unique to the liberal communitarian vision.

9. Office of the Actuary, Health Care Financing Administration, "National Health Expenditures, 1986–2000."

10. See George J. Schieber and Jean-Pierre Poullier, "International Health Care Expenditure Trends: 1987," *Health Affairs* 8 (1989), 169–177. This lower figure is justified economically by this relationship, but clearly not ethically.

11. Benjamin Barber, *Strong Democracy* (Berkeley, Calif.: University of California Press, 1984), p. 295. The most extended debate on vouchers has been in the area of public education. Some liberals have endorsed the idea as a mechanism to increase parent activism in education and to equalize choice among the rich and the poor. See Christopher Jencks and Judith Areen, *Vouchers: A Report on Financing Education by Payments to Parents* (Cambridge, Mass.: Center for the Study of Public Policy, 1970), and John E. Coons and Stephen D. Sugarman, *Education by Choice: The Case for Family Control* (Berkeley, Calif., 1978).

12. This point about a single funding source has been made by Norman Daniels, "Why Saying No to Patients in the United States is So Hard: Cost Containment, Justice, and Provider Autonomy," *New England Journal of Medicine* 314 (1986), 1380–83, and by Hiatt, *America's Health in the Balance,* p. 193.

13. See, for instance, Janet L. Bly, Robert C. Jones, and Jean E. Richardson, "Impact of Worksite Health Promotion on Health Care Costs and Utilization: Evaluation of Johnson and Johnson's Live for Life Program," *Journal of the American Medical Association* 256 (1986), 3235–40.

14. This view of progressively expanding participatory institutions is opposite to the one adopted by Barber, *Strong Democracy,* who argues that "the institutions [of direct democracy] offered here cannot be addressed piecemeal. Taken one at a time, they become more vulnerable to abuse and less likely to succeed in reorienting the democratic system" (p. 263).

15. Fein, *Medical Care, Medical Costs,* p. 200.

16. *Roe* v. *Wade,* 410 U.S. 113 (1973).

17. Society for the Right to Die, *Newsletter,* Fall 1987, p. 3. As a result of *Cruzan,* this policy is probably illegal.

18. The area of terminating artificial nutrition and hydration is relatively new; the first court challenges date from 1984 and 1985. In most cases, state courts have recognized and respected the hospital or nursing home's right to refuse to terminate these treatments; see *Brophy* v. *New England Sinai Hospital,* 398 Mass. 417 (1986). But the New Jersey Supreme Court in *Jobes,* 108 N.J. 384 (1987), forced a nursing home to terminate J-tube feedings for an incompetent patient because it had not informed the patient's family of its policy of refusing to terminate artificial feedings before the patient became a resident. It is not clear whether this decision will be upheld or followed in other jurisdictions; but it is certainly the exception.

19. Paul Starr, *The Social Transformation of American Medicine* (New York: Basic Books, 1982), pp. 315–320.

20. Ibid., p. 318.

21. Renee C. Fox and Judith P. Swazey, *The Courage to Fail,* 2nd ed. (Chicago: University of Chicago Press, 1978), pp. 219–225.

22. See J. S. Murray, W. H. Tu, J. B. Albers, J. M. Bunell, and B. H. Scribner, "A Community Hemodialysis Center for the Treatment of Chronic Uremia," *Transactions of the American Society for Artificial Internal Organs* 8 (1962), 315–318.

23. Gerald R. Winslow, *Triage and Justice* (Berkeley, Calif.: University of California Press, 1982), p. 14.

24. A. H. Katz and D. M. Procter, *Social-Psychological Characteristics of Patients Receiving Hemodialysis Treatment for Chronic Renal Failure* (Washington, D.C.: Department of Health, Education, and Welfare, July, 1969).

25. Harry S. Abram and Walter Wadlington, "Selection of Patients for Artificial and Transplanted Organs," *Annals of Internal Medicine* 69 (1968), 615–620.

26. "Scarce Medical Resources," *Columbia Law Review* 69 (1969), 620–692.

27. Because of Shana Alexander's 1962 *Life* article on the Seattle Artificial Kidney Center's committee for the selection of dialysis patients, "The God Committee," local control over patient selection for dialysis has been the subject of much scrutiny and criticism. Among the most extensive critiques has been that of David Sanders and Jesse Dukeminier, "Medical Advances and Legal Lag: Hemodialysis and Kidney Transplantation," *UCLA Law Review* 15 (1968), 357–413.

28. Fox and Swazey, *The Courage to Fail,* p. 225.

29. "Scarce Medical Resources," p. 642.

30. "Lobby to Seek Arizona State Funding for Transplants," *American Medical News,* December 4, 1987, p. 34.

31. Cited in Hiatt, *America's Health in the Balance,* p. 11.

32. Consumer Consultation Working Group, *Final Report* (Seattle, Wash.: Group Health Cooperative, July 11, 1986).

33. Alexander Leaf, "The MGH Trustees Say No to Heart Transplants," *New England Journal of Medicine* 302 (1980), 1087–88.

34. Hiatt, *America's Health in the Balance,* pp. xiii–xv.

35. Walter J. McNerney, "Control of Health-Care Costs in the 1980s," *New England Journal of Medicine* 303 (1980), 1088–95.

36. Hiatt, *America's Health in the Balance,* p. 212. See also Fein, *Medical Care, Medical Costs,* who writes: "The political climate has changed and there is a turning away from centralized government . . . The individual patterns found across the land are best understood and best addressed at a locus of control that is closer to those delivery systems and to the people

they serve . . . Multiple state programs are like a diversified portfolio: we will not do as well as we might if we bet on a single winning program, but neither will we do as badly if we were to commit a blunder" (pp. 199–201).

37. Fein, *Medical Care, Medical Costs,* p. 210.

38. Karen Davis and Cathy Schoen, *Health and the War on Poverty* (Washington, D.C.: Brookings Institution, 1978), p. 169, cite an example where "local medical societies sometimes fought the establishment of [neighborhood health] centers, refused to supply patient records, and worked to restrict hospital staff privileges for health center physicians."

39. Committee on Community-Oriented Primary Care, Division of Health Care Services, Institute of Medicine, *Community-Oriented Primary Care: A Practical Assessment,* vol. 1 (Washington, D.C.: National Academy Press, April 1984), pp. 103–104.

40. National Research Act, Public Law 9–348, July 12, 1974.

41. Code of Federal Regulations, Title 45, Part 46.107, March 8, 1983.

42. Health Research Extension Act of 1985, Public Law 99–158, November 20, 1985.

43. Information presented on the Group Health Cooperative of Puget Sound came from conversations with Elizabeth Anderson, Ph.D., staff ethicist of the HMO and management representative to the HMO's Ethics Council, and also from the Group Health Cooperative of Puget Sound, *Fact Sheet,* October 1987.

44. People can be affiliated with Group Health Cooperative in two ways: they can simply receive their medical care at the HMO, or they can buy a share for $100 and be voting members. The vote is distributed one per family unit. Of the 330,000 people affiliated with the Group Health Cooperative, about 60,000 are voting members.

45. Consumer Consultation Working Group, *Final Report.*

46. Davis and Schoen, *Health and the War on Poverty,* p. 170.

47. Ibid., pp. 168–170.

48. Ibid., p. 161.

49. Lisbeth Bamberger Schorr and Joseph T. English, "Background, Context, and Significant Issues in Neighborhood Health Center Program," *Milbank Memorial Fund Quarterly* 46 (1968), 291. See also Davis and Schoen, *Health and the War on Poverty,* chap. 6.

50. Harold B. Wise, Lowell S. Levin, and Roy T. Kurahara, "Community Development and Health Education: I. Community Organization as a Health Tactic," *Milbank Memorial Fund Quarterly* 46 (1968), 337.

51. Ibid.

52. Harold B. Wise, "Montefiore Hospital Neighborhood Medical Care Demonstration," *Milbank Memorial Fund Quarterly* 46 (1968), 297–307.

53. Davis and Schoen, *Health and the War on Poverty,* p. 177.

54. Daniel P. Moynihan, *Maximum Feasible Misunderstanding: Community Action in the War on Poverty* (New York: Free Press, 1969).
55. Davis and Schoen, *Health and the War on Poverty,* p. 200.
56. See, for example, Howard E. Freeman, K. Jill Kiecolt, and Harris M. Allen II, "Community Health Centers: An Initiative of Enduring Utility," *Milbank Memorial Fund Quarterly* 60 (1982), 245–267, and Davis and Schoen, *Health and the War on Poverty,* chap. 6.
57. Davis and Schoen, *Health and the War on Poverty,* p. 198.
58. Brian L. Hines, *Oregon and American Health Decisions: A Guide for Community Action on Bioethical Issues* (Washington, D.C.: Department of Health and Human Services, July 1985), p. 5.
59. Ralph Crawshaw, Michael J. Garland, Brian Hines, and Caroline Lobitz, "Oregon Health Decisions: An Experiment with Informed Community Consent," *Journal of the American Medical Association* 254 (1985), 3213–16.
60. Brian Hines, "'Health Priorities' Project Collects Data on Government Programs," *Oregon Health Decisions Reporter,* January 1988, p. 2.
61. Hines, *Oregon and American Health Decisions.*
62. See Daniel Callahan, *Setting Limits* (New York: Simon and Schuster, 1987), pp. 174–193.
63. For more details on the diseases cited here, see Eugene Braunwald, Kurt J. Isselbacher, Robert G. Petersdorf, Jean D. Wilson, Joseph B. Martin, Anthony S. Fauci, and Richard Root, eds., *Harrison's Principles of Internal Medicine,* 12th ed. (New York: McGraw-Hill, 1990).
64. David Kinzer, "The Decline and Fall of Deregulation," *New England Journal of Medicine* 318 (1988), 112–116.
65. InterStudy, *The InterStudy Edge.*
66. Donald R. Cohodes, "The Loss of Innocence: Health Care under Seige," in C. J. Schramm, ed., *Health Care and Its Costs* (New York: W. W. Norton, 1987), p. 76.
67. Fein, *Medical Care, Medical Costs,* p. 213.
68. "Government Gives Private Sector a Chance to Run Medicare Plans," *New York Times,* March 10, 1988, p. A1.
69. In February 1988, for instance, the Harvard Community Health Plan in Boston enrolled 360,000 members in nine major sites and twenty-two care settings. Similarly, Kaiser programs enrolled 5 million members in ten states; see InterStudy, *The InterStudy Edge.*
70. A similar endeavor has occurred when a fee-for-service multi-specialty group practice formed a community primary care practice. See Division of Health Care Services, Institute of Medicine, *Community-Oriented Primary Care: A Practical Assessment,* vol. 2 (Washington, D.C.: National Academy Press, 1984), chap. 9.

71. See Starr, *The Social Transformation of American Medicine,* chap. 6, and "How Pre-Payment Got Its Start," *Group Practice* 22 (December 1973), 17–19.

72. Davis and Schoen, *Health and the War on Poverty,* p. 198.

73. Clifton A. Cole, "Community Health Centers—Fifteen Years Later," *Urban Health,* April 1980, p. 40.

74. Division of Health Care Services, Institute of Medicine, *Community-Oriented Primary Care,* vol. 2, chap. 5.

75. See Davis and Schoen, *Health and the War on Poverty,* chap. 6.

76. Wise, "Montefiore Hospital Neighborhood Medical Care Demonstration."

77. See Davis and Schoen, *Health and the War on Poverty,* chap. 6, for a review of the complex issue of measuring the actual cost of neighborhood health centers.

78. *Federal Registrar* 52 (Sept. 30, 1987), 36716–21.

79. John E. Kralewski, Bryan Dowd, Roger Feldman, and Janet Shapiro, "The Physician Rebellion," *New England Journal of Medicine* 316 (1987), 339–342.

80. Michael Walzer, *Spheres of Justice* (New York: Basic Books, 1984), p. 311.

81. See Division of Health Care Services, Institute of Medicine, *Community-Oriented Primary Care,* vol. 2, p. 80.

82. Hines, *Oregon and American Health Decisions,* pp. 22–26.

83. This objection was raised by Daniel Callahan.

84. To object that justice requires that all American citizens should have access to the very same basic medical services implicitly suggests that there are sufficiently common elements among conceptions of the good life that can inform one compromise scheme of basic medical services for the United States. But this would have to be demonstrated, not just asserted. In particular, such a demonstration would have to suggest that there is a compromise scheme of basic medical services which the four different conceptions of the good life outlined in Chapter 4 would endorse. There is the trivial—and unreasonable—case of providing Presidential medicine to everyone. But even this conflicts with the relational conception of the good life. Hence it seems unlikely that the range of pluralism will be sufficiently narrow to permit one scheme for the entire United States.

85. Such arguments are made against another view in Norman Daniels, *Just Health Care* (New York: Cambridge University Press, 1985), pp. 20–23.

86. It is worth considering that there may be an economically objective way to determine what proportion of the GNP to allocate to medical care at

the political level by considering the precise empirical relationship observed in economically advanced countries between per capita gross national product and per capita medical costs; see Schieber and Poullier, "International Health Care Expenditure Trends: 1987." But it must be noted that while this provides an objective determination from an economic perspective, it remains to be justified politically. Indeed, there is no *a priori* ethical reason for a political community to adhere to the implicit determinations of justice espoused by the distribution of resources made in other countries.

87. John Rawls, "The Priority of Right and Ideas of the Good" (manuscript, August 24, 1987).
88. See Robert Nozick, *Anarchy, State, and Utopia* (New York: Basic Books, 1974), chap. 10. This objection was raised in various ways by Michael Sandel, Dennis Thompson, Arthur Applbaum, and Robert Rosen.

Conclusion

1. Dennis Thompson, "Political Theory and Political Judgment," *PS* 17 (Spring 1984), 193–197. A similar issue is raised and addressed by Norman Daniels in *Just Health Care* (New York: Cambridge University Press, 1985), chap. 9, when he examines how the principles he develops apply in a system without full compliance to justice.
2. An example of this can be found in Marcia Angell, "The Baby Doe Rules," *New England Journal of Medicine* 314 (1986), 642–644.
3. Tom L. Beauchamp and James F. Childress, *Principles of Biomedical Ethics,* 2nd ed. (New York: Oxford University Press, 1983), p. 8.
4. Charles Fried, *Right and Wrong* (Cambridge, Mass.: Harvard University Press, 1978), chap. 7, has suggested that lawyers should be friends of their clients. But, as others have mentioned, he fails to take this ideal seriously because he is not willing to see that such friendship might entail moral deliberation and changing a client's moral views. But this is precisely what should occur in a professional-client relationship and what is advocated here for the physician.

Index